Margaret Sanger
and first child, Stuart,
aged 6 months.

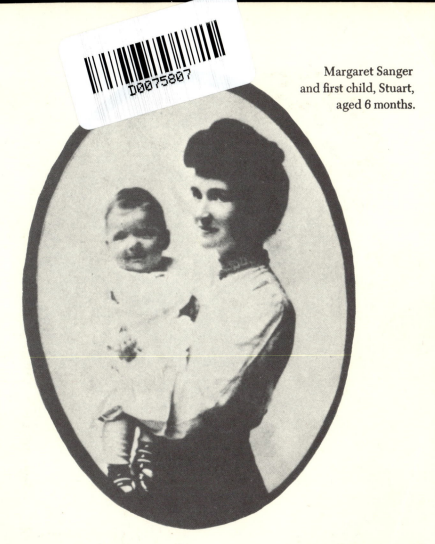

Mrs. Sanger, fighting to change
federal birth control laws, testifies
before congressional committee, May, 1932.

Margaret Sanger, guest of
Mahatma Gandhi, urges birth control
for India, February, 1936.

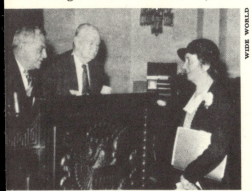

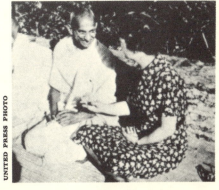

WIDE WORLD

UNITED PRESS PHOTO

THE MARGARET SANGER STORY

LAWRENCE LADER

THE MARGARET

SANGER STORY

AND THE FIGHT FOR BIRTH CONTROL

GREENWOOD PRESS, PUBLISHERS

WESTPORT, CONNECTICUT

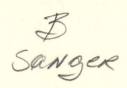

Library of Congress Cataloging in Publication Data

Lader, Lawrence.
    The Margaret Sanger story and the fight for birth
control.

    Reprint of the ed. published by Doubleday, Garden
City, N. Y.
    1. Sanger, Margaret, 1879-1966. 2. Birth control.
I. Title.
[HQ764.S3L3 1973]   613.9'4'0924 [B]   73-11855
ISBN 0-8371-7076-1

Originally published in 1955 by Doubleday & Company, Inc.,
Garden City, New York.

Reprinted with the permission of Lawrence Lader.

Reprinted in 1973 by Greenwood Press
A division of Congressional Information Service, Inc.
88 Post Road West, Westport, Connecticut 06881

Library of Congress catalog card number 73-11855
ISBN 0-8371-7076-1

Printed in the United States of America

10 9 8 7 6 5 4 3 2

For my grandfather,
HENRY M. POWELL 1867–1953

OTHER BOOKS BY LAWRENCE LADER

The Bold Brahmins: New England's War against Slavery
  (1861-1963)
Abortion
Margaret Sanger: Pioneer of Birth Control. With Milton Meltzer
Breeding Ourselves to Death
Foolproof Birth Control: Male and Female Sterilization
Abortion II: Making the Revolution

Lawrence Lader has been involved in the field of population control, as both author and activist, for twenty years. He has been
chairman of the National Association for the Repeal of Abortion
Laws, and has served on the executive committee of the Association for Voluntary Sterilization and on the board of Zero
Population Growth.

PREFACE TO THE REPRINT EDITION

This reprint of my 1955 biography of Margaret Sanger has been kept unedited and unrevised to preserve the mood and excitement of the times, and the portrait of Mrs. Sanger as the author knew her at the height of her career.

*After 1955, Sanger's work in the United States focused on one critical task—the development of a simple and safe birth control pill. For years she had goaded scientists to pursue such research and raised money for their laboratories. Finally, at the Foundation for Experimental Biology in Shrewsbury, Massachusetts, she found a team, headed by the late Dr. Gregory Pincus, which could carry on the basic research in female sex hormones and produce the pill as we know it today. Even before her death, she would see the pill revolutionize the practice of contraception, and broaden acceptance far beyond the limitations of traditional, mechanical techniques.

Margaret Sanger was consumed by another monumental vision—the building of a birth control movement overseas that would become the International Planned Parenthood Federation. As early as 1920 she warned of the disaster of population growth. By 1953, world population, one billion in 1830, had soared to 2.5 billion. And it was expected to reach 6.5 billion by the year 2000 even with a considerable decline in fertility. Only a highly organized world movement, backed by the skills and financial resources of the United States and wealthier nations, could prevent the progress of developing nations from being crushed under an avalanche of new births.

Margaret Sanger roamed the world, organizing one country after another—Britain, Ceylon, India, Pakistan, West Germany, and Japan into IPPF. The movement at first was organized from her suitcase. Then came a tiny office in London with a part-time assistant. Already ill and bed-ridden by 1961, she wrote Hugh Moore, an industrialist determined to put a solid financial base under IPPF, that she would come to New York's Waldorf Astoria

3

Hotel for a fund-raising banquet "if humanly possible, if I have to crawl, I will be there." One hundred thousand dollars was raised on the spot in her last public appearance.

That was the first year IPPF could announce a small working budget. By 1972, its budget had grown to over twenty-five million dollars, and the organization included 79 member nations with birth control assistance programs in over 100 countries.

One historic court test in her last years capped Sanger's long struggle against legal barriers to birth control. With some state laws still prohibiting clinics and free flow of contraceptive information, a group of Planned Parenthood officials in Connecticut carried a test case to the United States Supreme Court. In 1965, the Court declared that "privacy in the marital relation is fundamental and basic"—a sweeping triumph that not only wiped out the restrictive Connecticut law, but the law of any state still limiting the use of contraception.

Margaret Sanger spent her last years confined to bed at a Tucson nursing home. At eighty-seven she could no longer bounce back from repeated heart attacks, as she had done before. She died on September 6, 1966, and was buried in the cemetery at Fishkill, New York, near her former Willow Lake home. The next day a *New York Times* editorial called her "one of history's great rebels and a monumental figure of the first half of the twentieth century."

Sanger's fifty-year campaign, both for the individual's right to contraception and society's survival in the face of unchecked population growth, has continued to produce a world-wide impact. As a result of Roman Catholic pressure the United States government was fearful of sponsoring birth control as late as 1959, and first supported contraceptive research under President John F. Kennedy. Former President Dwight D. Eisenhower reversed his opposition in 1965, and with former President Harry S. Truman became cochairman of Planned Parenthood-World Population. President Lyndon B. Johnson eventually pushed through massive federal aid for family planning at home and overseas, and Congress has voted increasingly larger budgets to promote voluntary sterilization as well as contraception.

Within a few years of Sanger's death, federal, state, and local governments have formed an enthusiastic partnership with the family planning campaign. Even the Catholic hierarchy, opposed to any form of contraception but the rhythm method, has diluted its opposition in daily practice. Significantly, the majority of Catholic women not only use contraception, but have drastically reduced their family goals to an average of 2.75 children (compared to 2.35 for non-Catholic women). Births throughout the United States declined so sharply in 1972 that the fertility rate fell to 2.03 children per family—significantly below the "replacement level" of 2.1 children.

If Sanger's campaign for population control has achieved national acceptance through such organizations as Zero Population Growth, Inc. and the National Organization for Non-Parents, her influence on the Women's Liberation movement has been even more pronounced. In 1914 in the first issue of the *Woman Rebel,* she insisted that a woman could only secure "life, liberty and the pursuit of happiness" when she makes herself "absolute mistress of her own body." Fifty years later, the feminist movement finally focused its demands on Sanger's dictum. Without control over their procreativity, women could not achieve equality in employment or education, or free themselves from their traditional role as menial housewives programmed into a cheap source of breeding, child care and domestic labor. Only contraception and legalized abortion could prevent the married woman from being forced into deeper subservience by an unwanted child; the single woman from being terrorized by an illegitimate birth and social ostracism. The dependence of women on men would now be deprived of its essential prop.

In her vision of the revolutionary impact of birth control, Margaret Sanger predicted a "new woman" who would gain "the greatest possible fulfillment of her desires upon the highest possible plane." She wanted fulfillment for women not just in creative energy and careers, but in love and sex. The new woman would have to cleanse the social fabric of puritanical debris and inhibitions that had perverted our thinking for centuries. In this blueprint, Sanger became the precursor of the Woman's Liberation movement today. As a woman rebel, as a woman in love, as a perceptive scientific thinker who forced society to grapple with the most crucial issues of our time, Margaret Sanger had the relentless energy and tactical skill to stamp her vision on the world. The most remarkable part of her story is that her vision has become a reality within a few years of her death not only in the United States but in many other nations.

FOREWORD

by Abraham Stone, M.D.

A few rare men and women in a generation achieve true greatness. By virtue of their wisdom, their vision, their courage, the nobility of their character, they reach unusual heights and profoundly influence human destiny. To this select and unique group belongs Margaret Sanger.

Early in her life Margaret Sanger saw a vision—a vision of womanhood freed from subjection to uncontrolled fertility, a vision of every child a wanted and planned child, a vision of motherhood conscious and voluntary. With remarkable energy, courage, and steadfastness, she has dedicated her entire life to the realization of this dream.

Margaret Sanger coined the phrase "birth control," and today it is practically synonymous with her name. To her, birth control meant regulation, planning, the prevention of unwanted conception. This idea of control and planning has remained the basic principle of the National and International Planned Parenthood movements which have developed under her guidance and leadership.

From the beginning, Margaret Sanger felt that the prescription and evaluation of contraceptive techniques was primarily a medical problem. Although at first the doctors of the country were apathetic and even hostile to her ideas, it was she who carried on the fight for medical freedom in this field, the freedom for the doctor to use his conscience and his skill in this area of preventive medicine. In establishing the clinical center which later became known as the Margaret Sanger Research Bureau, she visualized it as an experimental center in public health. It was to be, she wrote, "a nucleus for research, a laboratory dealing with human beings . . . an experimental bureau designed to demonstrate its influence as a social need and prove itself as a health center."

The late Dr. Hannah Stone and I have successively been the medical directors of the bureau almost from its inception. We thus had the great privilege of coming in close contact with Margaret Sanger

7

over more than a quarter of a century. I also had the opportunity to travel with her on many of her international trips—to England, Sweden, Japan, India, Thailand, and elsewhere—and I have come to know her as a person. To know Margaret Sanger is to realize that she is not merely a rebel, a crusader, an indomitable fighter for a cause to which she has dedicated herself, but that she is also a *radiant rebel.* Her charm, her humor, the warmth of her personality, her disarming modesty, and her intuitive wisdom are sources of constant admiration and joy to those who know her. To me, her friendship has indeed been an inspiring and cherished privilege.

It is to the great credit of Margaret Sanger that she very soon realized the wider implications and significance of birth control. Starting primarily from the viewpoint of the need of birth control for the physical and mental well-being of the individual woman and family, she soon saw the world-wide significance of fertility control for the social and economic well-being of humanity, and for the stability and peace of the world.

In 1927, Margaret Sanger called together in Geneva the First International Conference on Population Planning. In spite of the fact that it was organized by her, the delegates attempted to ignore and suppress all questions of population planning, and carefully avoided even the mention of birth control. Recently, twenty-seven years later, at another World Population Conference called together by the United Nations and held in Rome in 1954, population planning and fertility control occupied an important part of the program, and were favored by most of the participating social scientists and demographers.

Rarely does a great pioneer live to see the realization of her dreams and vision. Margaret Sanger has done so. Abused, persecuted, prosecuted, and jailed, she has within her lifetime become recognized nationally and internationally as one of the great women of our age. Two photographs on the wall of the Margaret Sanger Bureau clearly symbolize this transition—one, taken in 1915, shows her standing in a courtroom before the bar of judgment, being prosecuted for the advocacy of birth control; the other, taken in 1949, shows her receiving an LL.D. degree from Smith College as a "leader in the world-wide study of population problems and pioneer in the American birth control movement." Such a striking change of social attitude within the lifetime of an individual is unique.

The dramatic life of this radiant rebel is described with admirable clarity and understanding in *The Margaret Sanger Story*. The writer, Lawrence Lader, has made a comprehensive study of the available data and approached the task with deep sympathy. Margaret Sanger's life is filled with dramatic events from her early adolescence in Corning, New York, to her latest journey to Japan in 1954. Mr. Lader has succeeded in weaving together the threads of her complex life into a colorful and absorbing pattern.

The story of Margaret Sanger is not only that of an individual woman. It is also the story of the birth and development of an idea and of a movement which is bound to play a vital role in the future destiny of mankind. It is the story of a woman who has already left a permanent imprint on human history.

THE MARGARET SANGER STORY

CHAPTER 1

The factory town of Corning, New York—it would soon claim the right to be called a city since its population had reached the ten thousand mark—was hardly the place to introduce any new and explosive ideas in the 1880s. Particularly the ideas of that agnostic freethinker, Colonel Robert G. Ingersoll.

But Corning's leading stonecutter, Michael Hennessy Higgins, who was well known both for the beautiful angels and saints he chiseled out of marble and granite for the local Catholic cemetery and for his support of unpopular social and political causes, was a stubborn man. An Anglo-Irish freethinker, he was convinced that Ingersoll's dogmas would bring the light of reason to the predominantly Irish Catholic workingmen of the city. He thereupon invited "Colonel Bob" to speak at Corning. Unfortunately the hall he rented for the occasion—the only one available—happened to be owned by the local Roman Catholic church.

A large crowd had already gathered outside the hall that Sunday afternoon when Higgins and Ingersoll arrived. Higgins was accompanied by one of his daughters, a striking little girl with wide-set gray eyes and two braids of auburn hair that bounced rakishly off her shoulders. It was a tense, expectant crowd. Many of the men had obviously come to jeer. Higgins pushed his way through them and tried the door. It was locked. It would never open that afternoon, for Father Coghlan, the local priest, had learned the name of the speaker. No matter that the rent had been paid—he had no intention of allowing an agnostic like Ingersoll within the church's hall.

A moment later someone cursed the names of Higgins and Ingersoll. A fist fight broke out. Then a shower of tomatoes, apples, and cabbage stumps descended on the two men. Higgins calmly mounted the steps and announced to his followers that the meeting would go on as scheduled—only transplanted to a clearing in the woods behind his house.

The little girl, who clutched the hand of Michael Higgins, was never to forget the look of disdain on her father's face as he pushed his way through the angry mob and called to his friends to follow him. Higgins was a tall, hard-muscled man with a massive head and a shock of flaming red hair. He held his head high as he led the procession to the woods. The little girl, running at his side, tried to hold her head just as high. It was late in the afternoon when they reached the clearing with the tall pines outlined against the radiance of the setting sun. Higgins stood on a tree stump, and in a ringing voice, introduced "Colonel Bob" to the small group which stood in a circle in the clearing.

The little girl felt a strange, wild excitement inside her as she watched her father. Much of what he said she did not understand. But she knew that for the sake of an idea he had defied an angry crowd. An idea was worth all that. Someday she too would stand up like her father and fight for an idea. Only her name then would be not Margaret Higgins, but Margaret H. Sanger.

2

Michael Higgins was born in Ireland and he never lost the rich brogue that embellished his Irish tales. His parents had immigrated to Canada, but he had run away from home at Lincoln's first call for volunteers—though forced to wait until his seventeenth birthday until he could join the Twelfth New York Volunteer Cavalry as a drummer boy. After the war, he had studied anatomy, medicine, and phrenology—not to practice them professionally but to perfect his skill in modeling when he settled down to make his living as a sculptor in marble and granite in Corning.

But the dominant interests of his life were politics, economics, and free thought—always of the most radical brand. He became an ardent advocate of Henry George and loved to read aloud passages from *Progress and Poverty*. He would roar with delight at each meaty sentence and make the children reread them—"to elevate the mind," he told them. Michael Higgins worshiped the mind. "The one thing I've been able to give you is a free mind," he announced with fine Irish oratory to his family. "Use it well and give something back to your generation."

At a time when the Higgins family was going rapidly into debt and needed its large supply of coal for the winter, Michael Higgins invited Henry George to speak at Corning's leading hotel and invited fifty of his friends to attend an expensive dinner in the economist's honor. Most of his guests were far more affluent than Higgins—but the Higgins family went without coal for months.

Higgins' principles often conflicted with the practical necessities of the home. He not only looked askance at private property but at the custom of locked doors. When he was the last to bed, the doors remained unlocked. In the middle of the night, his wife once stumbled over a tramp who lay sprawled on the kitchen floor, and rushed back to the bedroom, calling to her husband to put the man out. "Oh, let him alone," he muttered, turning over to go back to sleep. "The poor devil needs sleep like the rest of us."

His generosity was unstinted—though often, unfortunately, at the family's expense. Once when he went out to buy a dozen bananas for supper, he ran into a crowd of children. He promptly bought fifteen dozen bananas and distributed them all to his youthful admirers.

Michael Higgins was the one clear voice of rebellion in Corning, a small-town Socrates hemmed in by Victorian smugness. To his workshop every day came a large circle of friends in their off moments— cabinetmakers, cobblers, masons, and sometimes a few doctors and the local editor. The little Higgins girls, who often sat wide-eyed on a bench in the corner, wondered how their father ever got any work done. He loved to preach, to argue, to thunder his opposition to all dogma and cant. His own small library was one of the best in town, and he demanded the privilege of books for all through free libraries and free books in the public schools. He supported the right of full individual liberty for women as well as men, defended Susan B. Anthony and her campaign for woman suffrage, and considered Mrs. Bloomer's bloomers an admirable expression of feminine freedom—though his own wife and daughters never wore them.

The principal targets of his wrath were religious bigotry and blind obedience to religious dogma. "Try all religions," he would tell his children. "Study them. Understand them." Once when Margaret had finished her evening prayers and climbed on her father's chair to kiss him good night, he asked quizzically, "What was that you were saying about bread?"

"Why, that was the Lord's Prayer. 'Give us this day our daily bread,'" the little girl replied.

"Whom were you talking to?"

"To God."

"Is God a baker?"

Margaret was shocked. But she tried to defend herself with phrases she had heard from her elders. "No," she admitted, "but it means rain and sunshine and all the things which make the wheat."

"So that's the idea," Higgins laughed. "Then why don't you say so? Don't take anything for granted—even things that have been repeated for centuries. You'll only grow up when you begin to do your own thinking."

3

The city of Corning, where Margaret Higgins was born, the sixth of eleven children, was a grim setting for the child of a workingman in the 1880s. "I can never look back on my childhood with joy," she once wrote. Over fifty years later, she said, "Even when I'm passing through Corning at night by train, my body knows I'm there without my seeing it. I actually become sick to my stomach."

The Higgins house was in a pine woods at the edge of town. "Even today the smell of a pine bath or pine needles disturbs me," she said recently.

Margaret's mother, Anne Purcell Higgins, was a slender woman, straight as an arrow, with gray-green eyes that were set wide apart and wavy black hair that contrasted dramatically with her spotless skin. Unlike her husband, she had been born a Catholic—though she never attended church after marriage. Father Coghlan often came to call on Anne Higgins. He implored her to turn Higgins from his godless path, to come to church, to send the children to parochial school and insure the saving of their souls. Anne Higgins was torn by conflict. But she could not match the steel-like quality of her husband's dissent, and the Higgins household remained a center of rebellion.

Margaret and the other Higgins children, thereafter, were known as children of the devil. On their way to school, their classmates shouted names at them, stuck out their tongues, mocked them. From her childhood the mark of the rebel was on Margaret.

After Father Coghlan had failed in his mission to Anne Higgins, he became the outspoken enemy of her husband. Higgins' work had been almost entirely for the local Catholic cemeteries. Now his commissions for marble angels, which had been dwindling steadily for the past few years, were cut off entirely. Occasionally he received jobs on public buildings or other stonework in adjacent towns, where his reputation was still high. Then he would be away for weeks and sometimes come home with a thousand dollars in his pocket. Food was bought for the winter. All the children had new clothes. But it might be a year until he had another large commission. Meanwhile the family sunk heavily into debt.

"Christmases were on the poverty line," Margaret once wrote. The Christmas of the Ingersoll incident was worst of all. The day before Christmas the neighborhood children lined up outside the door of the parish house to await their gifts. Margaret joined the line unobtrusively—the desire for candy or a pair of gloves outweighing the risk of a heretic's presence. But the young parish priest spotted her and brusquely ordered her off the line.

4

The streets of Corning climbed steeply from the Chemung River, which divided the town. Huge glass factories on which Corning had made its reputation lined the riverbanks. All around them on the flatlands stretched the homes of the factory workers and the poor— by 1890, almost all emigrants from Ireland. Rolling clouds of smoke from the factory chimneys kept these homes under an almost perpetual blanket.

On the hills above the city lived the factory executives and the aristocracy of Corning. In their big white frame houses with verandas, gardens, spacious lawns, and often tennis courts, Margaret soon noticed that there were only two or three children. She was an excellent pantomimist, and on Saturdays and Sundays was often asked to these homes to entertain the boys and girls with fairy stories or dramatic monologues. Margaret liked to organize plays. She liked to direct: "You be the big bear, you be the wolf." She was a gay, vivacious child, too exuberant for bitterness, but too intelligent not to want to bring into her own life what she admired most in the rich.

The financial plight in which Michael Higgins continually floundered—even before he incurred the enmity of the Catholic Church— was directly connected, Margaret saw, with the size of his family. She was the sixth child—but a new baby seemed to come almost every year, one after another, adding to her father's debts. The stigma of the large family made so strong an impact on Margaret's mind that a few years later when she went away to school she hesitated to admit the full number of her brothers and sisters. "To me the distinction between happiness and unhappiness in childhood," she stated, "was one of small families and of large families rather than of wealth and poverty."

The family had already moved to the pine woods at the edge of town when Margaret was a little girl. The air was considered better for Anne Higgins' lungs. She coughed constantly. Consumption, people called it. Tuberculosis was considered a disrespectful word that implied poverty. Margaret would see her mother's frail body shaken by such violent fits that she had to lean against the wall to support herself. Yet the children kept coming. Throughout her youth, Margaret could remember her mother only as pregnant or nursing a new baby. Her strength was drained by each pregnancy, by the constant care of the children, the washing and sewing. Anne Higgins never seemed to have a moment to herself, never the time to walk with her husband in the evening or visit the local theater.

The whole thing seemed mixed up and senseless. How could a man who wanted to bring utopia on earth with Henry George and socialism inflict such hardship on his wife?

"Mother bore eleven children," Margaret wrote years later. "She died at forty-eight. My father lived until he was eighty." The contrast was inescapable.

Yet the paradox was that Anne Higgins never questioned the constant childbearing that drained her strength. Only Margaret seemed to feel her mother's subservience. Her father had taught her the meaning of rebellion too well.

Between Michael and Anne Higgins was a strong devotion—"an atmosphere in the home which reflected the love of our parents for each other which in some way made up for the lack of material comforts in our lives," Margaret wrote. The children never had to take sides with either parent. They knew that if they pleased one they pleased the other.

Although Michael Higgins took no responsibility for the daily chores of the household, in the realm of family illness, he reigned supreme. From Margaret's childhood, he was the only doctor the family had. He brought all the babies into the world. He nursed his wife through six weeks of pneumonia. He set and straightened a younger brother's broken leg. He carried Margaret through a serious case of typhoid fever, ivy poisoning, and all the childhood ailments.

His cure-all was "good whiskey," which "liberated the spirit." There was nothing, from a deranged system to a depressed mind, it could not banish. When a case of mumps turned into large ugly abscesses, he sterilized the blade of his jackknife over a flame, lanced the abscess, and cleaned the wound with whiskey. When Margaret's face was swollen with poison ivy, a doctor advised Higgins to paint it three times a day with iodine. But the pain gave her such torture that after a few days he abandoned this "outside" treatment and went back to whiskey. Margaret soon recovered.

Michael Higgins could express his devotion to his wife in subtle but powerful ways. When their four-year-old son, Henry George McGlynn (who had both the names of the economist and Father McGlynn, a rebel from the Church), died suddenly of pneumonia, Anne Higgins' grief was inconsolable. It was the first death in the family, the first child she had lost of her ten living children. All his attempts to comfort her seemed useless. She did not even have a picture of her handsome son to preserve his memory.

The next night after everyone had gone to bed, her father called Margaret and asked her help. At eleven o'clock, they went forth into the darkness with a wheelbarrow full of tools and a bag of plaster of Paris. They walked two miles to the cemetery where the child had been buried. As quietly as possible with his pick and shovel, Higgins dug up the coffin while Margaret was posted at the gate with a lantern to warn against intruders.

After the death mask was made, Margaret worked secretly for two nights with her father in his studio, helping him to break the mask, to mold and shape the cast. On the third day after supper, Michael Higgins quietly asked his wife to come into the studio. Tenderly he removed the cloth from the plaster bust and presented her with the likeness of her dead son. She said nothing, but wept quietly and gratefully for a few moments.

5

In the eyes of the local school children, Margaret was a heretic against the Church. In her own eyes, she was a heretic against the limitations of Corning. She was too young yet to know her course, but the moment of breaking free was inevitable. She felt some indefinable power growing inside her, mysteriously, often frighteningly. "I began to fear that power within myself which determined actions beyond my control," she wrote. "It seemed at times as if there were two 'me's,' usually together, but at times pulling apart. I often talked to that other 'me' and found her full of romance and daring. She urged me on to venture and action. She was intrepid, resourceful and very daring."

Subconsciously at first, and then more purposefully, Margaret examined the limitations of the role of women in the world around her. She was already beginning to test herself against a stern ideal of action—a testing that psychologists might call an assumption of the masculine role. She made herself do the things she dreaded most— go upstairs alone to bed without a light, go into the cellar without singing, go up into the rafters of the barn and jump into the haystack thirty or forty feet below. "When I had conquered all these dreaded feats," she wrote, "I felt more secure and stronger within myself."

The one thing she feared most, however, was to walk on the ties of the railroad bridge which spanned the Chemung River. Margaret had friends across the river on a large farm with tasty apples that she loved, but to get there she always walked three miles in a roundabout way across another wooden bridge for traffic and pedestrians. On the railroad bridge, there was not only the danger of falling through the space between the ties but the chance of meeting a train as you crossed.

"Nevertheless, I felt I must walk across that bridge. I trembled with fear as I got near the place, but the more afraid I felt the more determined I was to make myself do it . . . When about a quarter of the way across, I heard the singing of the steel rails! I knew a train was speeding towards me! I could not see it because a curve in the road was just beyond the bridge . . . Suddenly around the curve the huge engine emerged . . . I tried to hide behind an iron girder to protect myself from the force of its speed when my foot slipped and I fell through space, saved only by the fact that both arms had not been able to pass through . . . I bowed my head, shut my eyes and prayed to the engineer not to emit steam . . . There I hung I do not know how long until my terror subsided at the sight of a man, a friend of my father's, who was fishing on the bridge and who came to my rescue . . . He gave me a scolding . . . advising me to go straight back.

"I knew I never could go back home defeated. It was just as impossible to go back instead of forward as it was to stop breathing. Terrified though I was, bruised and bleeding as well, the remainder of that journey across the bridge was somehow easier than the first part . . . After this I felt almost grown up. I did not talk about it, but something inside me had conquered something else."

Many years later Margaret said, "I always hated weakness in myself or anyone else." At some point after she had crossed that bridge, she had begun to prove to herself that women too could have the strength to change the order of things.

This power, this fixed determination, showed itself constantly. Once she had to visit a friend at Clinton, Connecticut, and changed trains at New Haven. There she found that the last train that stopped at Clinton that evening had already left. She was stuck in New Haven for the night—with forty cents in her pocket. She asked for the station manager, marched boldly into his office, and protested vehemently against a railroad that could not organize its schedule well enough to include an evening train. He must have been impressed by the audacity of a mere girl telling him how to run his trains, for he smilingly ordered the next train which passed through Clinton to make a special stop for her—an occurrence that made her something of a heroine in that town.

The first incident of outright rebellion came at the end of her eighth grade at school. Someone had given her a new pair of gloves, the first new pair she had ever worn. They were hard to pull over her fingers. She delayed outside of school, stretching them over her hand. When she came into the room, she was three or four minutes late. The teacher, a self-important person who enjoyed mocking others, snapped at her, "So your ladyship has arrived." The class burst into laughter. Margaret sat down, hoping the teacher would forget her. But the taunting continued even after Margaret had opened her books and begun to work. Finally she stood up, tucked her books under her arm, and marched out of the room.

"I walked straight home to Mother and announced I was through with school, I'd never go back again," she wrote. "I knew that nothing on earth or in heaven could change me. I'd go to jail, I'd go to work, I'd starve and die; but back to that school and teacher I would never go . . . A family council was called. I was questioned as to my future . . . Did I think I had an education? . . . Was I prepared to earn my living? Questions were hurled at me. Taunts and insinuations and threats of factory life filled the air . . . I had only a few months to finish and then would be ready for high school. It made no difference if it had been an hour—I would never go back."

6

The result of the family council was that Margaret should be sent away to school. Her older sisters, Mary and Nan, had made the decision. A pattern had already been established. The girls were the strong, aggressive members of the family. Nan had ambitions for everyone. She plotted their course carefully.

Mary was tutoring in Buffalo in Latin and Greek—but she could master almost any subject or craft. She could do needlepoint, upholster a couch, shingle a roof, or tend a sick cow. Nan had postponed the study of sculpture to make a good living translating French and German. The two sisters pooled their funds to pay Margaret's tuition and clothes at Claverack College near the town of Hudson in the Catskill Mountains. Margaret would get room and board by washing dishes and waiting on tables.

The three years at Claverack were "epochal in my life," Margaret once stated. She had broken free at last from Corning. For the first time, she could grasp a world she had never known except through her father's teachings. Claverack was coeducational—about five hundred boys and girl in different wings of the same building. Here were gay and spirited girls who dressed in New York fashions and discussed the latest Broadway plays. Here were well-grounded teachers who could answer the questions of an exploring mind.

Even chapel was an adventure. Following her father's precepts at Corning, she had made the rounds of all the churches but accepted none. But in the Claverack chapel, which was Methodist, students were supposed to express their convictions. On Saturday mornings, they stood up to speak on the Bible, religion, politics, and social issues.

Many of the students dreaded making these speeches. Margaret looked forward to hers. At last, she could speak on the issue that consciously or unconsciously had been pushing her forward beyond the horizons of Corning—the quest of women for some new expression, for women's rights, for suffrage. She wrote long letters home to her father and got longer ones in return, crammed with facts about important women of history—Helen of Troy, Ruth, Cleopatra. She studied the lives of women poets and authors and heard for the first time the name of Mary Wollstonecraft, one of the first women rebels, a name that would sing in her memory.

When word got around that Margaret would speak on women's rights, some of the boys, following the usual attitude of the day toward feminine suffrage, ridiculed her with cartoons of women in trousers and smoking large cigars. Margaret ignored their jibes. She would steal out to the cemetery in the evening and there, standing on the monuments over the graves, recite the words of her speech again and again to the quiet dead. Here she could close her eyes. She could dream. Instead of tombstones, there were a thousand listeners, hanging on her every word. She was speaking for women. She had become a new voice in the world.

After suffrage, she supported free silver and William Jennings Bryan. She had heard the "Boy Orator" speak on the Chautauqua circuit and had been stirred by his wondrous phrases: "You shall not press down upon the brow of labor this crown of thorns." Most of the students were for gold. But Margaret arose in chapel to speak out in lonely splendor for free silver and Populist reform. "I wanted to help grasp utopia from the skies." she stated, "and plant it on earth."

One of the girls advised her later, "You'll never get a beau if you keep talking like that." But the intensity of her speeches never interfered with the obvious pleasure she transmitted to her audience. What boy could resist the flame of her auburn hair no matter what her subject? She both attracted a wide variety of beaux and proved herself an alluring actress in school plays—so alluring that the elocution teacher began to hint at an acting career.

At the next vacation, she announced to her family that she would become an actress. Everyone laughed except Mary. Devoted Mary— an angel on earth, Margaret called her later—was always willing to stand behind her younger sister. She gave Margaret the money to apply for Charles Frohman's dramatic school in New York. Photographs were taken; application made. Then the forms arrived for her to fill out—chiefly detailed information of the measurements of her calves, ankles, and hips. What importance were these things, transmitted coldly to some stranger, compared to the quality of her voice, her ability to act? It offended her sense of the dignity of a woman; it cheapened the dream. Margaret promptly threw the photographs and application in a drawer and forgot them.

In her last year at Claverack, Margaret's buoyancy, her ability to

organize everything from a class picnic to a singing class, made her
a natural leader. The girls often took walks with boys to out-of-
bounds spots and met them in town for tea. But it was Margaret
who concocted the boldest of these ventures. A group of girls were
to slip out of a window after hours and meet their special admirers
at a dance in town. All went well, and the dance was at its height
just before midnight, when the school principal, Professor Arthur
Flack, entered. The whole group was marched silently and uneasily
back to Claverack.

The next morning Margaret was summoned to the principal's
office. Without glancing at her, he said, "Miss Higgins, don't you
feel ashamed for getting those girls into trouble and making them
break the rules?" For a moment, she thought someone had told on
her. But he went on, "No, I didn't have to be told. I knew you were
the ringleader. I've watched your influence over others. It's a rare
gift you have. Think about it seriously because you'll use it often
in the future. You'll have to make a choice—use it to get yourself
and others into trouble or use it for constructive work which will
benefit everyone."

Margaret always remembered this conversation as a point in her
maturity. She had felt this strength growing within her. Now she
knew it had to be directed and controlled.

7

She had decided to attend Cornell College and become a doctor.
Still too young for admission, she took a job teaching primary school
at Paterson, New Jersey. They were hard, unrewarding months—her
class made up of eighty-four immigrant children, mainly Poles, Hun-
garians, and Swedes who could speak almost no English. Then at
Christmas time her father summoned her home. Her mother's illness
had become critical.

Anne Higgins was now so weak that she had to be carried from
room to room. She had been spitting blood during the last few
months. The high red spots on her cheekbones stood out startlingly
against her white skin. Doors and windows were kept tight shut, and
every crack stuffed according to the treatment of the time to keep
out the raw March air. Margaret labored day after day in the sick-
room—the contagious quality of tuberculosis was still unrecognized
—while her mother's coughing fits grew more intense.

Margaret had been invited to Buffalo for Easter, and her mother insisted she needed the change. Anne Higgins sent the younger children out of the house one by one on some errand or pretext. She had more difficulty with her husband, finally persuading him to go to the foundry for new stove bricks. Much against his will, he left the house, but had gone only a few blocks when some Celtic intuition forced him to return. Anne Higgins was gasping in death. She hated scenes. Knowing she was about to die, she wanted to be alone.

Margaret rushed home to find her father brooding and inconsolable, shut off from the rest of the family. His wife's death had changed him from a benevolent father into an irritating tyrant. "He who had given us the world in which to roam," Margaret wrote, "now apparently wanted to put us behind prison bars." Margaret, as the eldest daughter at home, took her mother's place—managing the finances, ordering the meals, paying the debts, and tending the younger children. Even months after the funeral, her father kept her chained to the house, protesting if she received the slightest attention of one of the town gallants who called on her.

Not that the young men of Corning held any interest for her. Their world stopped at the city limits. Their only conversation was hunting, guns, and dogs. They knew nothing of politics, social problems, or the theater.

After six months of paternal tyranny, Margaret, her younger sister, Ethel, and a friend decided to go to an open-air concert. They knew that their father had set a ten o'clock limit on staying out, and at the stroke of ten, they were running toward the house. But when they arrived, three minutes late, the lights were out and all doors were locked. They banged on the door for at least ten minutes. Finally it opened. Their father reached out and pulled Ethel into the house, muttering, "You're not to blame for this outrageous behavior." Margaret was left alone on the street in the chilly October night.

Too cold to sit on the veranda without a wrap, Margaret went to the house of a friend and was hospitably received. The next day, she borrowed the money to visit another friend in Elmira after telegraphing Mary and Nan. The closing of that door was the turning point of her early rebellion. It was almost a symbol—not just the closing of the door at home but the end of her life at Corning. She had already outgrown the city. Now she was on her way toward outgrowing her father, the man who had always stood as an Olympian ideal in her life. "Mentally I had developed beyond my age," Margaret wrote. "I could endure all hardships—anything but remain at home. I wanted a world of action."

Accepting the invitation of Esther Farquharson, a Claverack classmate, she went to New York. Esther's mother knew one of the board members of the new White Plains Hospital outside the city. Still intent on Cornell and a medical degree, Margaret decided first to become a nurse. She applied for admission, and a week later was accepted into the whirlpool of a probationer's life at a small suburban hospital.

CHAPTER 2

The training of a probationary nurse was hard and relentless. Margaret slept in the made-over servant's quarters, a tiny room under the roof of the old manor house which the hospital occupied. On each floor of ambulatory patients there was only one bathroom. There was no electricity, and there were no bells to ring for assistance. With no resident internes on duty, a nurse was on her own much of the time. She had to haul her own supplies. She had to make all the dressings and bandages, mix solutions, and sterilize equipment in two inches of boiling water at the bottom of a wash boiler.

The months she had spent nursing her mother now brought an additional penalty. She had developed tubercular glands and was running a temperature. She was operated on—but only two weeks later assigned to night duty, where she stayed for three grueling months.

It was almost a reprieve when she was transferred to a large New York hospital for her postgraduate course. The Manhattan Eye and Ear Hospital, then at Forty-first Street and Park Avenue across from the Murray Hill Hotel, had the latest surgical techniques and equipment and provided more off-duty freedom—even an occasional dance for the nurses and doctors. It was at one of these dances that her partner, a young doctor, was called out to the waiting room. He was building a house in Westchester and his architect had come to show him the blueprints.

"This is Mr. Sanger," her partner said to Margaret. Sanger was a dark, wiry man of medium height with intense, fiery eyes. The three of them pored over the blueprints, but every time she looked up she found that the architect's eyes were concentrated on her. She was on the night shift, and finally had to leave them to go back to the ward. Even hours later, she could feel the intensity of those eyes.

At seven-thirty the next morning, the end of her shift, she left the hospital for a short walk. Sanger was waiting there on the steps; he had been waiting all night. They walked together that morning and every morning after that. He swept into her life impetuously, impatient of conventions.

Margaret, who had shunned the juvenile attentions of the boys at Claverack and the dullards of Corning, was an "incurable romantic," she admitted. Sanger "had that type of romantic nature which appealed to me." Although an architect by profession, he was an artist by temperament. He worked on assignment for a number of leading architectural firms and participated in the design of some of the city's important buildings, including Pennsylvania Station. But his real interest was painting. He talked constantly about going to Paris to study. He had been saving money for years. Now they would go together. They would get married and go together, he urged breathlessly.

Everything he did was that fast. They would be walking past a store window. A scarf that matched her eyes would catch his attention, and he would rush in and buy it without a moment's discussion. He sent her flowers constantly, took her to the opera every night she was off duty. He seemed to have no conception of the importance of money. "All it can do is make you happy," he would say. After the years of debts and budgeting at home, this was a dazzling interlude for Margaret.

Sanger, in fact, symbolized certain of the ideals of her youth. Although his family was not wealthy, they represented the educated and comfortable world of the houses on the hill above Corning. His father, who had raised sheep in Australia, had met his mother in a small German town during his European travels. From them, Sanger had inherited his talent for painting and his taste for music.

Further, Sanger represented the mature intellect she had admired in her father. He was more than ten years older than she. He had a large circle of friends among musicians, writers, and artists. Moreover, he knew Eugene Debs, whom Michael Higgins had lionized. Sanger was the only man she had met outside of her father who could make social and political theories a meaningful and important adventure.

Like everything Sanger did, even their marriage on August 18,

1902, was impetuous. They were driving through the country when he suggested that they stop to visit a friend of his, a minister. Unknown to her, he had secured a license and insisted that the minister perform the ceremony on the spot. "He had everything arranged, the witnesses, the ring, the minister and a boy to hold the horse," Margaret wrote her sister Mary.

Sanger also wrote Mary to thank her for "your very kind assurances of good will," and added that if Michael Higgins "would think the way you do, everything would be plain sailing . . ."

Higgins did become very fond of Sanger in short order, but that first year of "plain sailing"—or what Margaret called their "world of rosy dreams"—was soon interrupted by illness. Her incipient tuberculosis flared up again. In addition, she was pregnant. The doctor ordered a complete rest in the high altitude of the Adirondacks. Although it was a severe drain on Sanger's savings, he insisted that she go to a small sanitarium near Saranac where Dr. Trudeau, a specialist in pulmonary tuberculosis, could attend her. She stayed there until late October, returning to their small apartment at St. Nicholas Avenue and 149th Street just before the birth of their first son, Stuart.

Sanger had made arrangements for his regular doctor to handle the delivery, or if he was not available, his assistant. But when Margaret's labor pains came in the middle of the night, neither doctor could be located. Sanger had to rush around the corner to find the nearest general practitioner. Due almost as much to this young doctor's inexperience as to Margaret's physical condition, the delivery was unusually hard but the baby was strong and healthy.

Margaret never became a confirmed believer in psychological analysis, but she admitted later that "the birth of my first son may have, and doubtless did have, a tremendous bearing on my activities [in birth control]." When she was in California in 1930, she received a personal note from the doctor who had attended her twenty-five years back, saying, "Someday I want to hear from your own lips just what bearing my lack of knowledge of obstetrics may have had upon this profound movement that is so essentially yours. It was a hard night for both of us."

"Something in that note," she wrote afterward, "affected me like a shot . . . I had to leave my work and go home. All that night I suffered with pains in the back and had all the symptoms of labor pains! And this twenty-five years after my son was born! It was extraordinary. I am not a hysterical person, yet it was all I could do to pull myself together for the next two days. The memory of that agonizing birth kept me in mental torture, and I felt again the physical pangs of those lingering hours . . ."

Out of the suffering of that night, as well as the suffering of poor mothers, bearing their seventh or tenth child, which she was to witness later as a nurse in New York, Margaret was to become the protagonist of motherhood, the voice of all women in their desire to bring a plan and reason into the chaos of reproduction.

The ordeal of that birth so overtaxed her limited strength that she had to return to the Adirondack Mountains. Still, the tuberculosis spread, and within the next eight months she had virtually lost interest in living. Dr. Trudeau urged that she be separated from all family responsibilities and come to live near his Saranac clinic. Two of his medical associates examined her. "What would you like to do?" they asked.

"Nothing."

"Where would you like to go?"

"Nowhere."

"Would you rather have the baby sent to your mother-in-law or your brother?"

She shook her head indifferently. Nothing mattered. She was not even interested in the baby. One of the doctors returned alone a few minutes later, put his hand on her shoulder, and shook her. "Don't be like this!" he exclaimed. "Do something! Want something! You'll never get well if you keep on this way."

She could not sleep that night. At last, she had been jolted out of her stupor. "It gradually dawned on me," she recalled later, "that preparations were really being made for a long and lingering illness and eventually death. I went to bed . . . I turned the problem over and over in my sleepless mind. 'I won't die! I won't!' I kept repeating to myself." At dawn, she dressed and packed her bags, then woke the nurse and told her to get the baby ready for the trip back to New York. She had decided to act. She was through with invalidism, stuffing herself with quarts of milk and dozens of eggs a day, swallowing huge capsules of creosote. She wanted to be home with her husband in an atmosphere of love. It was one of those decisive, almost mystical acts that were to occur at many other points of crisis or serious illness in her life, in which she would call upon some deep reservoir of strength to fight back against impossible odds.

Sanger met her at the station, soothed her fears, telling her that she had done the right thing. For a few months, he settled her at a small family hotel in Yonkers while she slowly overcame her rejection of food. They would build a home of their own in Westchester and start life anew, he insisted. Almost by sheer will power—though she remained under medical care all year—she roused herself from the depths of invalidism and soon was able to scour the countryside with her husband to find a site for their home.

At Hastings-on-Hudson, less than an hour from New York, they found what they wanted. On fifty acres of hillside overlooking the Hudson River, a group of doctors, schoolteachers, and college professors, calling themselves the Columbia Colony, had built a series of small homes with gardens and sweeping lawns—the kind of setting with sunshine and space to play that they wanted for their children. The Sangers bought an acre of land and rented a cottage while they set out to build that special home which every architect plans to infuse with his dreams. Using unadorned stucco tile, Sanger designed a spacious nursery—they were planning a larger family—opening on a veranda overlooking the Hudson, a studio, a distinguished colonial dining room, and fireplaces in every room, with an especially large one in the library.

Sanger was a fastidious architect. He would return in the evening after his work in New York to find that the workmen had committed some minor error that was a grievous insult to his ideas of perfection. After Margaret had fixed him a quick supper, he would rush over to their house to tear down some partition or paneling that did not fit his standards. At ten or eleven at night, the early-retiring neighbors would often be awakened by the terrifying blows of Sanger's hammer.

Sanger and Margaret, working by artificial light, applied the stain on the woodwork of the living room and library. For weeks, they toiled on the rose window, which was to crown the head of the staircase. Each leaden petal was painstakingly leaded and welded together. Their fingers were cut, their nerves often strained. But all the relentless effort that went into that window was to symbolize the beauty and permanence of their future.

During her recuperation, Margaret enjoyed the domestic trivia of suburban life. It was a closed-off world, where the most pressing problems were homes, gardens, and schools. The high point of each week was usually the trip to New York,when the mothers would bring their children in for a pair of shoes and a visit to the museums. Margaret and a neighbor, Mrs. John House, were not satisfied with the first-grade standards at the public school, and for a while undertook to teach their sons at home—each mother serving as instructress on alternate weeks. When Stuart and some of his friends began to ask, "Where do babies come from?" Margaret decided to prepare a special course. Using animals and the simple phenomena of nature as illustrations, she taught them the rudiments of sex biology—a small but important step toward the development of her own work in New York a few years later.

Margaret and four other mothers, striving to bring the intellectual life of New York closer to home, decided to form a women's club devoted mainly to literary meetings. They followed the reading lists of a Columbia University course, and at each meeting featured a talk by one of the mothers on Browning, George Eliot, or Shakespeare. Ironically enough, that same club, which achieved enough standing to join the General Federation of Women's Clubs, refused not many years later to allow Margaret to address them on the subject of birth control.

Sanger encouraged Margaret's efforts to write and often insisted on doing the dinner dishes while she worked on one of her papers. He was a devoted husband. "When he was paid for a big commission," Margaret recalled, "he brought me orchids and embroidered Japanese robes, which I had no occasion to wear, and filled the house with luxuries. This did not go with my practical sense. I protested, 'They're beautiful. Thank you, but can we afford them?'

" 'Certainly,' he answered, and out of his pocket came tickets for the opera or theater, his chief pleasures.

" 'But we shouldn't,' I remonstrated as I shuffled a sheaf of bills which were overdue, although I knew they would eventually be paid."

A neighbor, describing the Sangers years later, called them "a happy and affectionate family."

Late in February the house was almost finished, but they refused to wait until the last plaster had dried. One afternoon a moving van pulled up to the door and boxes, crates, and barrels were carted in. Four-year-old Stuart was put to bed early, and Sanger stirred a roaring fire in the furnace against the penetrating cold. Then they began to open the crates and boxes like eager children. Carrying her second baby, Margaret was exhausted hours before she wanted to stop.

They went to bed, happy in the midst of the half-opened crates which littered their home.

In the middle of the night, the German maid pounded on the bedroom door. "Madam, come! A fire in the big stove!"

Smoke already filled the house. Margaret took Stuart from his crib while Sanger raced down the stairs to call for help. By the time Margaret got to the stairs, the fire had crept halfway up, but putting a bathrobe over the child's head, she groped her way into the open air.

"It was a moonlit night in February," she described it. "It had rained earlier, and the rain had frozen into crystals on the branches of trees and shrubbery . . . In that setting of unreality the flames, as if directed by devilish intent, spurted only through our prize leaded rose window.

"I stood silently watching the effect of months of our work and love slowly disintegrate. Petal by petal, it succumbed to the licking flames . . . It had taken so long to weld those things together . . . This thing of beauty had perished in a few minutes.

"I stood there amazed, but I was certain of a relief, of a burden lifted, a spirit set free. It was as if a chapter of my life had been brought to a close . . . Somewhere in the back of my mind I saw the absurdity of placing all one's hopes, all one's efforts, involving as they did heartaches, debts and worries, in the creation of something external that could perish irretrievably in the course of a few moments. Subconsciously I must have learned the lesson of the futility of material things. My scale of suburban values had been consumed by the flames, just as my precious rose window of leaded glass had been demolished."

Fortunately the house was covered by insurance. Since only part of the inside walls were burned, they moved to a rented house near by while Sanger went over the walls and ceilings with his workmen, removing charred boards and making plans and specifications for rebuilding. In less than six months, the house was ready again. But although they covered every inch with new paint and stain, they could never quite get rid of the ineradicable odor which clings to a burned building almost like the smell of death. Whether she realized it or not at the moment, the fire marked the beginning of the end of her life as a suburban housewife.

Their second son, Grant, was born shortly after the fire; their daughter, Peggy, only twenty months later. For the next two years, therefore, Margaret was immersed in the daily routine of mother-hood. "I loved having a baby to tend again," she wrote, "and wanted at least four more as quickly as my health would permit." Unlike Stuart, who was stocky and sandy-haired, Grant was dark-haired, highly affectionate, and artistic in temperament. Margaret had par-ticularly yearned for a daughter, and they had almost completed steps to adopt one when Peggy was born. "She was vivacious, mis-chievous, laughing—the embodiment of all my hopes as a daughter," Margaret wrote. Sanger called his wife Peggy. Their daughter, who resembled her mother in so many ways, was given the same name.

Once the two younger children had passed infancy, however, Mar-garet's rebellion against the stagnation of Hastings reached the point where it could no longer be pacified. It was a period of strange dis-content and groping. "I was not articulate enough to express this even to myself," she wrote. All she knew was that she was tired of the "tame domesticity of the pretty hillside suburb." One of her neighbors at the time recalled her "fear of becoming kitchen-minded." She was devoting an increasing amount of time to her reading and writing—so much time that she often used only a safety pin on the children's clothes if a button fell off until a generous neighbor, who admired Margaret's ambition, took the children in tow and insisted on sewing the new buttons.

"A new spirit was awakening within me; a strong insistent urge to be in the current of life's activities," she wrote. Something that had been boiling in her since she had stood in the Claverack ceme-tery and shouted her demand for women's rights to the tombstones was finally trying to express itself. Part of this new spirit was politi-cal. She and Sanger were already entertaining leading intellectuals like John Spargo, who had written a biography of Karl Marx.

But politics was only a small part of a much larger awakening. In the writings of Havelock Ellis and August Bebel, in the demands of Charlotte Perkins Gilman for a new freedom for women, Mar-garet found an expression of her own longing to play some part in the social revolution that was changing the country. The longing was indefinable. But Margaret's deep mystical sense had already convinced her that she was born to live, to act, to rebel—Hastings could not hold her!

There were more practical reasons for moving to New York. Sanger was working on a commission in New Jersey that would last all year and the daily commutation across the river and up to

Hastings was too strenuous. Further, he was also feeling the pull of wider horizons. He wanted to devote at least six months a year to painting. A few years back, they had taken off the whole summer and gone to Dublin, New Hampshire, where a friend had loaned them his guesthouse and Sanger had stayed at his easel. Now in New York, he could be closer to the bubbling cauldron of modern art.

But what Margaret wanted most of all in New York was her independence. She had definitely decided to go back to professional nursing and earn her own money. Her marriage after ten years was approaching a turning point. They had both been happy. Yet Margaret was haunted by Sanger's lack of achievement. She was going through a period of disillusionment. Like Michael Higgins, her husband had been an Olympian figure. But he had not kept pace with her own growth. He had put her in a doll's house—the Hastings house—just as Ibsen's Helmer had done to Nora. But she could never be confined. Her strength had outpaced his; she was ready to break free and soar.

The fire in the house had provided the final rupture with the past. "I was never happy in that house again," she stated. "The first opportunity we had to sell it, we let it go." Within a month they moved to New York, to a large, rambling apartment on 135th Street near Eighth Avenue—closer than even Margaret realized to the precipice of events that would plunge a "frail, shy woman" into "turmoil, uncertainty and despair."

CHAPTER 3

On November 17, 1912, a startling series of articles, entitled, "What Every Girl Should Know," began to appear each Sunday on the woman's page of the *Call*, the leading New York Socialist newspaper. Their intention was to revolutionize "women's entire attitude towards sex." They called on each mother "to clear her own mind of prudishness and to understand that the procreative act is natural, clean and healthful," and proclaimed that "the sexual impulse . . . inspires men to the highest and noblest thoughts . . . and is the creative instinct which dominates all living things."

For twelve weeks, in language both frank and painstakingly scientific, the articles described the problems of puberty and adolescence, the changes taking place in a girl's body, the functions of ovaries, Fallopian tubes, uterus, and vagina, and finally the causes, prevention, and danger of the social diseases.

No textbook, magazine, or school had dared up to this point to give women the pertinent facts about their own bodies or the essential information that should be passed on to their daughters. The dead hand of Victorian morality, personified by a strange and powerful figure named Anthony Comstock, still gripped the country. Secretary of the New York Society for the Suppression of Vice, ruthless and fanatical, Comstock had adroitly pushed through a harassed Congress a few hours before adjournment in 1873 the censorship law which bore his name. As special agent for the Post Office Department, Comstock was empowered by the law to open any letter, package, pamphlet, or book passing through the mails and personally decide what was lewd, indecent, or obscene.

Despite the thousands of letters from women that flooded the offices of the *Call*, praising the articles and asking for reprints for their daughters and friends, Comstock and the Post Office Department stepped in and announced that the article on gonorrhea had violated the boundaries of public taste. The *Call* was notified that if it printed the next article on syphilis, its mailing permit would immediately be revoked. On February 9, 1913, the left-hand column of the woman's page was left completely blank except for the words: "What Every Girl Should Know. NOTHING! By order of the Post Office Department."

The author of this revolutionary series was Margaret Sanger. She had been in New York less than six months, but already she had fired the first shot in her rebellion that was not only a direct challenge to Comstock, but an open appeal to women to break with the past. She was now part of the exuberant movement that was sweeping the country. It could not be classified by names and labels. It was a hunger for change, a passionate upheaval against the dead morality and social and economic injustices of the last decades.

In the Midwest, it had brought Socialist mayors into office; in Chicago, that driving reformer, John Peter Altgeld. In Washington, it took the form of "trust busting." In the logging camps and mines of the West with the Industrial Workers of the World, and in the industrial cities and unions of the East with the anarchists, syndicalists, and Socialists, it came in more explosive shapes. But despite the conglomeration of labels, the everlasting divisions and splinterings within each group and party, all were welded together by an enormous hunger for revolt and what Granville Hicks called "a gaiety of great hopes."

The significant fact is that Margaret Sanger's articles on sex were published in the leading Socialist newspaper. This was only logical, for her first plunge into the radical revolt was through the Socialist party.

Local No. 5 of the Socialist party, which William and Margaret Sanger joined, had its headquarters only ten blocks from the Sangers' rambling old apartment on 135th Street. After its meetings, the members would often adjourn for beer to the Sanger living room. Margaret saturated herself in debate. Here were earth-shaking ideas that would change the world. Here were the parry and thrust of quick, decisive minds of men like John Reed, just out of Harvard but already a master reporter, and "Big Bill" Haywood, the I.W.W. leader, a one-eyed giant with a booming voice and an enormous head always cocked on one side, as if to get a better view of you.

Margaret Sanger was intrigued by this new political and economic radicalism—yet she was never really part of it. Rebellion for her was always seen through a woman's eyes. She came out of the main stream of the women's rights movements. Yet she was not satisfied with its limited platform. She was still searching for more basic answers.

From the first revolt of women at the Woman's Rights Convention at Seneca Falls, New York, in 1848, its leaders, principally Mrs. Lucretia Coffin Mott and Mrs. Elizabeth Cady Stanton, had hammered at the theme that men had established an "absolute tyranny" over women. Their first demands were suffrage and equal property rights, equal job opportunities and equal pay.

The first of these demands was won in New York when legislation gave women control of their own property and the right to make a will. By 1860, almost all northern states had passed similar laws. Many of these early women rebels became ardent abolitionists. Through the Women's Loyal League, Susan B. Anthony became a leading advocate of the Thirteenth Amendment, which turned the Emancipation Proclamation into law.

But it was the struggle for the vote that became the unifying issue for the feminists. In 1869, Miss Anthony teamed with her inseparable friend, Mrs. Stanton, to found the National Woman Suffrage Association. Into their camp came other leaders, like Amelia Bloomer and Lucy Stone—the first better known in history for her Turkish-style trousers gathered at the ankle, the other for keeping her maiden name after marriage.

By the turn of the century, women were making strong demands for economic equality. In 1870, only one and a half million women held jobs in the United States. By 1905, the number had swollen to five million. The older craft unions in the American Federation of Labor rarely concerned themselves with the new masses of immigrant women who were taking jobs. But the I.W.W. included women in its one big union for all. The Socialists gave some of them responsible positions. Women were becoming union officials and organizers, and the fight for equal pay and working conditions now took its place alongside the fight for the vote.

Margaret Sanger herself in these first months worked as an organizer and was responsible for bringing scores of the Scandinavian women workers in her area into Local No. 5 of the Socialist party. But neither the feminist movements nor the unions, she felt, went deep enough. What did a woman's refusal to wear a wedding ring

or her insistence on keeping her maiden name add to her basic quest
for freedom? The vote and equal pay were essential, of course.
"None of these demands, however," Margaret wrote later, "affected
directly the most vital factors of her existence."

This instinctive hunger to enunciate a new freedom for women
had been stirring inside her since childhood. It was a revolt both
against the subservient life at Corning and the death of her mother.
What could the vote, equal property rights, or feminism mean to a
woman who had been enslaved by the bearing of eleven children?
What use to her were these rights until she controlled the destiny
of her own flesh?

She saw that women needed a new vision—"not to preserve a man-
made world but to create a human world by the infusion of the
feminine element into all its activities." She had been reaching
toward this freedom during all her years of study of Havelock
Ellis, Freud, Bebel, and the new psychologists. "The most far-reach-
ing social development of modern times is the revolt of women
against sex servitude," she was to write. "When women have raised
the standard of sex ideals and purged the human mind of its un-
clean conception of sex, the fountain of the race will have been
cleaned."

Mabel Dodge, whose keen intellect and ample hospitality made
her Greenwich Village salon one of the intellectual centers of New
York, would be one of the first in the next few years to recognize
this new voice in the wilderness of Bohemia. "It was as if she had
been more or less arbitrarily chosen by the powers that be to voice
a new gospel . . ." Mrs. Dodge wrote in her autobiography.[1]

The Dodge salon was in her lavish apartment at Ninth Street and
Fifth Avenue. You walked up the red-carpeted stairway to the second floor, where the large living room, with its painted white woodwork and dazzling twinkle of Italian glasses on the shelves, was
always filled with a varied collection of trade unionists, actors, mys-
tics, anarchists, celebrities, and nonentities—"everybody touched in
the head with some wild little sacred excitement about life," Max
Eastman commented later. Huge slabs of beef and copious decanters
of whiskey and sherry always waited on the sideboard. The conversation and debate, often wild and excitable, lasted far into the night.

Although Margaret Sanger made only occasional visits to the

[1]*Intimate Memories* (New York: Harcourt Brace, 1933–37), Vol. III, pp.
69–71.

salon, Mrs. Dodge was quick to herald her as "the first person that I, personally, ever knew, who set out to rehabilitate it [sex]"—to make it "a scientific, wholly dignified and prophylactic part of right living . . ."

All during 1912 in the political cauldron of Socialist politics, Margaret Sanger studied the link between poverty, large families, and her dream of the "revolt of women against sex servitude." The laundry workers of New York—the "Irish Amazons" and their husbands—had gone on strike that winter without permission of Samuel Gompers and the American Federation of Labor. The hardest worked and most poorly paid men and women in the unions, they had reached the breaking point. One man described to Margaret Sanger his typical day: he rose at five, had ten minutes for lunch, the same for supper, and dragged himself home at eleven at night. It was shorter hours and higher wages the men demanded above everything else.

But when Margaret Sanger talked to the women in their dingy tenement rooms, she found an even more fundamental yearning. Dominating each was the relationship between her husband, her children, and herself. Many had five, six, or seven children crowded into their three-room apartments. Each new child pulled them deeper into the hopeless morass. The constant dread of more children was even more important in their lives than the question of hours and wages.

"Poverty and large families seemed to go hand in hand," Margaret pointed out at the next meeting of Local No. 5. "If the unions were fighting for better wages and shorter hours, they should be equally concerned with the size of the workingman's family."

In Lawrence, Massachusetts, that winter of 1912, the textile workers, whose wages and hours had brought them almost to starvation level, finally went out on strike. One of the girl pickets was shot by the police. I.W.W. leaders rushed up to take charge of the strike. City police and company police patrolled the streets. Lawrence was an armed camp, a grim, freezing town haunted by stinging winds and hunger as the workers' money dwindled and vanished.

Always before in these strikes, it had been the hunger of children that had broken the resistance of the workers. They were of seven nationalities but chiefly Italian. The Italians' union and radical leaders in New York, who had formed a strike committee, decided that morale could be maintained only if the children were brought from Lawrence to New York and placed in the homes of sympathizers. Because of her nursing skill, Margaret Sanger was a logical choice to lead this mission.

Taking off a week from her professional nursing, she caught the train for Boston on a freezing January evening and made connections there to Lawrence, accompanied by John Di Gregorio, secretary of the Italian Socialist Federation's defense committee, and Carrie Giovannitti. Even bundled in overcoats, they were numb with cold. At Lawrence, 119 children were huddled in a large hall. Mrs. Sanger insisted on an immediate medical examination. She found them emaciated, almost all with adenoids and enlarged tonsils, one boy sick with diphtheria who had been working until the day of the strike. Their clothes were in shreds, and although their parents worked in the richest woolen mills in the country, only four of them wore overcoats, and almost none woolen underwear.

The wind was so bitter that they had to run the children to the railroad station. They had not been provided with extra money for buses or taxis, so when they reached Boston the whole party made the long trek on foot from North to South Station. The children sang to keep up their spirits. Tramping through the streets and on the train to New York, they alternated between the "Marseillaise," the "Internationale," and other workers' songs, each singing in Italian, French, Polish, German, English, or whatever tongue he knew best.

In New York, thousands of men and women from the Italian Socialist Federation and other labor groups were waiting at the station. "Shouting, cheering, with tears in their eyes, hundreds of these men broke through the ropes." Margaret Sanger described the scene in an article she wrote for the *Call*. "Tearing off their own coats, they wrapped them around the cold and tired little bodies, placed them on their shoulders and marched on with the throng." The welcoming committee had arranged a parade to Webster Hall near Union Square. A band marched out in front, torches were lit, banners bellied in the breeze. At Webster Hall, the tables were piled with food and the hungry children snatched at it and stuffed it down.

During the next week, ninety-two more children were brought to New York. But as nation-wide attention became focused on the desperate condition of the Lawrence workers, Congress set up a committee to investigate the strike and its causes. Victor Berger of Wisconsin, the only Socialist member of the House, asked Mrs. Sanger to testify. She described the undernourished children, their illness, the pitiful condition of their clothes. From notes made on the spot, she told exactly how few children had overcoats or underwear. This was something new for a congressional hearing, not a union leader but a small, fragile woman telling in simple language about the needs of human beings. The testimony impressed the committee, and helped swing public opinion behind the workers, so that by the end of March the strike was eventually won. For one moment in those marbled committee chambers of Congress, Margaret Sanger had spoken as the voice of motherhood.

But the few dollars in wages, the shorter hours won by the strikers, she realized, were only a small step forward. What good would a few dollars be when these already hungry families with three, four, or five children had to feed another three or four mouths? What future would there be for these working mothers until they were able to control the size of their own families?

Not long afterward she received a telephone call from Anita Block, editor of the woman's page of the *Call* and wife of John Block, a leading Socialist. "Will you help me out?" she asked. "We have a lecture tonight and our speaker is sick."

"But I can't speak," Margaret protested.

"You've got to. There's no one else we can call on."

Margaret finally agreed, but she was so terrified she could not eat that night. What could she say to these working women who came long distances to the meeting seeking enlightenment after ten hours of work? She was no expert on labor or socialism. But at Lawrence she had seen how closely the intimate problems of family life were tied to the worker's future welfare. At last, she would bring some of these problems out in the open.

That night in the old second-floor meeting hall of Local No. 5, she rose fearfully to her feet. "Her face seemed to light up," an old associate said later, "as if some religious thing had come over it." Her wide-set gray eyes, the radiant auburn hair pinned in coils around her head, had a disarming simplicity. She spoke simply, directly, but a current of excitement poured from her, flooding the room.

They questioned her for an hour afterward. She had touched some deep problem here, she saw. She had been right. Motherhood, the size of the family were intimately connected with the problems of the worker. So great was the demand for more information that Anita Block scheduled additional lectures, and Margaret's audiences grew to seventy-five, then a hundred. Other clubs began asking her to speak. Anita insisted that the lectures should be made available to the whole readership of the *Call*. "Turn them into a series of articles," she told Margaret. Night after night, after she came home from long hours of nursing, Margaret sat up writing the articles—her first demand for a new and clean conception of sex—which became "What Every Mother Should Know," followed by a second series, "What Every Girl Should Know."

But it was among the swarming tenements of the Lower East Side that Margaret Sanger finally touched the core of women's emancipation. More and more her nursing calls seemed to come from this vast area of poverty below Fourteenth Street. She stayed there working till late at night, coming home exhausted, strained to the breaking point. William Sanger was worried, afraid that her incipient tuberculosis would break out again.

Fortunately Sanger's mother had come to live with them and take care of the children during the long hours Margaret was away from home. But the children too wondered what was happening to their mother. Grant, still too young for school, would clutch her by the knees and ask, "Are you going downtown?" She would nod and Grant would hold on tighter, saying, "I hate downtown."

It was the degradation of motherhood that haunted her. Here were thousands of working women, crowded like animals into their tenement flats. One block alone, bounded by Canal, Hester, Eldridge and Forsyth streets, held almost three thousand people, Italians, Jews, Irish, and Germans. From the Health Department records, she learned that there were over four hundred and fifty babies in that block—but only a single dilapidated bathtub in the backyard of each house. The infant death rate was horrifying—204 out of every 1,000.

She saw families of seven and eight children packed into three-room flats. Often these families took in extra "boarders" to help pay the rent. A single room would hold as many as six sleepers, the little girls forced to dress and undress in front of the men. In one Elizabeth Street tenement, forty-three families were jammed into sixteen flats.

Ten thousand apartments here were never touched by a ray of

sun. Their only windows were on narrow courts, airshafts no more than two feet wide, filled with the smell of garbage.

Over every building hung the moldy, indefinable smell of poverty, which even the sting of a nurse's antiseptics could not drive away. Many buildings had toilets only on every other floor. There was no garbage disposal, and women on the sixth or seventh floors often waited for days to drag their garbage down the rickety, unlit stairs. On one maternity case to which she had been called by an insurance-company doctor, she climbed up five flights to an airless room, but the baby had already arrived. A boy of ten had been his mother's only assistant. He had wrapped the placenta in a piece of newspaper and dropped it into the airshaft.

Most of her cases were confinements. They were frail, wasted women, often the mothers of five or six children. A few days after the baby was born and Mrs. Sanger was about to leave the case, these women would invariably ask the same question. "I couldn't stand another baby now. All the time I'm sick. There's no money. What can I do to stop another baby?"

The women pleaded with her: "Tell me the secret! Please!" When they grew bitter, they would say, "It's the rich that know all the tricks." But when she told them she doubted that the rich knew more than they did, they laughed at her and accused her of holding back information for money.

In their desperate attempts to prevent continued pregnancies, the women turned to any resort—herb teas, drops of turpentine on sugar, rolling downstairs, inserting slippery elm and even knitting needles and shoe hooks into the uterus. If they heard of a new remedy, they would hurry to the drugstore. A friendly clerk might say, "That won't help you, but here's something that might." But most druggists, fearful of breaking the law, refused to give advice.

Public abortionists flourished throughout the area. Going home at night, Margaret Sanger would pass lines of women, sometimes a hundred of them with shawls drawn over their heads, waiting on the street outside the abortionist's office as if they were standing in line for a movie. She learned the tragedy of these operations—a quick examination, the payment of five dollars, and then the woman would be sent out on the street. Usually the flow began the next day and continued for four or five weeks. Often these women had to be taken to the hospital for a curettage. Then she would learn that Mrs. Cohen "had been taken to Bellevue but never came back," or that

Mrs. Kelley "had sent the children to a neighbor and then put her head into the gas oven." It was senseless, horrible—a hundred thousand abortions each year, she heard, in New York alone.

But what could be done to stop it? The question kept her awake at night. She began to fear each trip to the Lower East Side. Often she had almost decided to stay away from the area entirely, but something kept driving her back. These were human beings. Their husbands worked ten or twelve hours a day as laborers, truck drivers, small shopkeepers to bring home a few dollars. Why should these women be old and broken at thirty or thirty-five?

She saw they were trapped in an endless circle. Poverty and childbearing were inescapably linked. Unless they could stop this endless chain of children, their lives were futile, wasted. "No woman can call herself free who does not own and control her body," Margaret Sanger was to write. "No woman can call herself free until she can choose consciously whether she will or will not be a mother."

But the issue went beyond poverty, beyond the Lower East Side. It was as old as history. Rich or poor, women had always struggled against this biological slavery. "The earning of her own living does not give her the development of her inner sex urge, far deeper and far more powerful in its outworkings than any of these externals," she stated. "The most important force in the remaking of the world is a free motherhood."

One final moment in the summer of 1912 changed her life unalterably. She was called one day to a Grand Street tenement, to another one of those endless tiny flats in a decaying airshaft building. A woman lay in bed, pale and wasted, a small, dark-haired woman still under thirty named Sadie Sachs. It was another case of attempted abortion. Jake Sachs, a truck driver, had come home the night before to find his wife unconscious on the floor, his three children weeping helplessly. He had called the nearest doctor, but septicemia had already set in.

The doctor and Mrs. Sanger struggled to save the woman's life. For two weeks in the July heat, she practically lived in that room. She had to carry food and ice up three flights. Waste had to be carted to the toilet downstairs. Jake did everything he could, but he had to be out driving his truck to pay the doctor's bills. So Mrs. Sanger stayed by the bedside, slowly nursing a little more life into the wasted face. At the end of three weeks, Mrs. Sachs was sitting up.

But as the doctor finished his last examination, she leaned over and whispered to Mrs. Sanger, "Another baby will finish me, I suppose." Margaret evaded a direct answer. But she drew the doctor aside at the door and told him that Mrs. Sachs was worried about having another child. "She ought to be," he snapped.

Then he went back to Mrs. Sachs. "Any more of this," he said, "and there'll be no need to send for me."

"I know, I know." Mrs. Sachs nodded. She raised herself slightly in bed. "What can I do to prevent another baby?" she whispered.

The doctor had worked hard to save Mrs. Sachs' life. But this question had no answer. He spoke quickly, almost laughingly. "You can't have your cake and eat it too, young woman. There's only one way. Tell Jake to sleep on the roof."

Then he was gone. Margaret turned toward Mrs. Sachs. But she was already weeping quietly. "He can't understand," she whispered. "He's only a man. But you do, don't you? You're a woman. Please tell me the secret."

Margaret Sanger stood there, helpless. What could she say? A woman's life depended on the answer, the lives of countless women everywhere. But she didn't know the answer. All she could do was make Mrs. Sachs comfortable, promise to come back in a few days, and wait by the bedside until she dropped off to sleep.

Even days later, Margaret Sanger could not erase the sight of Mrs. Sachs from her mind. And all she could do was make excuses to herself, put off going back day after day.

The days turned to months, and she still did not go back. Then the telephone rang, and it was Jake Sachs' desperate voice. His wife was sick again. Another attempted abortion. She took her nurse's bag and hurried downtown. The same familiar doorway, the same dingy stairs. In the bedroom, Mrs. Sachs was lying in a coma. The doctor worked desperately to save her, but it was too late this time. In ten minutes, she was dead. Mrs. Sanger folded the pale, wasted hands across her breast, the same hands that had stretched out toward her. Jake Sachs, "helpless in his loneliness, bewildered in his helplessness," she wrote later, "paced up and down the room, hands clenching his head, moaning, 'My God! My God! My God!'

"After I left that desolate house I walked and walked and walked; for hours and hours I kept on, bag in hand, thinking, regretting, dreading to stop; fearful of my conscience, dreading to face my own accusing soul. At three in the morning I arrived home . . .

"As I stood at the window and looked out, the miseries and problems of that sleeping city arose before me in a clear vision like a panorama: crowded homes, too many children; babies dying in infancy; mothers overworked . . . half sick most of their lives . . . made into drudges; children working in cellars; children aged six and seven pushed into the labor market to help earn a living; another baby on the way; still another; yet another . . .

"One after another these pictures unreeled themselves before me . . . I watched the lights go out, I saw the darkness gradually give way to the first shimmer of dawn . . . I knew a new day had come for me and a new world as well.

"It was like an illumination . . . there was only one thing to be done: call out, start the alarm, set the heather on fire! Awaken the womanhood of America to free the motherhood of the world! I released from my almost paralyzed hand the nursing bag, which unconsciously I had clutched, threw it across the room, tore the uniform from my body, flung it into a corner, and renounced all palliative work forever.

"I was now finished with superficial cures, with doctors and nurses and social workers who were brought face to face with this overwhelming truth of women's needs and yet turned to pass on the other side. They must be made to see the facts. I resolved that women should have knowledge of contraception. They have every right to know about their own bodies. I would strike out—I would scream from the housetops. I would tell the world what was going on in the lives of these poor women. I *would* be heard. No matter what it should cost. *I would be heard.*

"I went to bed and slept . . . the first undisturbed sleep I had had in over a year . . . free from dreams, free from haunting faces."

CHAPTER 4

That winter of 1913 Margaret Sanger challenged the laws of the United States Government. To spread the knowledge of contraception throughout the country, she had determined to test the Comstock law and risk imprisonment. Since its passage in 1873, no information on contraception had been sent through the mails or by interstate commerce. Druggists, hospitals, even doctors, were afraid to use the mails for contraceptive advice or take any action that might leave them open to prosecution.

Comstock even had his feminine associates write decoy letters, appealing for contraceptive help, to doctors all over the country. "There are cases where pregnancy means almost certain death to a woman," stated a contemporary article in *Harper's Weekly*. "In cases of Bright's disease, tuberculosis, and pelvic malformation, it is fraught with the gravest danger. Yet a doctor telling such a woman how to avoid pregnancy is liable to imprisonment." This was the type of trap Comstock had set for a tenderhearted midwestern physician. Two women decoys had begged him for contraceptive protection from their husbands, supposedly insane, and he had obligingly answered their request by mail. Comstock immediately had him arrested. Sentenced on both counts to the full ten years at Leavenworth penitentiary, the doctor was not released until seven years later, a broken man.

Where could Margaret Sanger find the contraceptive information to give to working women? When she called on doctors who she thought could help her, they asked her to leave their office. Druggists either furtively avoided her questions or sold her in great secrecy techniques that were unscientific and often blatantly harmful.

It was obvious that the visage of Anthony Comstock had cast its dread shadow over the land. Margaret's own friends warned, "Stop this foolish thing now before it's too late." She turned to the feminist leaders and suffragettes. Surely they would not be frightened by Comstock. But they too said, "Wait till we have socialism, economic equality! Wait till we have the vote! The Comstock law will be changed."

But how could she wait when millions of women needed this information? Drastic as it was to break the law, it was even worse to sit by and do nothing. "Shall we look upon a piece of parchment as greater than human happiness, greater than human life?" she wrote in explanation of her stand.

She began to search the libraries for contraceptive knowledge. She sat for hours in the Astor, the Lenox, the Academy of Medicine, poring through obtuse medical texts. She went to Washington to the Library of Congress. But there was only a brief pamphlet, written in 1832 by a daring Massachusetts doctor, Charles Knowlton, with information she could not accept as authoritative eighty years later. Even William J. Robinson, a New York doctor who had been preaching the need for contraception in his own heretical paper, *Medical Critic and Guide,* had never printed a specific technique.

These months of searching and frustration had left her close to exhaustion. She had become a stranger even to Sanger. He had grown more irritated lately at her long absences from the house; he complained that this search had become an obsession, and tried to hold her by childish devices that only served to force them farther apart. When the children came home from school, they would hunt for her, crying, "Where's Mother?" On those rare days when they found her, they would dance round, shouting, "Mother's home, Mother's sewing," as if sewing implied a little measure of permanence.

She decided with Sanger to take a cottage that summer of 1913 on the wind-swept dunes near Provincetown on Cape Cod. He was tiring of architecture and could concentrate for a few months on painting. She could have the children close to her. On the strip of beach in front of their cottage, they had sunrise breakfasts and sunset picnics, romped on the sand and swam day after day. "I wanted to feed, to bathe, to clothe them," she wrote later. "I wanted to bind them to me and allow nothing to force us apart."

"Big Bill" Haywood came to Provincetown that summer to rest after the exhausting months of the Paterson, New Jersey, textile strike. "Big Bill" and the other I.W.W. leaders had been the only labor people to grasp the immediate connection between childbearing and poverty. "Don't wait," he told Margaret. "Get your contraceptive information at the source. The women of France have been limiting their families for a hundred years. Go to France and get your answers."

Sanger was as anxious as Margaret to make the trip. At last, he could study painting in Paris. The trip seemed so urgent that they drew from the bank their combined savings. They may not have realized it at the moment but they were making a clean sweep of the past.

They sailed from Boston in October on a small, crowded cabin boat, landing first in Glasgow. Here she was to write a series of articles for the *Call* on Glasgow's system of municipal government ownership, considered one of the Socialists' principal achievements. The city's housing developments were fine new buildings. There were light, air, a minimum of rooms and cubic space allotted to each child in a family of up to three children. But what happens to the families with six children? she asked the officials. "They must live elsewhere," they said.

She found them in crowded tenement districts on the outskirts of the city, mainly near the shipyards, far from the municipal bakeries, laundries, markets, and tram services. Walking through these streets at night, she met hundreds of women in rags, dragging two or three little children behind them, calling out, "Bread, bread." What had municipal government ownership done for them? No system of government, no matter how well planned, she saw, could succeed without population control.

They pushed on to Paris and subleased an apartment on the Boulevard St. Michel. Sanger found a studio at Montparnasse. While the children were at school, she visited the working-class districts of Paris, searching for the facts on contraception.

"Have you just discovered this knowledge of contraception?" she would ask the French women.

"Oh no. *Maman* told me."

"Who told her?"

"*Grand'mère*, I suppose."

Since 1807, when the Code Napoléon had decreed that family property must be split equally among all children, the thrifty French workers and peasants had embraced the advantages of family limitation. Methods of contraception, she learned, were passed on from mother to daughter, generation after generation. Women prided themselves on their special formulas for suppositories and douches. Such knowledge was considered as essential to a girl as her ability to run the house.

It was the quality of children, not quantity, that counted now. The small family had become a recognized goal in social evolution. The syndicalists had made it part of their labor platform, distributing leaflets and books on methods of contraception. The English Neo-Malthusian movement, represented here by its newspaper, *Génération Consciente,* was a powerful influence in union ranks.

Day after day Margaret Sanger talked to doctors, midwives, druggists, working women. From each, she collected the best formulas for douches, the latest techniques in suppositories, sponges, and pessaries. At the drugstores, she bought the most efficient devices and stored them with her carefully recorded notes in her trunk—all to form the basis of her pamphlet, *Family Limitation,* which would usher in the birth-control movement in the United States not many months hence.

At last, she had found what she wanted. Every minute in Paris now was wasted. She had to get back. Sanger had put up with almost a year of her agonized frustration, her moods, the ceaseless conflict inside her between home and marriage and this thing that had taken over her whole life. Could she ask him to return to America now? He was passionately happy at his painting. He deserved this chance at a new career. Stay in Paris and paint, she urged. She would return alone with the children. On New Year's Eve of 1914, she said good-by to Bill and boarded the *New York* for home, neither of them aware that the swirling currents of history had irrevocably ended their marriage and made this parting final.

There was no other way. They had moved into separate worlds. Their twelve years together had been devoted, tender. Even now there was no open disagreement. But as this huge tide of revolt swept her forward, the rootless life of an artist had become impossible for her. Why not admit it? Their paths had diverged too far.

Once he had urged her interest in women's problems. He had been proud of her first success as a speaker. But in the last year her constant meetings with feminist leaders, the endless succession of strange associates who dropped into their home, planning and arguing till all hours of the night, had made him touchy and jealous.

She could not blame him. Yet there was nothing she disliked more than jealousy—all through her life she instantly rebelled when any man became over-possessive.

She could no longer be tied to the house, the details of domesticity. Her horizons had expanded far beyond Sanger's understanding. His strength could no longer match hers. She was soaring, unchained, into some untouched sphere. She would not only speak for American motherhood, be the voice of the new freedom. But she herself had to live as the synthesis of this new freedom—live as Shelley had once written, "as though to live and love were one."

Neither Sanger nor any man, for now, could hold her. A few years later she was to write Juliet Rublee, one of her oldest friends and associates: "Where is the man to give me what the movement gives in joy and interest and freedom?"

If this had an element of selfishness in it, it had even more of selflessness. Later in his effort to win her back, Sanger pleaded with her that "*no work* is so great that two should miss the sweetness of life." But he misjudged her, as many men were to misjudge her. Her work had become an obsession that was to rule out the strongest ties in life—sometimes even her children. Much as she loved Stuart, Grant, and Peggy, the misery, the need of a million other mothers and children now drove her onward as if she had become the single voice of all their hopes.

Back in New York and settled in a small apartment on Post Avenue near the upper tip of Manhattan, Margaret Sanger determined to bring her knowledge of contraception to the women of America through a new monthly newspaper, the *Woman Rebel*. It would be a brash, flaming paper, not only a scathing frontal attack on the Comstock law, but an inspiration to women to break any chains that limited their freedom. Its slogan would be: "No Gods, No Masters." The first issue in uninhibited language would define a woman's duty, "To look the world in the face with a go-to-hell look in the eyes."

She plunged ahead almost singlehanded. She was editor, circulation director, treasurer, bookkeeper. Outside of the slim savings left over from the sale of the Hastings house, which had been divided with Sanger, she had no financial backing. But what did money matter? "I don't really know how most of my ventures in this work were ever financed," she wrote years later. "I do things first and somehow or another they get paid for. I suppose here is the real difference between the idealist—or the 'fanatic,' as we are called—and the ordinary 'normal' human being."

She sent notice of the birth of her paper to half a dozen radical publications—the *Masses, Mother Earth,* the *Call, The Liberator.* At union meetings, she distributed hundreds of leaflets announcing the first issue of a paper ". . . for the advancement of woman's freedom . . . A paper dealing with the conditions which enslave her and the manner in which she is enslaved, by motherhood, by wage slavery, by bourgeois morality, by customs, laws and superstitions."

Gradually a small group of supporters formed around her: writers, clerks, laborers who would come to her house night after night to debate and plan the first issues. A new movement was being born, and it had to have a name. They ran over a list of possibilities, but quickly discarded such British and French importations as Neo-Malthusian, "family limitation," and "conscious generation." They tried voluntary parenthood, voluntary motherhood, race control, and birthrate control. None sounded right until someone suggested, "Drop the 'rate.' " Birth control had just the right implication, just the right ring to capture the American imagination.

The first issue of the *Woman Rebel* appeared in March 1914. No such collection of pyrotechnics had ever been collected in eight pages. Margaret Sanger lashed out at Comstock and announced she would break the law by publishing contraceptive information. She described the horrors of abortion and told how they could be eliminated if contraceptives were made available to all mothers. She pleaded with women not to bring into the world "a child we are not physically, mentally or financially prepared to accept or care for." Then she moved on to a more philosophic analysis of the new world women must make for themselves. Mary Wollstonecraft, an earlier rebel, was extolled for her "passionate demand that sex should be obliterated by the larger claim of woman to be considered as a human being." Woman can only get "life, liberty and the pursuit of happiness" when she makes herself "absolute mistress of her own body." This is the final freedom—when she wins the "absolute right to dispose of herself, to withhold herself, to procreate or to suppress the germ of life."

Birth control and the emancipation of women from sex servitude continued to be the focus of the next seven issues. The Comstock law, she accused, forced women to patronize "the profitable business of abortion quacks." The rich bought birth-control techniques from high-priced doctors while the poor were prosecuted for seeking the same information. The pages were crowded with ringing phrases: "A woman's body belongs to herself alone," and "Enforced motherhood is the most complete denial of a woman's right to life and liberty." But there was also a persistent appeal to the working class. "If you working women of the United States support the *Woman Rebel* in this fight for the freedom of your own bodies," she wrote in the June issue, "you will re-create the revolutionary spirit of your class." She attacked a wide range of enemies of working women, from the instigators of the Ludlow massacre to the churches, who "want to keep you in ignorance of your own body."

Even some of Margaret Sanger's allies in the radical movement like Max Eastman, editor of the *Masses*, considered the *Woman Rebel's* style "very conscious extremism and blare of rebellion for its own sake." The regular journalists, of course, attacked it ferociously, the Pittsburgh *Sun* ending its editorial with a single line: "The thing is nauseating." Yet this exuberant, often reckless paper struck a unique spark for thousands of women who had been waiting for this kind of uncompromising leadership. Emma Goldman, the anarchist leader, an unrivaled expert herself at fiery language, wrote admiringly to Margaret during her tour of the country that the paper was "the best seller we've got," and sold five hundred copies in Los Angeles alone. During its eight months of publication, she received over ten thousand letters, most of them from women pleading for specific birth control techniques. These women, and subscriptions secured through trade unions, supplied the *Woman Rebel's* basic circulation of two thousand copies each month. But copies even reached Europe, and such feminist leaders as Mrs. Pankhurst, Ellen Key, and Rosa Luxemburg became regular readers.

The inevitable counterattack from Comstock came on April 2. Just four weeks after the first issue had been published, Margaret Sanger found on top of her pile of morning mail a letter from the Post Office Department. "In accordance with advice from the Assistant Attorney General for the Post Office Department," it read, "you are informed that the publication entitled the *Woman Rebel* for March, 1914, is unmailable under provisions of Section 211 of the Criminal Code as amended by the Act of March 4, 1911."

"I reread the letter," she recalled. "At first, the significance of its contents did not register on my brain. I read it again, and yet again; and then I *knew* the fight was on." She had reached the edge of the abyss. The next step was the courts. But she had expected all this. "I had sensed with amazing accuracy the denunciation, misunderstanding, accusation, and ostracism which was to follow. I was prepared for anything. Nothing could come as a surprise."

Only time was important now. She had to publish as many issues, reach as many thousands of women as possible before the inevitable happened. Checking at the local post office, she found that only half the March issue, only the *A–Ms* had been confiscated. Margaret Sanger and a few friends sat up all night addressing a new set, and then tramped all over town in the early dawn, dropping a few issues in each chute to prevent the Post Office authorities' detecting and confiscating the whole mailing. Three more issues were banned by the Post Office Department: May, July, and August. Each time she wrote to the department, demanding to know which articles specifically ran counter to the law. Her questions were never answered.

The *Woman Rebel* had never actually carried one single line on contraceptive techniques. Its purpose was to stir, to agitate, to develop within women "a conscious fighting character against all things which enslave you." But for the readers who had been pleading for specific information, she decided to write *Family Limitation*. It was a simple, practical pamphlet, incorporating all the knowledge of pessaries, douches, suppositories, and sponges that she had collected in France, together with diagrams for their use. Its style was bare, scholarly, unemotional as any textbook. Yet its theme constantly returned to her basic gospel—a new and wholesome conception of sex, free from restraint and prudery. "A mutual and satisfied sexual act is of the greatest benefit to the average woman," she wrote. "The magnetism of it is health-giving."

Family Limitation was to be her final challenge to the Comstock law. "There was no rest, no contentment in my heart until every word had been set down in its proper place," she wrote later.

She took the manuscript to a printer, long known for his courage and liberalism. He read it carefully and turned pale. "That can never be printed," he said. "It's a Sing Sing job." She tucked the manuscript under her arm and went to the next printer, then the next—twenty of them in one week. It was always the same. The printer would call his lawyer, shake his head sorrowfully. "I'd like to do it, lady. But I got a wife and kids. They'd have me in jail in a minute."

At last, she realized it would never be printed by the regular trade. She had to find one individual through her contacts with the unions. The man was Bill Shatoff, a burly linotype operator on a foreign-language paper, later to become a highly honored builder of railroads in Russia, who agreed to set the type at night when his shop was supposed to be closed. The printing, binding, storing, all were done by five completely separate men, working on their own, unknown to the others. First she had thought of an edition of ten thousand. But as leaders in the wool, silk, and copper industries asked for large consignments of their own, she increased the run to a hundred thousand. Night after night she and a few friends worked in the storage room, wrapping, weighing, stamping. Bundles went to the mills of the East, the mines of the West, to Chicago, San Francisco, Butte, Lawrence, Paterson—all to be held until she judged the moment most propitious for release.

Family Limitation was to become the bible of the birth control movement. Eventually it was translated into thirteen languages, including Italian, Yiddish, Spanish, German, Japanese, Chinese, Swedish, and Finnish. Ten million copies were printed during the next few years and hundreds of thousands of other copies made by less conventional methods—"photographed, typewritten, mimeographed, even copied painfully out by hand so that the information could be spread from family to family," she noted later.

It had been many years since she had seen her father. Now news of the *Woman Rebel* and its suppression filtered back to Corning. A family council was called. Had Margaret lost her reason? Was she crazy enough to break a law openly? Coming so soon after her long struggle against tuberculosis, the verdict was that she was suffering a complete breakdown, probably a "nervous breakdown." Michael Higgins was dispatched to New York to take charge of his daughter and bring her home.

When Margaret outlined her plans to her father and analyzed her whole campaign for birth control, Higgins was appalled. How could a fine young woman like this talk about sex? Had her nurse's training coarsened her mind? Striding about the apartment, his mane of hair tossed dramatically across his forehead, he damned the *Woman Rebel*, thundered at Margaret as he had once thundered in praise of Henry George and Robert Ingersoll, argued and pleaded with her to give up this whole fantastic thing.

Then one hot August afternoon the doorbell rang. Higgins was reading his newspaper in the small study just off the living room. Margaret answered the door. Two men stood there, strangers. Was she the editor and publisher of the *Woman Rebel?* Yes. They thrust a legal document into her hands. She read it slowly, trying to keep herself from trembling. But in the morass of legal verbiage, one fact stood out—she had been indicted by the United States Government, indicted on nine counts that could mean a prison sentence of forty-five years if she was convicted on all.

They looked like decent, intelligent men. She asked them to come in and sit down. It would change nothing, but she wanted them to understand. For three hours, she poured out the story of birth control, told them about Sadie Sachs, the horrors of abortion forced on women by the Comstock law, the tragedy of thousands of mothers, useless, exhausted at thirty and thirty-five by endless poverty and childbearing. They nodded. It was all true, they admitted. The law was savage, unjust. But the law stood until it was changed, and under the law she had been indicted and nothing could change that.

When the agents had gone, her father came into the room quietly. He put his arm around Margaret. He had heard it all. There were no flowing speeches now, no fine Irish oratory. "You were right," he said simply. "Everything is on your side—logic, common sense, progress. If your mother had only known this, she would still be alive today."

Margaret Sanger was arraigned on August 25 at the old Post Office Building in downtown Manhattan. Assistant District Attorney Harold Content was determined to bring her to trial immediately. But Judge Hazel, probably influenced by a good word from the two federal agents, agreed to postpone trial to the fall term, six weeks off.

There was so much to do now, so little time. Peggy and Grant were visiting friends in the Catskills, Stuart was at camp in Maine. Not knowing where she would be by fall, she made careful arrangements for their schooling. The last two issues of the *Woman Rebel,* September and October, were rushed to completion. She was moving as if in a dream. Friends called on her with warnings, suggestions for seeking clemency from the government. One neighbor, a dancing teacher, even insisted on teaching her a series of dances and exercises that could be done in the limited space of a prison cell to maintain her health. Liberal lawyers like Theodore Schroeder and Leonard Abbott of the Free Speech League, goodhearted men with a reputation for defending the rights of trade unionists and freethinkers, insisted that they could get her off on some technicality if she would co-operate with the court.

Co-operate? They didn't seem to understand. Her own safety, a prison term were not the issues. It was the law that was savage and wrong. If she co-operated, she admitted that contraception was nothing better than obscenity and pornography. There would be no compromise. She wanted no prison term. But if it was the only way to demonstrate the bondage of women under this degrading law she would fight the law to the end. With her unerring sense of drama and belief in her destined role, she would become for all women the symbol of the new rebellion.

"If she could obtain that result by being burned at the stake," Isaac Russell wrote in the New York *Mail* shortly afterward, "why . . . that would be a cheap price to pay . . . For her rebellion against the law is rather complete, and she sees a distinct value in stirring up public sentiment by means of an act of voluntary martyrdom."

Her phone rang one morning. It was an officer of the court, an indignant, surly voice. Her case had been called that morning. Why had she failed to appear? Without a lawyer, she explained, she had no way of keeping track of the court calendar and thought that the court would notify her. She had better get a lawyer, the surly voice snapped, and ordered her to appear in court without fail the next morning.

The date was October 20. She walked into the U. S. District Court, Room 331 in the old Post Office Building. The voice of the clerk droned out one name after another. It was like an impersonal, relentless machine. Then she heard the clerk call out mechanically, "The People vs. Margaret Sanger." She felt suddenly alone. Into her mind flashed a huge map of the country, with thousands of pins to mark its cities and towns, and she stood alone against them all.

She walked down the aisle, one friend at her side, and faced Judge Hazel. Her case was not prepared. Could she have a month's adjournment? "Mrs. Sanger's had plenty of time," snapped Assistant District Attorney Content. The attitude of the court had stiffened sharply since her earlier appearances. Judge Hazel ordered her to get a lawyer immediately. The case would go on after the noon recess.

She remembered that Simon Pollock had represented the unions in the Paterson strike. She rushed to his office, and he agreed to take her case that afternoon and plead for another extension. But even that was futile. There would be no extensions on any grounds, Judge Hazel stated. The case was set for trial at ten the next morning.

"There's nothing I can do," Pollock told her. "You'd better plead guilty and let me make a deal with the D.A. so you'll only have to pay a fine."

Even Pollock didn't understand. She thanked him and told him she would call back later that afternoon. Then she went home. It was four o'clock. She had to make her decision immediately. Bill Sanger, uprooted by the war, had just returned from Paris. Although they lived apart, they were still good friends. The children's future was their common concern. Sanger rushed over to the apartment. "Give up the fight for now, Margaret," he begged. "Let Pollock have his way. Let him get you off with a fine." A few of her closest friends called. It was the same. Compromise, compromise, they urged. Don't throw everything away in this one desperate plunge.

She had to be alone to think. She had to get away from the apartment and its memories of the children and everything she held dear. She packed a bag and went downtown to a small hotel. Sitting in its impersonal sterility, she faced the issues. The one indisputable fact was that the attitude of the court had changed. Hysteria was growing in the country. The Germans were advancing toward Paris. The European war had taken over the headlines, crowding every other thought out of people's minds. Even civil rights was a petty issue now. What chance would she have to make the judge understand the importance of birth control? The whole thing was a nuisance to the government. They wanted her out of the way. If she went into court tomorrow, she would get at least a year in jail, probably five.

She was not afraid of jail. Not if it meant the chance to make a fight on the real issue of birth control. But if she went now, it would be under the false issue of "obscenity." What she needed was time, time to assemble the real facts on birth control and destroy once and for all the degraded status of obscenity which had been used to cloak it.

If she refused to face trial and went away for a few months, she could assemble the material and fight back. Going away was harder than staying. How could she leave the children? Would they understand? Would her friends even understand, her associates on the *Woman Rebel?* Where could she go? Europe probably. England or Holland, where the birth control movement had made strong headway. She called the railroad station. There was a train to Montreal in a few hours.

"The hours of that memorable night of doubt," she wrote years later, "could well be called a spiritual crucifixion. The torture of indecision—the agony of deciding one way and then reversing the decision—how those minutes flew! I sat perfectly still, my watch on the table . . . It grew later and later. I knew there was no turning back once I boarded the train. I wanted no one to influence my decision one way or another. It was like birth and death—that journey had to be taken alone. Gradually, decision came. About half an hour before train time I knew that I *must* go. I wrote two letters, one to the judge, one to the district attorney. I informed them both that I would not be at court at ten o'clock the following day, and reminded them that I had asked for a reasonable time to prepare my case . . . I had asked for a month's postponement, and their refusal had compelled me to take a year!"

Talking about these terrible hours in the hotel room, Margaret Sanger said recently, "They were my Gethsemane. How could I do it? How could I leave three adorable children? It sickens me even forty years later to think of that struggle within me. But there was no turning back. I had to fight this through even if it meant leaving children, home, friends, everything I held dear."

A half hour before midnight she finished the letters to the judge and district attorney. She arranged about the care of the children. They would live with Sanger, but Nan, who was working as an interpreter with a New York business firm, would look after them in the evening and week ends.

She boarded the train to Montreal. On the train, she wrote another letter, which was mimeographed by her closest associate and mailed to her friends and the subscribers of the *Woman Rebel.*

. . . My work in the nursing field for the past fourteen years has convinced me that the workers desire the knowledge of prevention of conception. My work among women of the working class proved to me sufficiently that it is they who are suffering because of the law which forbids the imparting of information. . . .

Shall we who have heard the cries and seen the agony of dying women respect the law which has caused their deaths?

Shall we watch in patience the murdering of 25,000 women each year in the United States from criminal abortions?

. . . Jail has not been my goal. There is special work to be done and I shall do it first. If jail comes after, I shall call upon all to assist me. In the meantime I shall attempt to nullify the law by direct action and attend to the consequences afterward. . . .

At Montreal, she boarded the *Virginian*, alone, without a passport, not knowing how many months or years it might be until she could return.

CHAPTER 5

When she was three days out at sea on a Canadian liner loaded with munitions, food, and Englishmen who were returning home for war service, Margaret Sanger sent four identical telegrams with a prearranged key word to her four closest associates. It was this message that released a hundred thousand copies of her pamphlet, *Family Limitation*, which had been secreted in storerooms and closets in a dozen cities. It was the final act that sealed her exile.

The *Woman Rebel* had challenged the Comstock law, but it was *Family Limitation* which openly broke it. This was the significant step that set her apart from the rebels who had come before her. They had talked contraception; she openly and defiantly now gave practical contraceptive information to any woman who requested it. An enormous wall had been built around the subject by law, by the government, by society. She went up to the wall and forced it to crumble before her.

She had moved step by step toward this moment for two years, propelled relentlessly, as if in some huge Greek drama. "It was as though I was born to this," she said later. "I had to be the protagonist of American mothers. I wanted to express their longings, ambitions and thwarted lives."

It was almost as if she had no choice. She was moved by intuition, keeping a pad by her bedside to make notes of those ideas that came to her so forcibly in her semi-wakefulness that they could not be denied. "I could no more stop," she said, "than I could change the color of my eyes."

Once aboard ship, she was cut off not only from her family and friends but even from her own identity. Because her case was extraditable, she had been forced to buy her ticket under an assumed name. She had only a few hundred dollars taken from her slim savings. She knew no one in all England. Worst of all, she did not even have a passport.

But her confidence was a radiant thing. One of the other passengers, a man with high contacts in British Government circles, agreed to vouch for her when they reached Liverpool. The efficient, unyielding immigration officers there told her sharply, "England is at war, madam. We're sending back people without passports every day, and we can't make an exception in your case." But her friend guaranteed that she would get a passport from the United States Government as soon as she reached London, and she was finally allowed to enter.

She waited in Liverpool for letters and messages from home while the raw, cold rain beat down incessantly. She stayed in her room—the icy streets outside only increased her loneliness—trying to fill the time by writing letters. "Piercing chills penetrated to the marrow of my bones," she wrote later. "I was homesick for the children, lonely for friends as I had never been in my life, before or since."

She had a letter to the local Fabian society, which met a few days later at the Clarion Café. There she was introduced to Lorenzo Portet, a Spanish syndicalist, whose friendship was to lighten her dreary weeks in Liverpool. Portet once had been the ally and was now the heir of Francisco Ferrer, whose schools had first brought modern, scientific education to Spain and who had been shot in the purge of Republicans in 1909. Portet carried on Ferrer's work. He assembled the latest scientific literature of France, Italy, and England and had it translated and distributed through his Barcelona publishing house. Now he was teaching at the University of Liverpool. Margaret saw Portet and the other Fabians regularly, and was welcomed at their meetings. She also made short trips to nearby Wales, to the homes of the smelting workers in their tiny stone cottages, where she studied the relationship of the size of the family to the standard of living.

But London was her objective. London was to be her base and the center of her studies, and when the mail from home arrived, she took the next train and was soon rolling through the endless chimney-potted suburbs of the capital.

She rented a small room on the top floor of a rooming house in Torrington Square, near the British Museum. There was no heat, only an undersized fireplace that usually stood empty because she could not afford the coal. Since even the use of the bathroom cost extra, she had a small jug of hot water placed outside her door each morning. This she mixed with the frozen water of the washbowl on her dresser and poured the chilly combination into the throne-like tub of tin in the corner of her room. Her funds were so short that she saved a shilling each week by going to the basement dining room for breakfast instead of having the maid carry her tea upstairs. When she had a few extra pennies, her chief luxury was to rent an empty room with a small fireplace on the floor below and enjoy its warm glow for the evening while she wrote. Even her diet was meager. "It was tea and toast for breakfast," she recalled, "and tea, toast and marmalade for dinner."

The first people she had to see in London were the Drysdales. For sixty years, this family had been the driving force behind the Malthusian and Neo-Malthusian movement which grew from the population theories of the Reverend Thomas Malthus. In 1854, Dr. George Drysdale's *Elements of Social Science* had proclaimed the necessity of population control. A few years later his brother Charles and the editor, Charles Bradlaugh, founded the Malthusian League. Charles had married Dr. Alice Vickery, a pioneer feminist who overcame the prejudices of the medical profession by getting her medical degree in Ireland and becoming Britain's first woman doctor. She alone of this generation of Drysdales was still alive, but the leadership of the movement, which had become the Neo-Malthusian League in 1877, was now in the hands of her son, C. V. Drysdale and his wife, Bessie.

Margaret Sanger sent a note to the Drysdales at their apartment in Queen Anne's Chambers and was immediately invited to tea. It was a harsh, rainy afternoon when she came into the gay living room, with its chintz-covered chairs and blazing fire. Suddenly all the loneliness left her. It was like being home again. They held out their arms to her, welcomed her excitedly, filled her with tea and cakes. Dr. Drysdale, a slender, fair, balding man in his early forties, and Bessie Drysdale, practicable and hospitable, hovered over her with constant attentions.

Other members of the Neo-Malthusian League, Dr. Binnie Dunlop, Olive Johnston, who had been the Drysdales' secretary for years, and the feminist leader, Stella Browne, had come to meet her. They made her describe every detail of the *Woman Rebel, Family Limitation,* and her fight against Comstock. Dr. Drysdale listened gleefully, striding around the room, rubbing his hands together, and exclaiming, "Would to God we had a Comstock law! There's nothing that stirs the British like a bad law."

With their encyclopedic minds and statistical files on population problems going back a hundred years, the Drysdales were the key to a whole new world for her. They urged her to use their private library, study their reports, and ground herself thoroughly in the historical development of the movement. At the same time, she could round out her work in the reading room of the British Museum. "The warmth of my reception that afternoon," she wrote, "strengthened me to face the future."

In the reading room of the British Museum, she reserved a permanent seat. She was there each morning when the doors opened at nine and rarely left till the gate closed at seven. There was no problem of fireplaces or coal here. In the warmth of the reading room she began to search hungrily through every document on the Neo-Malthusian movement, starting with Thomas Malthus's *Essay on the Principle of Population* in 1798.

It was the needs of motherhood and the deep, instinctual necessity to speak as the rebel voice of American women that had brought Margaret Sanger to this point. Now in these months of rigorous study, she was to fit together the varied scientific and economic patterns of history which had produced the earlier writers and leaders of the movement.

Malthus, "the gloomy parson" as he was called, had developed the first population theories from the standpoint of economics. The world's population, Malthus saw as early as 1798, was expanding in huge, geometric steps at a frightening rate—in some backwoods areas of America doubling every fifteen years. But the amount of cultivable land necessary to feed this population could not be multiplied. The natural checks of war, disease, and famine were diminishing. Population would soon be running so far ahead of the produce of the land that disaster was inevitable.

But Malthus was an economist, not a practical reformer. The only check on the birth rate he could offer was late marriage and "voluntary restraint." He candidly admitted that both were hopelessly ineffective.

It was Francis Place, tailor, labor leader, and political genius whose London library was to become the center of England's intellectuals, who first applied Malthus's population theories to the daily lives of human beings, particularly the trade unionists.

Place had written his revolutionary pamphlet ninety years before the *Woman Rebel*. Yet the problem he faced, Margaret Sanger saw, was the same as that of her own family in Corning. The father of fifteen children, Place rebelled against the yoke of large families around the necks of the worker. In *Illustrations and Proofs of the Principle of Population,* published in 1822, he advocated the use of contraceptive techniques by every workingman.

But what were these techniques? Place was no scientist; he offered none. While his theories were immediately supported by such utopian reformers as James Mill, Robert Owen, Jeremy Bentham, and John Stuart Mill, it was not until Owen's son tackled the problem a few years later that the practical aspects of human biology were linked to the needs of family limitation.

It was America, Margaret Sanger was amazed to find, where the first book on contraception actually appeared. Robert Dale Owen grew up in the United States, where his father had come to found the utopian community of New Harmony on the banks of Indiana's Wabash River. Later a highly influential member of the U. S. House, Robert Dale Owen published his *Moral Physiology* in 1830. It was an epoch-making book, not only because it described three techniques of contraception for the first time, but because it based the need for contraception in the combined happiness of husband and wife. Contraception, Owen proclaimed, would improve the quality of marriage and the status of women, reduce prostitution, and create a eugenically sounder race.

Two years later, in 1832, Charles Knowlton, for the first time, applied the knowledge of the medical profession to contraception. Until Mrs. Sanger's own pamphlet, *Family Limitation,* Knowlton's book would remain unequaled for its revolutionary impact. Although only a few hundred copies of *Fruits of Philosophy* were printed at his own expense, here for the first time the theories of modern psychological science became part of family limitation.

Knowlton analyzed the financial and mental strain of the large family on both father and mother. He described the overbreeding of children as a significant factor in the mother's health and a cause of early death. Most important of all, his book was a detailed study of four methods of contraception: the condom, and coitus interruptus, which he opposed, and two preferred methods, the use of a saturated sponge in the vagina, and the use of chemical solutions by syringe.

Why hadn't this book swept the country in 1832 instead of disappearing into obscurity? Margaret Sanger searched for an answer. To begin with, it faced an unbreakable wall of Puritan morality. Knowlton was fined and served three months at hard labor in an East Cambridge jail. But the answer was far more complex. In a country of rapidly expanding frontiers, population growth was no problem. In both agricultural and factory areas, children were a family asset. The enormous industrial expansion after the Civil War created a huge labor shortage that even unlimited immigration could not fill. Somewhere around the turn of the century—and only sociologists who faced the problem after Mrs. Sanger were able to fit these complex factors into a meaningful pattern—the rise of trade unions and humanitarian reforms began to counteract the exploitation of child labor. The increasing standards of the middle class, and eventually of labor, the improvement of education, and technological changes which lessened the importance of masses of cheap labor—all these factors gradually worked against the large family.

In the United States, therefore, Knowlton, the first prophet of scientific contraception, was ostracized and forgotten. The only interest in contraception came in spasmodic bursts from the eugenicists like John H. Noyes and the Oneida Community, where the selective breeding of children was a major objective. "We are in favor of intelligent, well-ordered procreation," Noyes stated. Later such eugenic pioneers as Moses Harman and Ezra Haywood went to jail for suggesting that contraception could improve the quality of the race. A few spokesmen for women's rights like Frances Wright and Victoria Claflin Woodhull, and a few philosophic radicals like Colonel Robert Ingersoll preached the subject briefly. Even at the turn of the century, Dr. William J. Robinson's occasional articles on contraception in *Medical Critic and Guide* were a lonely phenomenon—and never part of the main stream of sociological and humanitarian reform.

The strangest factor of all, Margaret Sanger found, was that Knowlton's book, forgotten in America, became, in 1876, the tumultuous center of England's Neo-Malthusian movement. It had sold quietly in England all these years until a "disreputable Bristol bookseller" was suddenly accused and convicted of selling an obscene book. To make this a clear-cut case of the infringement of the rights of free press, Charles Bradlaugh, one of the Malthusian leaders, and his associate, Annie Besant, published their own edition of the book, notified the police, and were arrested. The trial, which lasted four days and was held before the Lord Chief Justice on the Court of Queen's Bench, dominated the headlines of every English paper. Bradlaugh and Annie Besant conducted their own defense. Convicted at first of defaming the public morals, they immediately appealed the case to a higher court and won.

The victory had major repercussions. First, it established in England once and for all that contraception was not to be considered obscenity. Second, it focused such attention on the family-limitation movement and the book that between Bradlaugh's arrest and the trial *Fruits of Philosophy* sold 125,000 copies, another 185,000 in Bradlaugh's edition, and 50,000 to 100,000 copies in other editions. Finally there was an indisputable tie-up between the trial and the growing acceptance of contraceptive techniques and the sudden drop of the birth rate in England after 1878.

At almost the same time as the trial, a young Englishman living in Australia, Henry Havelock Ellis, bought a copy of Dr. George Drysdale's *Elements of Social Science* and came under the spell of its explosive ideas. For the next forty years, he was to explore what he called "the central problem of life"—sex—and raise it from the depths of superstition and ignorance in which it had been buried. His monumental work, *Studies in the Psychology of Sex,* as well as many other books, had made him probably the world's leading authority on the subject.

After weeks of concentrated study at the British Museum, Margaret Sanger was having tea at the Drysdales' one blustery December day in 1914 when Stella Browne announced that she would introduce her to Havelock Ellis. No other individual at this point could have been of greater assistance to Mrs. Sanger's studies. An appointment with Ellis was like the fulfillment of a dream.

Havelock Ellis, like Freud, was a titanic explorer in an unmapped world. "Sex," he stated, "lies at the root of life, and we can never learn to reverence life until we know how to understand sex." The seven volumes of the *Psychology of Sex* revolutionized human thinking about a vast area of knowledge—*Sexual Inversion, Erotic Symbolism, Sex in Relation to Society,* to mention a few titles—and freed it from the dark obscurity of the ages.

Even as a medical student in obstetrics in 1884, Ellis saw that the prevention of conception was a fundamental corollary of sex knowledge. "Only by the regulation, limitation, and if necessary, prevention of conception in the light of our gradually increasing knowledge of heredity," he wrote, "can we hope to raise satisfactorily the general level of the race."[1]

Margaret Sanger had not only read the *Psychology of Sex* avidly during her years of study and probing; it was undoubtedly one of the major influences in her own newspaper articles, "What Every Young Girl Should Know," and "What Every Mother Should Know." "The new world of my dreams," she wrote, "was being constructed on the ideas Ellis put forth in his works." For her, he was a prophet, and even more. He was in her own words "a god-sent liberator."

Shortly before Christmas, Ellis had written her a note asking her to come to tea. With kindly foresight, he had given her exact directions on how to reach 14 Dover Mansions in Brixton across the Thames. "I climbed the stairs to his apartment," she said later, "and full of shyness and uncertainty, lifted the big brass knocker. Ellis himself opened the door. His tall, straight, slender figure, his great shock of white hair, his massive head and wide, expressive mouth— all blended into one overwhelming impression that here was a veritable god."

He led her into the living room and they sat before a small gas fire. The two candles on the mantelpiece flickered over his face, giving him the aspect of a seer. The blue eyes seemed sad, almost morbid. Yet there was often a sharp twinkle behind the bushy eyebrows. The face combined an open honesty with a peculiar aloofness. There was a thoughtful, preoccupied, deliberate air about him, touched with some strange light from another world. "A great god Pan with distant relations among the Satyrs," someone once described him.

While Ellis was preparing tea in the kitchen, he left her to look over his library and an assortment of recent clippings from America which he thought would interest her. That, she soon found, was always his way. He would enter into the life of the other person in little details; he would remember, for example, the kind of bread, fruit, or olives you liked, often walking miles to find them.

Soon he returned with a large tray of tea, cakes, bread and butter, and they ate and talked. His voice had a thin, high-pitched quality of its own—probably the result of years of virtual isolation in the Australian bush and in his London study, where he practically

[1] *Philosophy of Conflict* (Boston: Houghton, 1919), pp. 133–34.

cut himself off from the world. Small talk, she found, was virtually impossible for him. He said the important things or remained silent. "No other human being," she wrote later, "could be so silent and remain so poised and calm in silence."

They entered each other's lives slowly, almost reverentially. She described her battle with the Comstock law and he cautioned her and advised her. He believed so deeply in the cause of birth control that he wanted her to avoid any mistake. The impetuous, burning strength that poured out of her seemed to touch a depth in him that had not been reached in years. His calm wisdom nourished her with a rare combination of intellectuality and affection. "I felt as though I had been exalted into a hitherto undreamed of world," she wrote later.

"The second visit," Ellis stated,[2] "sufficed to bring us into a relationship of friendship. I may say of affectionate friendship, later combined with admiration and gratitude . . . Both in emotional attitude and mental outlook we had much in common. . . . I had rarely known a more charming and congenial companion and I had never found one so swiftly."

They met constantly after that. Ellis's days at the British Museum were Tuesdays and Fridays. He would leave notes at her seat listing helpful articles or outlining some new aspect of birth control that she was studying at the moment. His pockets always bulged with notes. Whether on a bus or walking the street, as soon as a thought came to him he jotted it down, passing it on to her later.

They went to concerts together and lunched regularly in the small restaurants around Soho. "Unless I was especially invited to lunch," she said later, "I never imposed but always paid my own share of expenses, whether for carfare, in a restaurant or in a taxi." Often they dined in his flat in the combination kitchen and dining room, warmed by the coal stove, where he liked to do his work. He was proud of being able to lay a fire with fewer sticks and less paper than an expert charwoman. He had learned to cook while teaching school and living alone in the Australian bush, and once told her that he would rather win praise for the creation of a salad than an essay.

Ellis's apartment had four rooms, one of which was set aside for his wife, Edith. She was on a lecture tour now in America, but she preferred her farm in Cornwall to London, while Ellis liked to be in

[2] *My Life* (London: Heinemann, 1940), p. 429.

the city and hear it throbbing around him even though he remained aloof from it. Whenever Edith came to London, her room was waiting, everything as she had left it. Her house in Cornwall had a special room for him. Either of them could board a train on a moment's impulse and be home in London or Cornwall in a few hours.

After one of the Sunday concerts in January at Albert Hall which they attended regularly, Ellis clipped off a lock of his flowing white hair and Margaret wrapped it carefully in the concert program and preserved it with her letters from him. On the days they didn't meet, he wrote her regularly, for he refused to have a phone in his house. His letters were usually short, at first checked by a certain restraint. On January 9, 1915, after reading the issues of the *Woman Rebel* she had given him, he exclaimed, "You know, I think you are splendid!" But then he went on to warn her, "It's no use, however, being too reckless and dashing your head against a blank wall, for not one rebel or many rebels can crush law by force. It needs skill even more than it needs strength."

But by January 13 he was no longer confining his comments to her work. "I think we should agree on the subject of love," he wrote. "I think that *passion* is mostly a disastrous thing . . . It's always felt for the wrong person. Indeed, its very intensity seems due to a sort of vague realization that there's nothing there. But I cannot say that I think that love is anything but good, and good for everything including work. I mean by love something that is based on a true relationship and that has succeeded in avoiding the blind volcano of passion. . . . To secure the peaceful and consoling and inspiring elements of love—and to escape the other—seems to me a very desirable and precious thing indeed, and by no means a common thing. . . ."

It was on this mold that they built their relationship. It was a harmony of minds and acts and feelings that went far beyond the physical, a sort of higher music that wove the books they read and walks they took together into a symphonic tapestry, into what Ellis called, and used as the title of a book, the dance of life itself. For him the dance of life achieved its ultimate beauty through the art of love.

"You darling woman," he wrote her on February 2, his birthday. "How wicked of you to send me that lovely present—the most beautiful present I have ever received—and the precious rose which is now before me in a little vase and has almost as delicious a fragrance as

the woman it comes from and which I mean to preserve for
always . . ."

They spent a final day together just before she left on a short trip
to Spain, and he wrote her: "It was a very lovely day and has left
me many thoughts and memories that are all beautiful to last till
you come back and much longer." The day she left he wrote:
". . . you said in your last letter before leaving that I was to miss
you. But I began to miss you even before you had left . . ." And in
a succeeding letter addressed to Spain, he ended: "With a good night
kiss! You are and always will be very loved to me."

They were vastly different yet so perfectly complementary—this
gaunt, lonely philosopher like "a tall angel," as a friend described
him, and this fiery woman who was all grace and spirit and about
whom Ellis himself had written: "I know you are not happy unless
doing something daring . . ." Her mind, which had worked by leaps
and bounds, he guided carefully into scientific channels. The reading
she did each day at the British Museum, the facts she unearthed, she
discussed later with him, learning slowly to put all the pieces into
perspective in the total struggle of women for sexual emancipation.
The Drysdales gave her the economic basis of birth control through
the eyes of Malthus. Ellis taught her to see birth control through
eugenics, through the family, through society, and finally as a conscious and deliberate cultural step in the higher development of man.

And what was Margaret Sanger doing for him? Ellis was fifty-five
when they met, and there is no doubt that he already felt that for
him the dance of life was running down. She flashed into his world
with the furious energy and courage that had carried her through her
early battles into exile. She touched him with her fire, and at a time
when he probably needed most a living expression of all that was
beautiful and feminine, she epitomized his dreams like those "sweet
and feminine and daring women" he described in *Impressions and
Comments*.[3] ". . . I feel my heart swinging like a censer before
them, going up in a perpetual fragrance of love and adoration."

Edith, on the other hand, still liked to think of Ellis as a philosopher and poet, essayist and editor—a role he had not played actively
since he edited the *Mermaid Series of Old British Dramatists* in the
1880s. She never completely accepted the importance of sex psychology. For her it was suspect and tainted.

The change Margaret Sanger had wrought in Ellis was shown in

[3] (London: Constable, 1921), Second Series, pp. 130–31.

Edith's reaction on her return. "What have you done to Havelock?" she demanded. "I left him shy and modest. I come home to find him egotistical."

As early as January 27, Edith's shadow began to touch their relationship. "As for me," Ellis wrote Margaret, referring to a quotation about his wife, "I still love all that I have loved, and even if I have loved another I should still love you."

Ellis himself wrote frankly to Edith about Margaret. "It was not my habit to practice deceit," he stated in his autobiography, "but here I never even felt the need of secrecy." But Ellis had misjudged Edith's health and the rising, almost hysterical tension stirred in her by the American tour. ". . . Your letter about M. came. I laughed and cried together," Edith wrote him on March 4.

All through that winter Ellis's repeated letters about Margaret were "the way in which in some degree—to which degree it is not possible to unravel—I innocently contributed to the tragic procession of events which filled the following eighteen months . . . It was absurd that my letters, which came from a heart so devoted to her should produce an earthquake, but in the exalted state into which she had been wound up it now seemed to her that the earth rocked."

". . . It was for Edith the very fact that my new comradeship was of the soul rather than of the body that made her feel she had been dispossessed in my heart," Ellis wrote.

Edith was quickly approaching a point of morbidity. On February 4, she wrote him: "Of course I got a fearful jump when I realized there is another. . . . It is a kind of strange realization which makes it still easier for me to die. I want to die, and yet I am at my zenith. . . ."

In a later reference to Oscar Wilde's epigram, ". . . each man kills the thing he loves," Edith claimed that she had been "killed in March." By April 22, her letters reached a despairing wail: "My own precious boy, Oh! Child!—oh, my darling!—I'm aching and aching." On April 29: "Havelock darling—I feel that the foundations of the deep have gone if you are merged in someone else . . ."

A news item on Margaret's work with Ellis, printed in the *Call*, only aggravated Edith's morbid fears. For the first time, Ellis cautioned Margaret: "Edith, who will be back about the middle of May, sends me a clip from the New York *Call* about the case in which it says you are in London, 'working with H.E.' I think, dear, you will agree with me it is better not to mention me in your letters home as everything you may chance to say becomes public property at once, and makes mischief and sets inquisitive people on the prowl."

To quiet Edith's fears, Ellis wrote her a long letter deprecating Margaret. ". . . It is of course quite ridiculous to refer to me as 'merged in someone else.' . . . M. is quite nice and a very pleasant companion, but she has no power to help or comfort me . . . It takes me years to get really attached to a person. . . . Only *one* person has really hold of my heartstrings, for good or for evil. . . ."

But this letter never reached Edith until her return to London and it did nothing to forestall the "tragic procession of events." Ellis had been her "foundation," her protector, had, in fact, married her in the days of the Oscar Wilde scandal to shield her from the public. Now Margaret seemed to have shaken the whole structure. Already sick with diabetes and close to a nervous breakdown, Edith sunk into a severe depression. She tried swallowing morphine tablets, but meekly submitted to an emetic. A few weeks later she considered suicide by jumping into the well outside Ellis's window but lacked courage to go through with it. Confined to a nursing home, she locked herself in the lavatory one day and threw herself from the window—suffering, however, nothing more than a sprained ankle.

Alternating with these severe depressions, Edith began to concoct grandiose schemes for her return to America for a lecture tour in conjunction with Ellis. "There was the desire to make clear to the world," Ellis explained in his autobiography, "that in spite of the doubts that she nervously imagined 'had spread abroad,' I stood openly behind her in close association . . ." But the trip was a monstrous impossibility, not only because of Edith's health but Ellis's dread of lecturing or even appearing in public.

Edith, who had clutched Ellis so desperately all these months in her frenzy to stay afloat, now became convinced that she was useless to him. Margaret had not seen Ellis since Edith's return, but Edith kept insisting on pushing them together. "I'm really angry with you for not coming here," she wrote Margaret from her farm on August 27. ". . . I'm sure you have some subtle idea of not hurting me or something. . . . Hope you two to be as much to each other as ever you care to be and hope you care a little for me too . . ." On November 7, while Margaret was traveling on the continent, Edith wrote Ellis from Cadgwith: ". . . Your letters make me ache for you, for none of us except M., and she is away, seem much good to you."

At the height of this period of mounting hysteria, Edith insisted that she divorce Ellis and that he marry Margaret. Ellis protested as gently and firmly as possible. But Edith had a "Deed of Separation" drawn up. It stated that Edith "may at all times hereafter live separate and apart as if she were sole and unmarried" and that Ellis could not use any "force or restraint to her personal liberty." "A strange deed," Ellis described it. ". . . perhaps one of the strangest ever drawn up." Edith thereupon took her own flat in London with another woman, but kept a special room always empty for Ellis—a symbol of love and rejection that provided the last desperate note to these sad months.

Despite Edith's separation agreement, marriage between Ellis and Margaret was impossible. They had discussed it objectively; and of all the men who loved Margaret in these years, Ellis certainly came the closest to holding her. But the birth control fight had taken over her life so completely that no other element could enter it more than momentarily. As soon as she finished her studies abroad, she had to return to face trial. The Comstock law had to be defeated; the birth control movement spread to every corner of the country. With the constant upheavals of her life, even the possibility of prison, she could never give Ellis the comfort and daily attention he needed —something he got years later from Madame Françoise Cyon.

Ellis, for his part, could not marry again while Edith lived. (She died of a chill on September 18, 1916.) Margaret had swept into his life with a radiance and fire that woke him to a new understanding of his own power; she had brought him a feeling of importance; raised him to an eminence that would soon, through her help in placing him in American magazines, illuminate the minds of audiences he had never reached before. But they would not see each other again for five years, although they wrote each other devotedly, sometimes passionately, every week. "As you know, I am likely to go on feeling nearer and nearer to you in absence or in presence, and I trust you will always understand that," Ellis wrote her on September 1, 1915. Margaret Sanger said later, "I have never felt about any person as I do about Havelock Ellis."

CHAPTER 6

The more statistics Margaret Sanger studied day after day in the reading room of the British Museum the more she realized that the focal point of all birth control information was in the Netherlands. The maternal death rate here was the lowest in Europe—a third of that in the United States. Its major cities had the world's lowest infant death rate. Most significant of all, the birth rate over the last twenty-five years had been cut almost in half. These significant statistics, she found, could be attributed in large part to the chain of clinics, founded in 1878 by Dr. Aletta Jacobs and Dr. Johannes Rutgers, where mothers were taught the techniques of contraception. They were the first birth control clinics in the world.

Dr. Jacobs, the eighth child of a poor physician, had fought her way into medical school to become Holland's first woman doctor and found the first free clinic for poor women and children in Amsterdam. The decline in stillbirths, abortions, and venereal disease was soon so apparent in the neighborhood of the clinic that thirty-four Dutch doctors determined to extend its work and organized the Dutch Neo-Malthusian League. In 1883, dissatisfied with the antiquated techniques, Dr. Jacobs and a German gynecologist, Wilhelm Mensinga, developed the diaphragm pessary, which was eventually adopted throughout the world.

With the Jacobs clinic as a model, Dr. Rutgers and his wife began the systematic training of midwives and nurses in contraception, and they in turn went out to set up new clinics all over the country. Such impressive benefits in public health had been produced in these thirty years that Queen Wilhelmina had recently presented the Neo-Malthusian League with a royal charter and medal of honor.

Here at last, Margaret Sanger exulted, was a government—unlike the United States, whose lawmakers lumped contraception with pornography—honoring birth control as a constructive force in society. Here at last was the living, practical evidence which she could study and bring back to America.

Making the hazardous Channel crossing despite submarines and floating mines, she reached The Hague and called on Dr. Rutgers at his house. A tiny square window in the upper part of the door opened mysteriously when she rang the bell. A face, weazened but intensely alert, appeared in the aperture. She explained her mission and Dr. Rutgers invited her to take breakfast with him at a nearby café.

They sat in the sun until noon, nibbling brioches and sipping the good Dutch coffee. A smiling, kindly man, he listened sympathetically while she described her battles with the Comstock law. But the hardest was still to come, he told her. Of course, he would help. He would put all the resources of his clinics at her disposal.

Each day for the next two weeks, she came to his office. The first startling lesson she learned was that fifteen different types of contraceptives were being used in Holland—each woman carefully examined for the type that fit her best. For Margaret Sanger this opened up a revolutionary aspect of birth control. She saw for the first time that clinical birth control depended on the skill of the doctor or nurse. If Dr. Rutgers prescribed a diaphragm, there were fourteen different sizes of the Mensinga diaphragm alone. Each woman had to be fitted for the exact size which would give her the most effective contraception and then instructed carefully in its use.

Within a few days, Mrs. Sanger had advanced so far in her training that despite the barriers of language, Dr. Rutgers allowed her to advise and fit patients herself. Before the week was over, she had handled seventy-five patients. "There was a determined social responsibility in the attitude of these peasant women coming into The Hague from surrounding districts," she wrote later in her pamphlet, *Dutch Methods of Birth Control.* "It seemed like a great awakening. Contraception was looked on as no more unusual than we in America look upon the purchase of a toothbrush."

Each day after leaving Dr. Rutgers, she went to the Central Bureau of Statistics with a translator to check the specific accomplishment of clinics in each city against the health trend in the country as a whole. In all areas surrounding Holland's fifty clinics, she found a significant improvement. The lower birth rate had improved labor conditions and wages. More children were going to school. Prostitutes were fewer, the venereal disease rate lower. From the eugenic standpoint, Dutch army records indicated a marked advance in physical stature and health.

One factor, she discovered, was sometimes as decisive as the birth rate in the health of family and the community. That was the spacing of children. For the total population could increase slowly without endangering the nation's standards as long as children were spaced enough years apart to protect the health of the mother and allow those already born to be assimilated carefully into the community.

Although Margaret Sanger could not get an interview with Dr. Jacobs, her trip to Holland had revolutionized her whole thinking and would determine the future course of the birth control movement in America. Her suitcase was jammed with contraceptive research and statistics—concrete proof to put before the American courts that a controlled and directed birth rate was beneficial, not just to the individual mother but to the whole nation. The fight for birth control, she knew now, was far more than a fight for free speech, far more than pamphlets and lectures to indoctrinate the public in its principles. It must be rooted firmly in science, in the medical profession. Once she had broken through the wall of ignorance in the courts, in the press, in society, the long-range campaign for birth control would have to be brought to America through the clinic and the doctor.

When she returned to London, it was spring. Dr. Vickery, even at eighty the indomitable grande dame of the Neo-Malthusian movement, dressed in purple or gray, with a prim white collar and wispy bonnet, found lodgings for her in a private home next to her own ivy-covered house at Hampstead Gardens. One of Dr. Vickery's friends, Edith How-Martyn, insisted that the story of Margaret's fight against Comstock and her trip to Holland should reach as large an audience here as possible. A few days later Margaret was informed that she had been booked for a speech at Fabian Hall on the afternoon of July 5.

Before representatives of almost every civic and social organization in London, Margaret Sanger for the first time in England gave the movement a new emphasis. She introduced the words "birth control," which from that point on gradually replaced the more classical terminology of Neo-Malthusianism. Instead of the inexorable economic laws of Malthus, she insisted that the movement could best be carried to the people on the human level—the mother, her health, her sexual emancipation. She gave a detailed report on the workings of the Dutch clinics and thus laid the foundation for the clinical approach to birth control, which was soon to be adopted by the Drysdales and their associates.

By the end of summer, Margaret Sanger's studies in England, Holland, France, and Spain, and her constant search for contraceptive information had reduced her small funds to the vanishing point. To supplement the savings she had brought to Europe, Leonard Abbott of the Free Speech League and friends in New York and Canada occasionally sent small donations. But at the end of August, Abbott wrote: "I am sorry that I have not been able to send you more money, but the fund collected is almost exhausted. . . ."

Then Lorenzo Portet, whom she had met in Liverpool, told her of an opening in his publishing house. The job would be to select appropriate books in English, aimed at a working-class audience, and particularly at women, for translations into French and Spanish. The salary was good. And since it would give her the opportunity to continue her contraceptive studies and—despite the complications of Edith's illness—keep her as close as possible to Ellis, she was strongly attracted by the plan.

The main obstacle was a subtle, persistent fear that something was wrong with Peggy. Her sister Nan and Sanger had been taking good care of the children and wrote her regularly of their health and progress at school. Yet she was guided to a large extent by her strong mystical intuition. It seemed to be innate to her Celtic blood. She was often influenced by dreams and kept a notebook by her bedside to record them and discuss them later with Ellis, who shortly before had published one of the first authoritative analyses of the subject, *The World of Dreams*. But her mysticism had deeper connotations that are difficult to pin down because she herself subscribed to no organized dogma. She had close attachments to one Rosicrucian group in New York. All through her life she had a strong affinity to Indian mysticism, yet accepted no specific gospel. What emerges then is a deep, transcendental belief in her own destiny, in her own role as the voice of motherhood, which had created in her the overwhelmingly urgent mission to unloose the force of love throughout the world, and in so doing, to cleanse it and regenerate it.

Night after night she would hear Peggy's voice, waking her out of a deep sleep, the same troubled cry ringing in her ears: "Mother, Mother, are you coming back?" A day or so later she would receive a letter from New York that all the children were well. She would laugh at her fears then, but somehow they crept back, always connected, strangely enough, with the number 6. It was almost as if 6 had been stamped on her brain. She tried to convince herself that the 6 referred to six o'clock, sixpence, or any other amusing combination. But gradually in the early-morning drowsiness of her mind, she saw distinctly a picture of a calendar on the wall with November 6 encircled.

When Portet's publisher asked her to sign a contract to stay in Paris, she agreed—but only if the date of agreement was postponed till after November 6. "All I know," she said, "is that something is going to happen on that day that will affect my whole future." They both laughed, as worldly people will laugh at these things. But the contract he drew up was dated January 1, 1916.

All during this time, she had been keeping close contact with the trend of public opinion toward birth control in the United States. In June, Abbott had written: "The whole atmosphere, so far as the subject of birth control is concerned, is changing for the better . . . Your arrest and imprisonment (if you are imprisoned) will not go by in the dark. Everybody in the country will know what is happening."

Then in August, she received a long report from an I.W.W. leader who had just returned from a four-month speaking tour of the country. "Everywhere there was the greatest possible interest in your work, your plans. . . . In Chicago five hundred short extracts of *Family Limitation* were published, and one girl told me the women in the stockyards district kissed her hands when she distributed the pamphlets." The report ended with an urgent plea that Mrs. Sanger return immediately and launch a nation-wide speaking tour sponsored by several radical groups.

Added to these factors favoring her return was the news of William Sanger's arrest. He had left Paris for New York just before Margaret's exile. On December 18, 1914, a stranger, who introduced himself as Mr. Heller, had visited his studio on Fifteenth Street, pleading that he was poor, that he had a large family, and wanted a copy of *Family Limitation*. Sanger told him he was sorry. Mrs. Sanger and he had agreed that they would carry on their work independently. Besides, he did not even know where the pamphlets were kept. But the man pleaded so pitifully that Sanger rummaged through the desk and finally found a copy in the drawer.

"I thought no more of it," Sanger wrote to Margaret, "until the

same man called again last Tuesday and wanted to know where
your books could be bought. I told him of a store on Grand Street.
"A few minutes later a grey-haired, side-whiskered, six-foot
creature presented himself and said: 'I am Mr. Comstock. I have a
warrant for your arrest.' He was followed by that man, Heller, bearing a search warrant. . . .

"He (Comstock) seemed anxious to enter into a discussion of the
case, saying that any statement I made would not be used against
me. I refused to discuss it, saying I wished to consult my attorney.

"He replied that lawyers are expensive and only aggravate the
case; and, patting me on the shoulder, said he advised me like a
brother, to plead guilty, and he would recommend to the court that
I be given a suspended sentence.

"I refused to entertain any such plea.

"I told him that, although I was in Europe when the pamphlet
was written and circulated, I believed in the principle of family
limitation. . . .

"I was arraigned and bail was fixed at $500. I was in that filthy
jail for 36 hours until bail was finally procured . . . There is every
possibility of getting one year's imprisonment and $1,000 fine. . . .

"It was also mentioned that *if I would give your whereabouts, I
would be acquitted.* I replied that they would wait until hell froze
over before that would occur. . . ."

After innumerable postponements, the case came up in September
before Justices McInerney, Herbert, and Salmon. On the morning
of the trial, the New York *Globe* quoted Sanger as saying, "This
pamphlet written by Mrs. Sanger is nothing more than a clean,
honest statement any doctor or trained nurse would give to their
patients . . . The truth is never obscene."

At the start of the trial in a crowded courtroom, Sanger began to
read a typewritten statement. "I admit that I broke the law, and yet
I claim that in every real sense, it is the law and not I that is on trial
here today."

Justice McInerney interrupted him curtly. "You admit you are
guilty and all this statement of yours is just opinion. I'm not going
to have a lot of rigamarole on the record. In my opinion, the pamphlet is not only indecent but immoral. It is not only contrary to the
laws of the state but contrary to the laws of God. Any man or
woman who would circulate literature of this kind is a menace to
the community."

In the remaining minutes of the trial, Justice McInerney interrupted Sanger and his lawyer continually, and finally pounded his gavel to announce that all argument was ended. The law provided a choice of fine or prison sentence. "One hundred and fifty dollars or thirty days in jail," proclaimed the justice.

Sanger jumped to his feet, his right hand raised in emphasis. "Then I want to say to the court," he shouted, "that I would rather be in jail with my self-respect and manhood than be free without it."

"At this," the New York *Times* reported, "the storm that had been gathering in the crowded courtroom broke. It began with a volley of handclapping and ended in a medley of shouts and cries. Men and women stood on the benches and waved their hats and handkerchiefs . . . The justice ordered attendants to clear the courtroom. Policemen charged the crowd but it was hard work, and required ten minutes to empty the room." Sanger was taken off to prison to serve his thirty days.

When Margaret received Sanger's letter, she rushed across the lawn to Dr. Vickery's house. Dr. Drysdale was there also and listened to her read the letter, his hands clenched in anger, his face flushing redder as he heard the flagrant procedure of the trial.

This news erased all indecision from her mind. It was always such bigoted injustice that drove her forward, almost as if each blow against the emancipation of motherhood was aimed directly at her, as if between her and all motherhood existed a mystic unity which made it imperative for her to fight back against each new attack.

Furthermore, it was fantastic that Sanger, who had never taken the smallest part in the birth control movement, should be imprisoned for her fight. His conduct at his arrest and trial had been flawless, even heroic. In the back of his mind, he had undoubtedly hoped that this imprisonment would act toward healing the breach between him and Margaret.

With Sanger in prison, she now felt an imperative need to return to the children. She was overwhelmed with loneliness for them. She wanted to hold them in her arms, be close to them night and day. The dread symbol of that number 6 on the calendar loomed ever larger in her mind.

Without further delay, therefore, she booked passage home, and late in September sailed from Bordeaux. It would be a dangerous crossing. Memories of the recently torpedoed *Lusitania* filled every passenger's mind as the ship moved into the fog-shrouded ocean.

"In darkness, with lights dimmed to avoid attracting the attention of German submarines, the ship plowed through the Atlantic," Margaret Sanger wrote later. "My own thoughts were as black as the night. Nervous tension crackled in the very air. The ship was carrying me onward, onward, to disaster, to prison, to inevitable sorrow . . . A queer sense of presentiment of evil was with me almost incessantly. When I succeeded in catching a few hours' sleep—mere minutes they actually seemed—I would wake out of unpleasant dreams. One of them was of attempting to walk through a crowded street, against traffic. The mechanical, automaton-like crowds were walking, walking, walking, always in the opposite direction. I was crowded to the curb and had to walk cautiously. They were impossible to fight against. And then suddenly in my dream the people turned into mice; they even smelt like mice. I awakened and had to open the porthole to get the smell of mice out of my nostrils."

At last, the lights of Staten Island blinked through the gray autumn mist on the morning of October 4, 1915. The old ship sidled alongside the dock on West Fourteenth Street. There was no one to meet her, no one waving from the dock. But a wild happiness grew inside her as she looked on American faces again, heard the rough accents of the porters and the fast-talking cab drivers, breathed in the crisp autumn air. To prolong the exultation, she picked up her one small bag and started to walk. She would soon be home at last, surrounded by the children. Passing a newsstand, she glanced at the display of magazines. There on the cover of *Pictorial Review,* one of the most respected magazines of the day, was the title of a leading article—"Birth Control." It was a strange, wonderful irony to be welcomed home, not by friends or relatives but by a phrase of her own creation on the cover of a magazine— welcomed home by the words which had sent her into exile!

CHAPTER 7

There was a whole year to make up in a few days, a year in which Stuart had grown into a husky, broad-shouldered boy, talking of nothing but sports, sports and Uncle Bob. Bob Higgins had been a football star at Penn State University. Stuart idolized him; Stuart carried a football under his arm around the house, made phantom plunges toward an unseen tackler, and told endless stories of his own football exploits at school.

Grant was more serious, a little shy, a little winsome. He and Peggy, always inseparable, had been attending a country day school in the neighborhood. Exuberant, mischievous Peggy. Her laughter always filled the house. She had a round, sweet face, the face of a glorious imp. Margaret Sanger took her and Grant shopping at Wanamaker's one day, and Peggy wandered off, got lost, and walked confidently into the office of one of the executives. Where did you come from, he asked the lost child? "From Paris," she retorted. Of course, it had been two years ago, but she liked the look of shocked surprise on the man's face.

Even laughter had to be measured. The shadow of the indictment hung over Margaret Sanger, the shadow of time slipping away. She sat down and wrote two letters, one to Judge Hazel, the other to Assistant District Attorney Content, notifying them of her return. "You state that after a week or ten days with your children," Content wrote back on October 13, 1915, "you thought it might be well to go over the pros and cons before your case is called for trial, and I think that is a very sensible suggestion."

She was neither afraid of trial, nor would she minimize its dangers. Sanger had just been released from jail, haggard and underweight, his eyes old and sunken in a youthful face. He had received a thirty-day sentence by pure trickery! If Sanger, with no previous connection with birth control, had been given this kind of justice, what could she expect after returning from exile, the leader of the movement, facing the far more severe federal indictment?

It was a time to fight, a time to find the means of bringing the issues of her case to the country. She began to formulate a strategy. Its first requirements were friends, money, and organized support.

The National Birth Control League had been organized in her absence and was now under the leadership of Mary Ware Dennett, Clara Stillman, and Anita Block. Her secretary had turned over to them all the files and mailing lists, mainly taken from the subscribers of the *Woman Rebel*. Except for Mrs. Block, a Socialist editor, they were mainly workers in the suffrage and feminist movements.

She wrote them and asked for a frank estimate of the support they would give at her trial. She received an answer from the secretary, Mrs. Stillman, telling her that the executive committee would meet the following week to make a decision. If Mrs. Sanger would be at Mrs. Stillman's home that afternoon, she would get its answer.

She went there with high hopes and was ushered into the sumptuous living room. Mrs. Dennett spoke for the group. The answer was short. The National Birth Control League, she stated, was aimed at changing the laws. It disapproved of Margaret Sanger's tactics. It could not support a person who had broken the laws.

Here was the same empty formula! Polite phrases like the "wrong tactics" and "lawbreaking." Women were forced to abortions, dying by the thousands because of this law. They would go on dying until this law was challenged and beaten. Speeches wouldn't do it; pretty phrases wouldn't do it. There could be no retreat, no compromise.

She decided to turn to the doctors. When Dr. Abraham Jacoby had recently been elected president of the New York Academy of Medicine, he had supported the principles of birth control in his acceptance speech. With this stimulus, Dr. Robinson had established a small committee at the Academy to investigate the subject. Mrs. Sanger wrote him now to ask what assistance the committee could give her. His reply was evasive. It had met only once, and he was not sure it would ever function. As a group, the doctors were obviously frightened. Robinson himself enclosed a check of ten dollars to help in the expenses of her trial.

Whom did that leave standing with her? Only the Free Speech League and a few radical allies who were raising a small defense fund. And that was for the trial—not her own living expenses. She had returned from Europe almost penniless. Nan had been wonderful, not only taking care of the children, but contributing to Margaret's personal finances. Her sister, Mrs. Ethel Byrne, also a nurse, became increasingly concerned. Why shouldn't Margaret return to nursing for a while? There was a profitable and easy maternity case coming up. "The woman asked for me," Ethel said, "but I'd rather you had it." Margaret shook her head—nothing could deflect her from her course. "Would you mind telling me," Ethel demanded, "how you intend to make a living?"

"I've cast myself upon the universe," Margaret said. "It will take care of me." She was not being facetious. Her faith in the necessity of carrying on the fight was so absolute that nothing could shake it.

Three days later, in her morning mail, Ethel received a letter from a friend in California who did not know where to find Margaret but was certain Ethel could reach her. "Please give the enclosed forty-five dollars to Margaret Sanger from her sympathizers," the letter read.

Ethel handed the money to Margaret, commenting wryly, "Here's your check from God."

The newspapers of September 21, 1915, carried the strange story of Anthony Comstock's death. He had caught a chill at William Sanger's trial a few weeks before, a chill that had now proved fatal. For forty-five years, this fanatical and twisted mind had forced its conception of good and evil upon the country, and then at the end had been deprived of its final vengeance. Comstock had sworn to harry Mrs. Sanger through the courts. Now this had eluded him.

But Comstock's death did not change the law. Nor did Margaret Sanger have time to examine its effect on the trial. With terrible suddenness, her own Peggy, the bubbling, irrepressible Peggy, was stricken with pneumonia.

Mrs. Sanger moved her daughter to her apartment, and later transferred her to a hospital. For the next two weeks, she never left the child's room, eating and sleeping by her side. Ethel moved in to help with the nursing. They had doctors in constant attendance. But there was no penicillin, there were no mycin drugs then to cut the fever. After the first week, Peggy no longer responded to treatment. Her resistance was failing rapidly.

Almost overnight this child of spirit and laughter became a silent face on the pillow. Most of the time, she lay in a deep sleep, opening her eyes only at rare moments. Once she looked at her mother and whispered, "Are you back? Are you back from London?"

"I'm right here, darling."

But the child did not seem to hear and kept repeating, "Are you back? Are you really back?"

The words were almost the very words Margaret Sanger had heard in London in the dim moment between sleep and waking when that strange symbol, that number 6, had forced itself on her mind. She tried to ignore the memory but it came flooding back with frightening clarity.

These were the most terrible hours of Margaret Sanger's life, and even forty years later they remain buried deep inside her. The mystic link between her and her daughter was the greatest reality of her life. Peggy summed up the beauty, the touch of heavenly laughter that made the meaning of all Margaret Sanger's work for motherhood complete. It was as if through Peggy she was able to touch the longings and hopes of all mothers, that through her daughter she was able to express her dream for the triumph of the feminine spirit.

The link between them was so intense that even before Peggy drew her last breath that night, Mrs. Sanger saw her child's spirit leave her body and float in dazzling-white, cloudy majesty before it left the room. The heart beat on a few minutes longer, but Peggy had gone.

It was hours later before Mrs. Sanger realized that the date of her daughter's death was November 6—that strange, overpowering number that had come to her again and again in her London premonitions.

No single event has had a greater impact on Margaret Sanger's life. It was to be many years before she could describe those days. "Grief so dulled my faculties that I was unable to think," she wrote. "I was numb in feeling, dumb in expression, and went about as in a sleep from which I did not even wish to awaken . . . The bottom seemed to have fallen from the very earth itself. A great gulf of loneliness set me apart from the rest of the world. It separated me from everybody and everything—from facts—from sunshine, night and day."

From the depths of her agony, Margaret Sanger struggled to grasp the meaning of that last hour when Peggy's spirit had appeared to her. Previously she had never been influenced by any specific religion or cult. Now she became unalterably convinced of the unity of life and death. She said later, "I went out to find the answer—where was Peggy?"

Someone had placed under her hotel door a leaflet that announced a talk on the evolution of women by a Persian swami at the Engineers Club. Margaret Sanger went. She knew no one there and believed that no one knew her. After the talk, they sat around the table in a semicircle while the swami led a mystical prayer. The room was dark and someone was holding each of her hands. Just before the lights went on, a woman at her left squeezed her hand hard and whispered, "You have had a terrible sorrow."

"So has everyone here," Margaret Sanger replied.

"Yours is for a child, a little girl," said the woman. "She just passed before me and kept repeating, 'Mother, stop grieving. You mustn't grieve any more.'"

The lights went on. Margaret Sanger turned toward the woman to question her further. But she had disappeared.

The terrible loneliness remained. "For two years at least after her death," Mrs. Sanger wrote, "it was impossible for me to sit across from a child in a train, in the New York subway, or in a streetcar. Tears would flood my eyes, and I would move swiftly away to another seat or another car, or even leave the subway at the next station, to the amazement and distress of those who happened to be with me."

The mystic link between her and her daughter has remained unbroken. Although she applied herself occasionally to Indian philosophy, Rosicrucianism, and astrology, she drew eventually on her own strength, a vast mystical reservoir that she attributes to her Celtic background, but is more encompassing and indefinable. It springs from the strength of all motherhood—as if she were born to express the essence of this strength, and her daughter, being a part of her, remains inextricably linked, whether in life or death, to the cosmic whole.

"Deep in the hidden realm of my consciousness," Margaret Sanger once stated, "Peggy has never died . . . and in that strange, mysterious place where reality and imagination meet, my little girl has grown up to womanhood."

2

When news of Peggy's death reached Assistant District Attorney Content, he immediately notified Leonard Abbott that the trial would be postponed. Margaret Sanger refused and demanded it be placed on the calendar for December. Three days after her daughter's death, she told Marie Howe, a leading feminist, that she would attend the meeting planned in her defense at the Park Avenue Hotel on November 20.

Although Dr. Morris H. Kahn wrote that "as her physician, I forbid her to undertake her defense in court at present as her physical condition does absolutely not allow it," Margaret Sanger drew some supreme strength from the people who flocked to her side. News of Peggy's death reached the country through the papers. Lumberjacks in the north woods, miners from West Virginia, bereft mothers, men and women from all walks of life wrote consolingly to her and even sent their small contributions, a dollar bill, sometimes five, for her trial. "Money came pouring in beyond my understanding, not large amounts, but large for the senders, and oh such tender, sympathetic letters!" she wrote. "I had never known until then that the loss of a child remains an unforgotten loss to every mother during her entire lifetime. Women wrote of children dead some twenty-five years before, for whom they were secretly mourning. They sent me pictures of dead babies and locks of hair; and, as if it were a fresh outlet and relief to their troubled souls, they wrote page after page of their own sorrows. This fresh contact with the source, contact with the motive power which had taken me out of my maternal corner two or three years before, renewed my desire and gave me the strength to carry on."

Always, Margaret Sanger seemed to stand alone. Now, even more than before Peggy's death, friends and advisers pleaded that her health on top of everything else made an open court fight impossible. Get her off with a suspended sentence, they told Leonard Abbott, one of her chief advisers. "I should advise Margaret Sanger to plead guilty . . ." wrote James P. Warbasse.

"I do not see that any principle is sacrificed by pleading guilty to a breach of the *law*," wrote Bolton Hall, a leader in the single tax movement, to Abbott.

"My personal feeling is that she has made all the sacrifices she can afford," Gilbert E. Roe, who had defended William Sanger, advised Abbott, "and that she ought to be willing to get out of the matter as easily as she can."

Even Max Eastman, then editor of the radical *Masses*, insisted that she strive for a legal compromise and arranged for her to see

Samuel Untermyer, an eminent lawyer who had won the commenda-
tion of liberals by his fight on the trusts. Untermyer received her in
his office amidst dozens of American Beauty roses. With his piercing
eyes and head too large for his body, he appeared to her like a
disembodied brain. He was efficient, courteous, sympathetic. After
discussing the case with her, he telephoned Content and asked him
to come to the office. "What are you trying to do, Harold?" he demanded. "Persecute this frail woman, the mother of a family?"

"We don't want to persecute her," Content replied. "We want her
to promise to obey the law."

"Why, of course she'll promise not to break any more laws,"
Untermyer assured him.

When Content had left, Untermyer said genially, "You see, we've
fixed that up. All you have to do is write me a letter saying you
won't break the law again."

But she couldn't promise that. The law specified obscenity, and
she insisted she had done nothing obscene.

Untermyer took down one of his ponderous books and studied it.
"The evidence," he said finally, "is that you have violated the law.
It seems to me that pleading guilty would let you out of your
troubles without loss of dignity and prevent your going to jail."

"I'm not concerned about jail," Mrs. Sanger insisted. "Going in
or staying out of jail has nothing to do with it. The question is
whether I have or have not done something obscene. If I have not,
I cannot plead guilty."

Untermyer stood up, coldly formal now. They had reached the
end of the interview, she knew. He could not understand her viewpoint. Few of her friends did. Compromise was all they seemed to
want. She did not seek martyrdom, but she refused to have the issue
of women's freedom buried in a morass of legal maneuvering.

She arrived then at one of her flashing, intuitive decisions. She
would dispense with a lawyer. She would make her stand against
the federal government alone. In one crucial act, she would dramatize the real issues at stake so that women everywhere could grasp
them immediately. To her supporters in England, she wrote: "I decided to plead my own case without counsel, as the ideas I have
sought to promulgate are not within the range of the psychology
of men lawyers."

It was not heroics but sound strategy. Only by switching from
the role of pleading defendant to that of fighting woman rebel,

speaking as the voice of all women, could she fire the imagination of the country.

New support came almost immediately. A group of women petitioned Judge Henry D. Clayton, who was to preside, to have the trial before a jury and to have half the jury made up of women. For the first time in the birth control movement the list included such socially distinguished names as Mrs. O. H. P. Belmont, Mrs. Lewis Delafield, and Mrs. William A. Colt, as well as Mrs. Mary Beard, the historian, and Miss Helen Todd, a leader in suffrage and social reform.

Dr. Marie Stopes, whose book, *Married Love*, Mrs. Sanger had helped to promote here, now gathered nine of England's most brilliant names on a letter sent directly to President Woodrow Wilson. ". . . Not only for the benefit of Mrs. Sanger, but of humanity we respectfully beg you to exert your powerful influence in the interests of free speech and the betterment of the race," wrote H. G. Wells, Professor Gilbert Murray, Arnold Bennett, Lena Ashwell, Dr. Percy Ames, William Archer, Edward Carpenter, Aylmer Maude, and Dr. Stopes. Such names could not be denied attention. The letter was reprinted in hundreds of newspapers.

Margaret Sanger, in fact, was quick to realize that by daring to go into court alone, she had taken on a role that caught the fancy of most newspaper reporters. Such liberal journals as the New York *Evening Globe*, the *New Republic* and the *Day Book* were already giving full coverage to the trial. But John Reed, then an editor of *Metropolitan Magazine* and always a loyal supporter, was trying to break down the reserve of the New York *Times*, which up to then had never used the words "prevention of conception" in its columns. "They are very sympathetic with your case . . ." he wrote her.

It was a casual newspaper acquaintance who convinced Margaret Sanger to make her most ingenious move of all. Since the public had come to think of all women crusaders as Amazonian, craggy-jawed, and repellent, why not have a portrait taken of the one dazzling exception to this rule? Underwood and Underwood studios, therefore, was appointed to take a picture of her and her sons. Stuart, with his square-cut features, looked vigorously athletic. Grant, his hair cut straight across the forehead in Little Lord Fauntleroy bangs, glowed with childish warmth. Mrs. Sanger, her careworn face dominated by wide-set, tender eyes, wore a simple blue dress and white lace collar. It was a typical American family group that immediately caught the attention of most newspaper editors. The picture was reprinted hundreds of times during the trial, and probably won her more sympathy than any other single act or speech.

Even those liberals and feminists who a few weeks before had damned her tactics as too radical were now converted to admiration by her daring. Two members of this group, Henrietta Rodman and Alice Carpenter, gave a tea for her, and from this event sprung the idea for a dinner the night before the trial on January 17, 1916, a dinner at the Brevoort Hotel at which Rose Pastor Stokes would be toastmaster and Margaret Sanger and Dr. Abraham Jacoby the featured speakers.

It was a startling affair. "Probably New York, 'where nothing is new,' never had a night-before-trial dinner before," said the Boston *Post.* The guest list included over two hundred impressive names. From the liberal and intellectual world came Walter Lippmann; Herbert Croly, the editor of the *New Republic;* Miss Fola La Follette, daughter of the distinguished U. S. Senator; John Reed; Richard S. Childs, and Miss Rachel Crothers. The medical profession was represented by Dr. Mary Halton, Dr. Ira S. Wile, Dr. A. L. Goldwater, and Dr. William J. Robinson. Most significant of all was the turnout of liberal-minded women from the most rarefied social circles of the city—Mrs. Willard Straight, Mrs. Ogden Reid, Mrs. Lewis Delafield, Mrs. Frances Brooks Ackerman, and Mrs. Thomas Hepburn, who as Kathy Houghton had been a friend of Margaret in Corning and whose daughter Katharine was to become a distinguished actress.

Margaret Sanger's speech was short, but it caught the audience and brought waves of applause rolling through the cavernous old dining room of the Brevoort. The moment she sat down, a dozen women leaped to their feet to announce their support. From a table almost directly in front of her, she heard a woman announce that she was speaking for the National Birth Control League, that the league was aiding Mrs. Sanger at the trial and needed immediate funds. Amazingly enough, she recognized the speaker as Mary Ware Dennett, one of the executive committee members who had "disapproved of her tactics" only a few months before. At the last moment, the league had jumped on the bandwagon.

When Margaret Sanger arrived at the Federal Court Building at nine the next morning, "friends jammed the court and overflowed by two hundred into the corridor," reported the New York *Telegram.* The congestion became so serious that the U. S. marshal had to order the doors closed. The *Evening Globe* was impressed by the make-up of the crowd—"members of the Cosmopolitan and Colony clubs as well as the humbler sociological organizations." It noted that "twenty expensive motor cars, manned by liveried persons, filled the street around the building."

Perhaps the most impressive aspect of the trial was the number of newspaper reporters and photographers who showed up—"nearly as many . . . as at the trial of Police Lieutenant Becker, who supposedly had the previous record," stated the New York *Mail.* "The table that ordinarily is more than ample for the few reporters," said the *Evening Globe,* "was wedged tight with representatives of newspapers . . ." Even Mrs. Sanger's apparel came in for comment. "The defendant," reported the Brooklyn *Eagle,* "was dressed in somber black, but the severity of her costume was somewhat relieved by a pair of white 'spats.' She wore a black felt hat, a sort of semi-opera hat formerly worn by members of the other sex." She told reporters she had brought it back from England.

The trial was scheduled for ten o'clock but Judge Clayton and Assistant District Attorneys Knox and Content did not arrive till ten-thirty. Mr. Knox immediately stood up and threw a bombshell into the courtroom by asking the bench to adjourn the case for a week. Mrs. Sanger, acting as her own lawyer, protested strongly. But Judge Clayton overruled her and agreed to the postponement.

The crowded courtroom, which had been awaiting Margaret Sanger's fiery defense, was suddenly deflated. Once on the street, however, her supporters crowded around her and, reported the *Telegram,* "proposed three cheers, which were given with a gusto that woke the echoes for blocks around the Federal Building." The next day the Washington *Post* gave its capsule analysis of the whole proceedings: ". . . one of the most unique trials in the history of the United States."

On January 24, Knox and Content asked a second postponement to February 18. It was now apparent that the government was using every possible method to delay the trial. Despite the earlier pessimism of her supporters, Margaret Sanger was on her way toward a startling strategic victory. "You can gain nothing by trial," Samuel Untermyer had written her on December 6, 1915. "You cannot even gain publicity in these days when the papers are crowded with international news . . ." Yet with the headlines proclaiming the dismal news of the German onslaught on Verdun, she had not only succeeded in rallying a strong band of feminists, intellectuals, and liberal-minded socialites around her, but was capturing front-page headlines herself in almost every major paper in the country.

The extent of this sudden publicity can be gauged from the headlines on January 20 in the Los Angeles *Record*. In only slightly smaller type than the four-inch banner on the wreck of the California Limited was the second-deck headline: "Form Birth Control League in L.A." The February 1916 issue of *Pictorial Review*, analyzing the mail response to its October 1915 article on "What Shall We Do about Birth Control?" reported that 97 per cent of its thousands of letters were favorable. An editorial in the Chattanooga *News* summed up the general newspaper coverage of the trial. "There is strong sentiment throughout the nation in favor of Mrs. Sanger . . ." it commented. "However the case comes out in New York, the courts will not be able to stop talk of birth control."

This same conclusion must have been shared by Judge Clayton and the District Attorney. The case had now reached a strange impasse. The more the government delayed, the stronger the support that rallied behind Margaret Sanger from petitions, letters, and newspaper editorials. On February 15, the New York *Sun* reported: "Mrs. Margaret H. Sanger appeared at the Criminal Branch of the United States District Court yesterday to make her weekly demand that she be placed on trial . . . The Sanger case presented the anomaly of a prosecutor loath to prosecute and a defendant anxious to be tried." The *Sun* also noted "the Government's reluctance to be used as an instrument in giving publicity to sex theories at this time." Margaret's ability to gather the support of public opinion obviously rankled Assistant District Attorney Content. "We were determined that Mrs. Sanger shouldn't be a martyr if we could help it," he stated later.

The trial came to a sudden and startling end on February 18. Through U. S. District Attorney H. Snowden Marshall, the government issued a nolle prosequi, dismissing the case. Nothing had actually been settled as to whether birth control material in the mails would still be classified with obscenity. "The quashing of the indictment settles nothing," stated a New York *Globe* editorial. "The right of American citizens to discuss sociological questions according to their convictions is just where it was before—subject to the mutton-headed restrictions of some post office clerk and the complaisant persecution of a Federal district attorney."

In actual fact—though not in the courts—Margaret had won a strategic victory of incomparable importance. Fighting virtually alone, she had overnight forced the issue of birth control out of the realm of obscenity and made it a public issue on the front pages of the country. Her will to fight after the impact of Peggy's death, this spirit of defiance which she somehow transmitted to people everywhere, had given men and women the courage to stand up and speak out on an issue that had always before been confined to whispers. Most important of all, she had challenged the federal indictment and forced the government to retreat. Instead of being jailed, she was now a nationally known figure around whom a movement was being born.

"Victory and vindication!" Margaret Sanger wrote. "This dismissal stands as evidence of the power of public opinion and active protest."

Immediately she dispatched a letter to thousands of supporters, labor groups, women's committees, and subscribers to the *Woman Rebel*, announcing her intention to carry the birth control fight to the country. "I am touring to the western coast, leaving New York City the 1st of April . . . Write at once and tell me the capacity of the largest hall . . . Let us make your town alive with interest on this subject, for it is the pivot around which all our social problems swing."

CHAPTER 8

From a quick glance at the headlines in the spring of 1916, it would appear that Margaret Sanger was making her way through the country by fire and sword. 1,200 ALMOST IN RIOT OVER MRS. SANGER, announced the front page of one St. Louis paper. "Mrs. Sanger is a splendid and admirable woman but a little too strong for Chicago," an officer of the Women's City Club told the *Commercial Tribune*. In St. Louis and Akron, her speeches were halted when two theaters rented for her were locked by their managers. In Portland, Oregon, she was jailed.

Actually such headlines were misleading. The explosions that followed Margaret Sanger across the country were set off by social and religious forces and not by Mrs. Sanger, who carefully stayed within the law and refused to give specific contraceptive information from the lecture platform. The opposition, however, used extralegal methods to stop her public appearances. Of all forms of bigotry, nothing roused her to greater anger. From her father, she had inherited an unshakable devotion to the basic constitutional freedoms. She still carried the scars of prejudice from her childhood in Corning when meeting halls had been denied Michael Higgins and she had become almost a heretic in the eyes of other children. She had been too young to fight back then. But now each show of bigotry brought her Irish blood to instantaneous heat, and in such moments there was nothing she liked better than a fight. "Thank God for the Irish blood that insists on living in you," Eleanor Fitzgerald, a friend, had written at this time. Another associate, Dr. Marie Equi, described her aptly as a "little bunch of hellfire."

The paradox was that despite the headlines, which seemed to picture Margaret Sanger in perpetual combat, she remained essentially a shy woman. It was an effort for her to meet new people and work with the organizing committees at each stop. She traveled alone. She stayed out of the public eye except at meetings. She disliked public speaking, and the very act of facing an audience caused her fear that was close to physical pain. All these physical factors were aggravated further by her extreme loneliness for Peggy, which even the frantic pace of her trip could not obliterate. "People, meetings, trips, talks, books, nothing healed the aching heart and loss but time," she wrote later.

Before she left New York, she wrote out her speech carefully. She would go on the roof of the small hotel on lower Lexington Avenue where she stayed and shout it hour after hour over the chimney pots of the city. She learned every word by heart, always afraid that if she skipped one word she would lose her place and be unable to continue. Then she tried it out on small groups in the suburbs.

Even after this preparation, she never lost her fear. "I used to wake up early in the morning, sometimes before it was light," she wrote later, "and feel a ghastly depression coming over me. I realized it was the impending lecture which was so affecting me, and I waited in trepidation for the hour." When she reached the platform, her knees would shake violently. She was almost sick each time until the moment when she got to her feet and spoke the first words.

Almost always her audiences were startled at the sweet, frail woman who addressed them. They had expected that anyone who could fight down the federal courts would be a hardened campaigner cut from the same mold as the professional suffragettes and feminists who had been covering the speaking circuit for years. But Margaret Sanger wore bright dresses with lace at the neck. Her voice was soft, and there was a delicacy and conviction in her words that made each speech almost a testament to motherhood.

"The greatest issue," she told Kenneth W. Payne in his syndicated column, "is to raise the question of birth control out of the gutter of obscenity, where my opponents have put it, and get it into the light of intelligence and human understanding."

A few paragraphs from her original speech—now a series of tattered yellow pages preserved in the Library of Congress and bearing the penciled notation, "given 119 times in one year"—show how she sought to put across this ideal in words that combined both power and beauty.

The opening sentence immediately made the audience feel her concern for children and the home: "The first right of every child is to be wanted, to be desired, to be planned with an intensity of love that gives it its title to being."

She could lift women toward her vision of a rare new world: "Birth control is the keynote of a new social awakening, an awakening of the parent towards a responsibility for its offspring, an awakening of the individual towards the consequences of his act. It is not only a welfare and economic expedient. It is a great social principle."

A moment later, she would be cutting and slashing at the tyranny of law, the hypocrisy of society: "To see those pale-faced mothers . . . their faces pinched and wan from overwork and worry, crowding forward, eager to face the torture of abortion rather than condemn an unborn child to poverty—to see this was enough to make one's blood boil with rage at the hypocritical silence of the medical profession who cater to the whims of the rich but ignore the tragedy of the poor."

Finally she could catch the hearts of women and make them beat to the revolutionary dream of birth control and the shaping of a new society: "Even as birth control is the means by which woman attains basic freedom, so it is the means by which she must and will uproot the evil she has wrought by her submission. . . . The most important force in the remaking of the world is a free motherhood!"

Margaret Sanger opened her tour in Pittsburgh, and then moved to Cleveland for two speeches, one at the First Unitarian Church. Its minister, Reverend Minot C. Simons, probably the first supporter of birth control from religious ranks, nailed up a poignant slogan on the church bulletin board after the first meeting: "The Noblest Motherhood is Conscious and Voluntary." Both Pittsburgh and Cleveland formed birth control leagues, and Mrs. Sanger stayed in each city a few days to help organize them. She laid out a basic plan of enlisting key members—a lawyer to investigate the state laws on birth control, at least one doctor to supervise the clinic, representative citizens from labor and social-welfare groups, and progressive-minded philanthropists who could give the essential financial aid to each new league. Once this work was done, she put the new league in touch with Mrs. Dennett's National Birth Control League. She had no organization of her own and had no desire to become entangled with internal problems.

In Chicago, despite the hundreds of letters she had received from the stockyards district in Hungarian, Bohemian, Polish, and Yiddish as well as English, she met unforeseen resistance. Hull House and other social agencies had done noteworthy work there. But they had also developed social workers concerned with their own prestige, who had built up an actual wall around the district. No new people or organizations could enter without their approval. The stockyards women were virtually cut off from advanced ideas. When a few of these key social workers notified Margaret Sanger that they were "not interested" in birth control, she suddenly found herself unable to hire a hall anywhere in the district.

But several young working women came forward to hold a meeting for Margaret Sanger. They hired a large hall just outside the district. She had leaflets and posters printed and distributed throughout the factories and stockyards. She contacted every union and radical group. The turnout of fifteen hundred people was an overwhelming victory.

She was scheduled to speak at the Minneapolis Public Library, but Dr. Mabel Ullrich told her that the Twin Cities were the most conservative in the country. "You won't get six people," she prophesied. If she could get six, Margaret Sanger wrote back, she'd go. When she arrived in the hall the night of the meeting, there were only a dozen people in the huge room. Dr. Ullrich had been right. Mrs. Sanger was introduced by an embarrassed chairman, but just as she started to speak dozens, then hundreds, of people poured in. Soon the hall was jammed and a hundred extra chairs had to be set up. Not till later did she find out that the announcement of her meeting had only appeared in the evening papers and had not reached the workers and farmers in outlying districts until suppertime. The words birth control had captured their imagination and brought them out in droves.

Frederick Blossom, manager of the Associated Charities of Cleveland, whom she had met there earlier and who had become one of her first supporters, telegraphed her in Minneapolis. A polished, clever, highly educated man with a Ph.D. degree, he had already recognized the shortsighted policy of alleviation practiced by the charity groups and grasped the social revolution that birth control promised. Could she speak at the National Social Workers' Conference then being held in Indianapolis? he asked. He could not get her a place on the regular program but guaranteed a special session for her. Since she had nearly a week before her next scheduled meeting in St. Louis, she decided to come.

Blossom's charming and ingratiating personality, later to play a sizable role in birth control, was perfectly fashioned for this type of organizing. Much of his charity work in Cleveland had been to cultivate the rich. He was smooth, tactful, never giving inflammatory speeches or scaring off potential supporters, as Mrs. Sanger was apt to do. Notices were posted throughout the hotel where the conference was being held, announcements left in every delegate's mailbox. Blossom himself went from session to session, carefully winning the support of delegates.

Although the meeting was held at four in the afternoon while the regular round-table discussions were going on, she packed the big amphitheater. People squeezed on window sills and radiators or sat on the platform. Despite opposition from a small minority, the great mass of delegates gave her their backing. These social workers would soon go back home to every state and carry her ideas to the urban areas better than any other missionaries. "This will kick the football of birth control straight across to the Pacific," Walter Lippmann wrote.

In St. Paul and Milwaukee, Margaret Sanger organized new birth control leagues. In Detroit, nine hundred members were signed up in two days. Then came St. Louis and the first violent explosion of the tour. Her supporters had engaged the Victoria Theater for the evening of May 21 and paid for it in advance. There had been rumor of boycott, but nothing specific. Mrs. Sanger and her party arrived at a quarter of eight. The street was blocked with people, the theater in total darkness, the doors locked.

Next morning's lead story in the St. Louis *Post-Dispatch* explained that "protests from Catholic priests and laymen against Mrs. Sanger's lecture on birth control resulted in the announcement of the management that she would not be permitted to speak at the theater." But it took a half hour of desperate telephoning that night before she found out that the Victoria's manager, threatened with a boycott, had locked the theater and fled to the country. Meanwhile, almost fifteen hundred people had gathered outside. The air was filled with catcalls, hisses, and cries of "The Catholics run the town" and "Break down the door!" Margaret Sanger was in an open car driven by Robert Minor, the cartoonist, and accompanied by Roger Baldwin of the Civic League, and Orrick Johns, the poet. Minor urged her to give her speech from the car. Without hesitation, she climbed on the back seat, raised her hand for silence, and began to tell the story of a twenty-one-year-old mother with three children who had come to her hotel room that very morning to plead for birth control information. Before she had finished two sentences, a police sergeant grabbed her arm and stopped her.

"Margaret Sanger abandoned the story," reported the *Post-Dispatch* the next morning, "but cried to the crowd, 'We're not in St. Louis. We're in Russia!'"

The crowd demanded she go on. But fearing a riot, the driver started his engine and drove off.

This was the first open use of extralegal pressure by the Catholic hierarchy. In a sense, she welcomed it. She was too keen a strategist not to realize that as soon as her opponents used unfair tactics to block freedom of speech, thousands of new supporters would be drawn to the movement purely on the basis of defending its constitutional privileges. Once the Victoria boycott happened, she exploited it to the fullest. She immediately announced that she was suing the theater's manager for five thousand dollars for breach of contract. Besieged by reporters, she made ample use of the newspaper columns to make St. Louis aware of the sinister implications of such boycotts. The city's editors to the last man now leaped into the fray.

"We do not know exactly what Mrs. Sanger's ideas are," the *Post-Dispatch* said in an editorial, "but we do know that her opponents are doing their ingenious best to confer immortality upon them. We also know they are giving St. Louis the worst kind of advertising an American community can get." The St. Louis *Globe-Democrat* warned that "to throttle free speech is to provide it with a megaphone." *Reedy's Mirror* printed a cartoon of the Capitol of the United States with a papal crown on it and highlighted the danger to the country if any religious group was allowed to dictate its opinions. "No idea let loose in the world has ever been suppressed," it said in a lead editorial. ". . . Her exclusion from a theater here set people to thinking and talking about her message who might otherwise never have heard of her."

Regarding the boycott as a blot on St. Louis, the Men's City Club invited Margaret Sanger to speak at a luncheon the next day. "It packed the City Club to suffocation," *Reedy's Mirror* reported. Not even Theodore Roosevelt's recent speech there, it was said, drew as large an audience. Although forty Catholic members of the club resigned in a body, a hundred new members promptly joined.

She was welcomed warmly in Denver, where the women already had the vote and knew how to use it. For the first time, she was received by a city's ranking officials. Judge Ben Lindsey, whose advanced theories on juvenile delinquency and family life made him one of the most controversial figures in the country, presided at her meeting. The primarily professional audience was unique for her—wives of doctors, lawyers, officials, and clubwomen.

In Texas, a Beaumont cowboy sang the praises of her campaign in a sprawling poem which began:

> *The fire of your gentle soul*
> *Has started waves of Truth to roll.*

In Los Angeles, police officials, instead of censoring her speech, as in Indianapolis and St. Louis, welcomed her at the railroad station. In the Northwest, her audience was crowded with old-time radicals—Wobblies, Socialists, freethinkers, and single taxers, who cheered her lustily but peppered her with questions on such diverse subjects as free silver, Henry George, and Marx. Many lumberjacks, who had been among the first subscribers to the *Woman Rebel,* came to greet her, thrusting out calloused hands and crying: "Put it there, Margaret. I'm behind you."

The enthusiasm of most of these western audiences was pictured in a dispatch from the Oakland *Tribune.* "They came in droves," it reported on June 15. "They came in swarms into the ballroom, where a few chairs were lined across the front of the room. As each came she seized a chair with mechanical precision and planted it forcibly as near the front of the platform as the laws of space would permit. Within a few minutes the Hotel Oakland ballroom miraculously filled."

In Portland, Oregon, Margaret Sanger realized that *Family Limitation,* which had been written hurriedly in 1914, needed revision. The time was especially appropriate, for in Portland she had the assistance of Dr. Marie Equi, a pioneer doctor of Italian ancestry who had cared for the cowboys and Indians while the Northwest was being opened, often riding all day in the saddle to reach a patient.

Mrs. Sanger was naturally pleased to have *Family Limitation* distributed as widely as possible, and had never copyrighted it. Often Wobblies, lumberjacks, or transient farmers printed or mimeographed copies and picked up extra money selling them to their

friends as they moved from place to place. Now a Portland automobile mechanic asked her if he could make reprints of this second
version and sell them at her next meeting. She had no objection.
Birth control information was not illegal in Oregon.

But as soon as the mechanic and two associates passed through
the aisles with their pamphlets, the police arrested them. Mrs.
Sanger wanted to testify in their behalf. Since she had scheduled
meetings in Seattle and Spokane, the trial was postponed a few
days until her return. In the meantime, the Mayor and City Council met in secret and passed a city ordinance against the pamphlet.
This clandestine maneuver on the part of five men so outraged Dr.
Equi and a group of Portland's women that they issued a leaflet
demanding: "Shall five men legislate in secret against ten thousand
women?"

Margaret Sanger adhered to the principle of immediate counterattack. As soon as she returned to Portland, she called a protest
meeting. This time she distributed the pamphlets herself and called
on ten women to volunteer their help. Four of them, including Mrs.
Sanger, were immediately arrested and taken to jail.

Hundreds of women followed her through the streets. "Some told
the police that they also had distributed the pamphlets and demanded to be arrested," reported the San Francisco *Call* the next
day. "The police locked the jail doors to keep them out." The four
women spent the night in jail, refusing to ask bail. "Let those who
put us in take us out," Margaret Sanger snapped.

The trial was held the next day. Two well-known lawyers volunteered to defend them. Mrs. Sanger had not consulted them. They
simply took the responsibility on their shoulders as citizens. Both
the original and revised pamphlets were put on trial and both were
judged "obscene." All seven defendants were found guilty. The men
were fined ten dollars, which the judge said need not be paid. The
women were not fined.

The case stirred such a furor that fifteen men walked through the
streets with signs reading, "Poverty and Large Families Go Hand
in Hand," and "Poor Women Are Denied What the Rich Possess."
Not only was a large new birth control league formed but thousands
of letters supporting Mrs. Sanger flooded the local newspapers.
Thousands of new requests came to her for copies of the pamphlet.

The Portland victory climaxed her three and a half months' tour,
during which she had created organizations from coast to coast.

Her meetings had attracted such attention that the press was forced.
to give her regular front-page space. In three and a half months,
she had made birth control one of the most fervently debated issues
of the day.

She should have been elated, but she wasn't. She came back to
New York in a state of exhaustion and almost psychological numb-
ness. She had driven herself relentlessly. She had allowed herself
so little time for rest that she later recalled with touching poign-
ancy, one short interval between the endless round of getting off
trains, introductions, and talking to committees. Someone at the
end of her San Francisco lecture had simply pulled her into a car
and swept her away to a hidden spot where the sun broke through
a forest of huge trees. "There she left me for fifteen minutes," Mrs.
Sanger wrote later, "in the midst of a cathedral of great redwoods,
with the sky overhead and myself alone. I have never forgotten the
peace and quiet."

Her ceaseless round of speeches had been like a mystical immer-
sion. Never before outside of New York had she touched the women
of the country directly. Now they flocked to the platform to shake
her hand and talk to her after each lecture. They telephoned her
hotel. Couples even came to her room at seven in the morning on
their way to work or late at night, knocking timidly on the door and
begging for a few minutes of her time. Many of them brought
bunches of daisies or wild flowers as tokens of their thanks. They
would go to any resort to attend one of her meetings. Although the
admission charge was kept low—usually twenty-five cents to cover
the cost of the hall and Mrs. Sanger's train fare—one woman without that amount had even left her wedding ring at the box office for
security until she could return the next day with the money.

But much as it forwarded the movement, the trip only intensified
her own frustration. What had she really done for these women?
She had stirred their hopes, given them a new vision. But what they
wanted most of all was specific information. A pamphlet wasn't
enough. The thousands of letters she had received on the trip—over
a thousand from St. Louis alone—cried out with the needs of these
women.

"I have born and raised six children and I know all the hardships
of raising a large family," wrote one mother. ". . . I have 3 daughters
that have 2 children each and they say they will die before they have
any more and every now and again they go to a doctor and get rid

of one and some day I think it will kill them but they say they don't care for they will be better dead than live in hell with a big family and nothing to raise them on."

A midwestern mother wrote: "There is a woman in our town who has six children and is expecting another. Directly after the birth of a child she goes insane, a raving maniac, and they send her to the insane asylum. . . . After about six months they discharge her and she comes home and is in a family way again in a few months. Still the doctors will do nothing for her."

Still another woman wrote: "In a few months I will again be a mother, the fourth child in less than six years. While carrying my babies am always partly paralyzed on one side. Do not know the cause but the doctor said at last birth we must be 'more careful,' as I could not stand having so many children. . . . I wonder if my body does survive this next birth if my reason will."

No speech, no pamphlet, Margaret Sanger knew, could help such desperate need—nothing but an organized chain of birth control clinics in every major city. That was the only possible goal now. She had to start by opening a clinic in New York that would be a model for the rest of the country.

The risk was tremendous. Section 1142 of the New York State law declared that *no one* could give information to prevent conception to *anyone* for *any* reason. On the other hand, Section 1145 stated that physicians could give prescriptions to prevent conception for the cure or prevention of disease. Two attorneys and several doctors assured her that this exception referred only to venereal disease. The intent was to protect the man and actually permit promiscuity. She would have to open a clinic as a test case and fight to include the rights of women in the law.

But where could she open a clinic? How could she find a doctor? Where would she get the money for rent and supplies? The obstacles seemed insurmountable.

Then three women from the Brownsville section of Brooklyn, each the mother of four or more children, came to her hotel room. "They told me of their own hardships, poverty and misery," Mrs. Sanger described the visit later, "of their own helplessness, their struggles to make ends meet. One woman said that she had just recovered from an abortion from which she had nearly died. Another abortion would 'take her off.' 'Then what will become of my children?' she moaned. They rocked back and forth in their chairs as they related their miseries, every tragic event told so simply as each woman re-counted her experience, scarcely able to allow the friend to finish before she took up the story of her own sufferings.

"When they had finished that hour's recital of misery, agony and hopelessness, I felt as if I had been through it all myself. I wanted to scream out, to do something. I remember hearing the story of a man in Spain who had become so desperate over the injustice of innocent prisoners that he took a revolver and fired it at the first person he met on the street. Innocent persons, of course, he had killed, but it was his only protest, the only way the poor creature had of expressing his indignation. I understood this man that day after those women left me."

A few hours later the telephone rang—a woman's voice. She had just come from California and had brought a check for fifty dollars to Margaret Sanger from Kate Gartz of Los Angeles. Where should she send it?

In one blinding flash, the whole dream seemed to take shape. She would go where these women needed her. The check would pay the first month's rent. Tomorrow she would organize the first birth control clinic in America and it would be located in Brownsville.

CHAPTER 9

Through the raw October winds, in what she later called "those passionate, dangerous and menacing days," Margaret Sanger tramped the streets of Brooklyn to find the right location for her clinic. The risk she faced now was more acute, more immediate than anything before. This would not only be a test of the law in a theoretical sense. Contraceptive techniques would be explained and demonstrated directly to mothers. Every hour the clinic remained open she would be making a direct challenge to the police. A raid, arrest, imprisonment were almost certain. "But if a woman must break the law to establish her right to voluntary motherhood," she wrote in the first issue of the *Birth Control Review*, "then that law must be broken."

Margaret Sanger did not consider her action a matter of lawlessness. The law was archaic, a degradation of motherhood outdated hundreds of years before. It had been replaced by a higher law, the law of the sacredness of life.

She envisioned the founding of the clinic as a point in history toward which such great scientific minds of the nineteenth century as Darwin, Huxley, and now Havelock Ellis had led. Down through the centuries, men had fought the tyranny of nature, harnessed rivers and floods, pierced the darkness with electricity, conquered the air with wings. Yet we had never controlled the most fundamental fact of life—procreation. The tyranny of uncontrolled reproduction was the greatest tyranny of all. "At a certain stage in the higher development of man, without ceasing to be natural," Ellis wrote on June 18, 1916, "the evolutionary process becomes conscious and deliberate. It is then that we have what may be properly termed birth control."

The founding of this clinic, therefore, would mean that an American woman could consciously and deliberately go forth to get personal and specific information that would make her the mistress of her own instincts and her own body. The clinic would be the first concrete realization in America of an evolutionary philosophy soon to change its social history.

Mrs. Sanger and Fania Mindell, who had come East from Chicago to help her, searched the vacant stores of Brownsville for a suitable location at a rent they could afford. At last, at 46 Amboy Street, they found two first-floor rooms in a sea of tenements huddling together as if for warmth. The landlord, Joseph Rabinowitz, was friendly and let them have the rooms for fifty dollars a month. The community, part Italian but predominantly Jewish, was apt to be tolerant of new ideas, particularly where the health of mothers was concerned. There would be less chance of broken windows, less hurling of insults on a street like this.

Now that Margaret Sanger had the start of a clinic, the two women doctors who had talked so enthusiastically about it a few months back suddenly withdrew their support. Their fears were understandable. A doctor serving the clinic would not only jeopardize her private practice but face the possibility of censure by the medical organizations and even the loss of her license. The recent case of Dr. Mary Halton had been sufficient warning. "Dr. Mary," as she was known to the poor and oppressed whom she especially befriended, had been on the staff of Grosvenor Hospital and conducted an evening clinic there. To one of her patients, who had been operated on for glandular tuberculosis, she prescribed a cervical pessary. A few nights later, when the patient came back for a refitting, "Dr. Mary" was out, and her horrified substitute immediately brought the case to the hospital board. "Dr. Mary" insisted that contraception had to be given this woman to prevent endangering her life. The board disagreed and demanded her resignation.

Mrs. Sanger interviewed every possible candidate in New York and wrote to her associates throughout the country. But she could find no doctor who would take the risk. Yet she insisted that the clinic open. Her studies with Dr. Rutgers in Holland had qualified her to give contraceptive instruction. Her sister Ethel Byrne could assist her. It would not make as useful a test case of the law, but it was better than waiting.

She immediately drew up a letter to the District Attorney of Brooklyn announcing the opening of the clinic. Then without waiting for a reply, which never came, she began the final preparations. Rabinowitz, their hospitable landlord, spent hours painting the walls a sparkling white—to make everything "more hospital-looking," as he put it. There was only a small budget for furnishings, but Fania knew Yiddish and could bargain with the local shopkeepers. They bought chairs, desks, flooring, curtains, and a stove. They even added an examination table, although the clinic would not conduct individual contraceptive fittings until a doctor was secured.

Meanwhile, Mrs. Sanger had five thousand handbills printed, each carrying the announcement in English, Yiddish, and Italian:

> MOTHERS!
> *Can you afford to have a large family?*
> *Do you want any more children?*
> *If not, why do you have them?*
> DO NOT KILL, DO NOT TAKE LIFE, BUT PREVENT
> *Safe, Harmless Information can be obtained of trained*
> *Nurses at*
> 46 AMBOY STREET
> *Near Pitkin Ave.—Brooklyn*
> *Tell Your Friends and Neighbors All Mothers Welcome*
> *A registration fee of 10 cents entitles any mother to this*
> *information*

They went through the neighborhood day after day, tucking the handbills into mailboxes, climbing up five flights of stairs to put them under doors. They walked through the endless lines of cramped, unpainted houses. It was one of the city's most congested areas, packed with what Mrs. Sanger called "a fatalistic, stolid and tragic army of New Yorkers." "Early in the morning," she wrote, "weary-eyed men poured from the low tenement houses . . . bound for ten or twelve hours of work. At the same time, or earlier, their women rose to set in motion that ceaseless round of cooking, cleaning and sewing that barely kept the younger generation alive." Everywhere unkempt children swarmed in the alleyways and played in the rubbish heaps—tragic incarnations of the specter of overpopulation.

The clinic was ready by the middle of October. In the outer room, bright with paint and new curtains, Fania would take each mother's case history and distribute copies of *What Every Mother Should Know*. Remembering how the scanty records of the Dutch clinics had made it difficult to analyze the social and economic impact of birth control on the community, Mrs. Sanger was determined to keep a complete record of every patient—name, address, age, number and age of living children, miscarriages, abortions, husband's job and salary, and other related factors.

In the inner room, Margaret and Ethel would demonstrate to seven or eight women at a time the principles of contraception. There were models of the cervical pessary and other techniques, with charts and drawings of how they were to be used. Ethel had a delicate, chiseled face and aub irn hair even more flaming than Margaret's. She had taken no previous part in the birth control movement, but she was a nurse of long experience. A devoted radical, with a mind like a steel trap, she considered birth control a part of the whole progressive revolt. Fired more by the dramatic role she could play in this unique experiment than by a long-range understanding of the movement, she threw herself almost passionately into what she considered the first real blow for women's freedom.

The opening day was October 16, 1916, a day bright and crisp after long rain, a day that stands as a significant turning point in social history.

At seven in the morning, they were dusting the furniture and adding the last touches. The registration cards were carefully stacked on the reception-room desk, the demonstration materials and pamphlets waiting on the shelves of the inner room. Would the women come? Not all the laws of New York State could have kept them away.

Before they had finished dusting, Fania called, "Come outside and look!" Halfway to the corner people were standing in line, at least a hundred of them, some shawled, some hatless, their red hands clasping the cold, chapped, smaller ones of their children. Some women were alone, some in pairs. Some came with their neighbors, some had infants clasped in their arms or had brought their married daughters. Some had come without telling their husbands. A few husbands brought timid, embarrassed wives, apologetically dragging a string of little children. All day long and far into the evening, they came in increasing numbers. A hundred women and forty men passed through the doors that first day, but Mrs. Sanger was nowhere near the end of the line when she had to close. The rest were asked to return in the morning.

The next day the Yiddish and Italian papers carried the story of the clinic. Women came, clutching scraps of paper with the clinic's address, clipped from the morning editions. In the next week, they came from as far away as Massachusetts, Connecticut, Pennsylvania, New Jersey, and the far end of Long Island. Each woman was asked the same questions for the record—number of children living and dead, number of abortions, of miscarriages. "These everyday questions," Mrs. Sanger told Elizabeth Stuyvesant in an interview for the Boston *Journal*, "touched a spring that let loose a flood of experience so real, so deep that you felt you were looking at life for the first time. So much cold truth, so many hopeless facts to show how little there was in life for these people, such heartbreaking confidences in response to a word of sympathy, that you came, at the end of a day, to wonder how the world could go on with so much sadness in it.

"They told us of so-called homes with two rooms and one window, with two beds for a family of seven, of years of heavy toil by fine, hopeful men and women with, at the end, only sickness, funerals and debts—stories of wives broken in health, husbands broken in spirit and always the helpless tale of children that were not wanted but came in never-ending numbers."

Newly married couples told of the tiny flat they had chosen, of the husband's low wages, of their determination to make their marriage work if only the children did not come too soon. A gaunt skeleton of a woman stood up one morning in the waiting room and said impassionately, "They offer us charity when we have more babies than we can feed, and when we get sick with more babies for trying not to have them, they just give us more charity talks."

"One woman of thirty-five," reported the Brooklyn *Eagle*, "told Mrs. Sanger: 'I have seven children. Just now I am wondering how I am going to get shoes for them. My husband earns fifteen dollars a week when he works, and he is a good man to me. I do not know what we would do if another baby came.'"

Despite the opposition of the Church, Mrs. Sanger's records showed that Roman Catholics, as well as Protestants and Jews, came to the clinic in almost exact proportion to their numbers in the community. She asked one Catholic woman what she would say to the priest when he learned she had been to the clinic. "It's none of his business," she answered indignantly. "My husband has a bad heart and works only four days a week. He gets twelve dollars, and we can hardly live on it now."

The woman with her nodded. "When I was married," she broke in, "the priest told us to have lots of children. I had fifteen. Six are living. I'm thirty-seven years old now. Look at me. I might be fifty!"

For Mrs. Sanger, the most tragic cases were the expectant mothers who came to her in the desperate hope of finding a way to rid themselves of pregnancy. Often they threatened suicide. One Jewish wife, after giving birth to eight children, had gone through two abortions and an uncounted number of miscarriages. Exhausted not only from cleaning and cooking for her family but taking in extra work at night from sweatshops making hats, she was at the end of her strength, in a state of morbid hysteria. "If you don't help me," she cried, "I'm going to chop up glass and swallow it tonight."

It was the faces of women like this who followed Margaret Sanger home at night and haunted her sleep. Her clinic had come too late to keep these women from the precipice. All she could do to save them was give the little attention and devotion in her power—talk with them, try to make them understand how much their husband and children needed them. "One more child won't make that much difference," she insisted. "Promise me to have this one and do nothing rash."

There were even a few gay moments. The grocer's wife on the corner, the widow with six children who kept the lunchroom up the street dropped in regularly to wish them well. The fat old German baker, whose wife passed out handbills for the clinic at the door, was always sending donations of doughnuts. Whenever the pressure got so severe that Margaret, Ethel, and Fania could not get out for a meal, they were sure to hear Mrs. Rabinowitz call downstairs, "If I bring hot tea now, will you stop the people coming?" Each day the postman delivered his customary fifty to a hundred letters from mothers wanting information, and always quipped, "Farewell, ladies. Hope to find you here tomorrow."

On the ninth day, while Margaret Sanger was out interviewing a doctor whom she hoped to get as medical director, a large, hard-faced woman, calling herself Mrs. Margaret Whitehurst, came to the clinic. She said she was the mother of two children and did not have the money to support more. She asked for literature and contraceptives. Fania, who had a strong intuitive instinct, immediately called Ethel aside and warned her that this was a policewoman. But Ethel was impulsive and said, "Bring her in anyway." She talked freely with the woman, even outlined the future plans and objectives of the clinic. Instead of the usual ten-cent fee, the woman insisted on paying two dollars. When she left, Fania took the bill and pinned it to a wall with the note: "Received from Mrs. —— of the Police Department as her contribution."

The next afternoon, October 26, the waiting room of the clinic was jammed. "There had been a steady stream of applications for information all day," reported the Brooklyn *Eagle*, "and at 4 o'clock, the closing hour, the women were still arriving." At this moment, Mrs. Whitehurst pushed her way into the clinic and walked up to Margaret Sanger. "I'm a police officer," she snapped. "You're under arrest."

Immediately three plain-clothes men from the vice squad, Detectives Boylan and Mooney and Sergeant Barry, barred the outside door and posted a policeman in front of it. The raid was carried off with almost mock grandeur by these veteran practitioners. They served their warrants efficiently on Margaret and Fania—Ethel was out at the moment and was not arrested till later. They herded the women patients into line like inmates of a brothel and gruffly took each name and address. Always fearful of the police, a number of the women began to cry. Some carried infants in their arms, and in a minute, the clinic was a bedlam of screaming voices. Mrs. Sanger went from mother to mother, assuring them that only the organizers of the clinic were under arrest and that they could return home in a few minutes. But it was half an hour before she could finally persuade the police to release them.

All literature, contraceptive supplies, and even the 464 case histories of the patients were confiscated—a tragic breach of ethics since these women had confided the most intimate details of their lives. Mrs. Whitehurst further insisted that the examination table be packed into the police van. "We were not surprised at being arrested," Margaret Sanger wrote later, "but the shock and horror of it was that a *woman,* with a squad of three plain-clothes men, conducted the raid and made the arrest. A woman—the irony of it!"

Mrs. Whitehurst's calloused manhandling of the patients goaded Mrs. Sanger's anger to the bursting point. The next day, the New York *World* gave its version, obviously through the eyes of the police, of the raid's somewhat startling climax.

Enraged when she was told she was under arrest, the police say, Mrs. Sanger turned on Mrs. Whitehurst and cried:

"*You dirty thing! You are not a woman!*"

"*Save all that sort of thing to tell the judge in the morning,*" retorted the woman detective.

"*No, I'll tell it to you now. And you have two ears to hear me, too.*"

"*Mrs. Sanger,*" interrupted Sergeant Barry. "*Please put on your hat and coat and come quietly with us to the station house.*"

"*I don't know about that,*" she countered with a laugh. "*I think if you want to take me to your old station house, you'll have to drag me there.*"

Mrs. Sanger's Irish blood, easily a match even for four Irish members of the vice squad, may well have exploded into such language—though her words would certainly have been more imaginatively chosen. Her own version of the scene, however, is far less lurid. "The patrol wagon came rattling up to the door," she wrote later. "I had a certain respect for a uniformed policeman—you knew what they were about—but none whatsoever for the vice squad. I was white-hot with indignation at their unspeakable attitude towards the clinic mothers and stated I preferred to walk the mile to the court rather than sit with them. Their feelings were quite hurt. 'Why, we didn't do anything to you, Mrs. Sanger,' they protested. Nevertheless, I marched ahead, they following behind."

Margaret Sanger was held for the night in the Raymond Street jail. The stench of the mattress nauseated her. The blankets were stiff with dirt and grime. Cold as she was, she refused such disease-infected covering. Lying on top of the bed, she wrapped her own coat around her. The one clean object in the cell was her towel, which she draped over her face and head as a partial protection against the roaches and bugs which came out of the walls. In the middle of the night, a rat jumped on her and she cried out, sending it scuttling away.

In the morning, a group of women, a committee from some society for prison reform, came through the cells, peering into them as if the inmates were animals in a cage. A gentle voice cooed at her, "Can we do anything for you?"

The other prisoners sat primly in their cells, looking as innocent as possible. But Margaret Sanger stood up. "Come in and clean up this place," she cried. "It's filthy and verminous."

Although the committee departed hurriedly down the corridor, she refused to let the issue drop. When reporters came to interview her about the clinic raid an hour later, she insisted that the taxpayers of Brooklyn be told how badly their money was being squandered on the Raymond Street jail.

Released on bail that afternoon, she immediately returned to Amboy Street. Pending the decision of the court, she decided to re-open the clinic. A few curious bystanders were standing at the door. She told them the news. Within an hour, the waiting room was crowded again with mothers. Let them arrest her. Let them come for her again. Even if she only had a few days, she could get the desperately wanted information to a few more women.

This time the police closed down the clinic for good. They forced Rabinowitz, the landlord, to sign ejection papers, despite the one-year lease, on the grounds that Mrs. Sanger was "maintaining a public nuisance" in violation of Section 1530 of the Penal Code. What final irony! In Holland, a clinic had been cited as a public benefaction. Here it was a public nuisance!

This time the police, not the vice squad, came to arrest her. They did not bother the patients, and Margaret Sanger and Fania walked quietly to the patrol wagon. A large crowd had already gathered at the door—women with baby carriages, women with children clinging to their hands, shopkeepers, almost everyone who lived in the neighborhood. There were no cries, no panic. The crowd stood there quietly, motionless, as if the one spark of hope they had counted on had been quenched for good, leaving them drained and empty.

"As I sat in the rear of the car and looked out at that seething mob of humans," Margaret Sanger wrote, "I wondered and asked myself *what* had gone out of the race. Something had gone from them which silenced them, made them impotent to defend their rights. I thought of the suffragists in England, and pictured the results of a similar arrest there. But as I sat in this mood, the car started to go. I looked out at the mass and heard a scream. It came from a woman wheeling a baby carriage, who had just come around the corner, preparing to visit the clinic. She saw the patrol wagon, realized what had happened, left the baby carriage, rushed through the crowd to the wagon and cried to me: 'Come back! Come back and save me!' The woman looked wild. She ran after the car for a dozen yards or so, when some friends caught her weeping form in their arms and led her back to the sidewalk. That was the last thing I saw as the Black Maria dashed off to the station."

CHAPTER 10

Faced with a long prison sentence, Margaret Sanger now saw the necessity of realigning the whole strategy of the birth control movement. Previously her voice had cried out to "the working women, the factory workers, the women of the labor unions and the unskilled workers," she wrote. "These were the people to whom my work was directed and for whom I was fighting. I felt that I was the protagonist of the mothers of the child laborers and of the wives of the wage slaves."

But now she realized "how helpless they really were, these mothers." They had not fought in the streets when the police closed their clinic. In England, suffragettes had barricaded themselves behind windows and doors, invaded the grounds of Buckingham Palace, forced the police to arrest them by the hundreds when their leaders had been arrested, and fought back even in prison. In Brownsville, however, the mothers stood mute and helpless. They were not yet a revolutionary force. The majority of them foreign-born, uneducated, and even illiterate, they could not even count on leadership from the Socialists or the unions. The Socialists (with a few exceptions like Debs) had never united on birth control as a major issue. The unions kept their sights on wages and hours; they wanted no part of the problems of women.

What was the answer? "To make club women, the women of wealth and intelligence, use their power and money and influence to obtain freedom and knowledge for the women of the poor," Margaret Sanger wrote. ". . . The women of leisure must listen. The women of wealth must give. The women of influence must protest."

This was a major shift in her strategy, resulting partly from growing disillusionment with the inaction of working women and her belief that a long court battle made more influential support a necessity. These women of influence could carry the birth control fight to the newspapers, the medical societies, the pulpits, and the clubs, to every center of influence in the country. More and more during the past year, she had depended for support on such women as Mrs. Pinchot, Mrs. Delafield, and Mrs. Juliet Barrett Rublee. Now for the first time, they co-ordinated their individual efforts for Mrs. Sanger's defense in an organized committee, the "Committee of 100."

"We desire to help in forming a body of public opinion which will lead to the repeal of all laws, Federal and State, which makes the giving out of information on the subject of Birth Control a criminal offense and which class such information with obscenity and indecency," proclaimed the committee in its credo. Its signers formed an illustrious group: Mrs. J. Borden Harriman, Mrs. Charles Tiffany, Mrs. Lewis L. Delafield, Mrs. Robert M. La Follette, and a few men like Rabbi Stephen Wise, Professor James Harvey Robinson, and Dr. L. Emmett Holt.

The credo's author and chairman of the committee was Juliet Rublee. She was both wealthy in her own right, and the wife of George Rublee, a prominent international lawyer who had been appointed to the Federal Trade Commission by President Wilson. After hearing Margaret Sanger speak on birth control at a small meeting, she was so moved "that I suddenly realized it had become the most important thing in the world to me." A strikingly handsome woman with dark hair and a gift for the exotic, which led her to combine bright greens, reds, and yellows in her dress and always wear a tinkling abundance of heavy silver jewelry, she now poured all the resources of her home, money, and contacts into the movement. She brought many prominent doctors to her house to meet Mrs. Sanger and secured the invaluable support of Dr. Holt, a nationally respected pediatrician and the author of *The Care and Feeding of Children*. Through her husband, she was soon to enlist such prominent families as the Paul Cravaths, the Dwight D. Morrows, and the Thomas Lamonts, who would give birth control new stature.

Even in legal strategy, Margaret Sanger saw that the Brownsville case could no longer be fought along the dramatic and revolutionary lines of her federal indictment when she had stood alone in court as her own lawyer. Now she was challenging Section 1142 of the New York Penal Code, contending that its prohibition against contraceptive information was unconstitutional. There was little hope of winning such a ruling from a lower court. The case would probably have to be fought all the way up to the United States Supreme Court, and this needed a lawyer who not only believed in birth control but had the background and skill to carry on a long and tortuously complex defense. The man she secured was Jonah J. Goldstein.

"J.J.," as his friends called him, was a rising Tammany Democrat. His strong sense of social consciousness came from his boyhood on the Lower East Side, where he had been influenced by Mary Simkhovitch, founder of Greenwich House, and Lillian Wald, the founder of Henry Street Settlement. Handsome, dark-haired, swarthy-skinned, and shy, he had become a lawyer in 1907, and in 1911 was appointed secretary to Alfred E. Smith, then majority leader in the New York State Assembly. Here he demonstrated his social vision by pushing a bill to require the physical and mental examination of children in the Children's Courts. He was also a club leader in the Educational Alliance and the University Settlement House, and later the organizer of the Jewish Big Brother Movement.

Goldstein's Tammany connections—he eventually became a distinguished judge and Republican candidate for Mayor of New York —would ordinarily have made his birth control affiliation somewhat ludicrous. Tammany and the Catholic hierarchy in New York saw eye to eye on most matters. But Tammany's leaders excused this transgression because of the large fees they supposed he was receiving from the birth control organization. Ironically enough, the actual fact was that in four years as Margaret Sanger's lawyer he never asked a penny for his work.

The Brownsville clinic case was heard before Magistrate Steers on October 30, November 3 and 6, and then set for trial on November 22. Goldstein guided Margaret, Ethel Byrne, and Fania Mindell through the tortuous legal maneuvers—the request for transfer to the county court and trial by jury, which was denied, the request for writ of habeas corpus, also dismissed. Goldstein explained patiently that they had to take every step that the law allowed if the case was to be pushed to the Supreme Court. But Mrs. Sanger rebelled constantly. During one day of courtroom parrying, she was in her seat when the judge entered and the clerk cried, "Hear ye, hear ye! All rise." She stayed seated. "For God's sake, help me," Goldstein whispered to her. "Stand up just this once."

"I thought this was a court, not a church," she snapped.

Her insistence on her own direct methods often brought surprising results. Goldstein had previously objected to having the trial set in the November session because Judge J. J. McInerney, who had expressed violent anti-birth control opinions when he was on the bench during William Sanger's conviction, was due to preside. This objection, however, was overruled. She immediately addressed an open letter to the judge:

In those birth control cases at which you have presided, you have shown all thinking men and women an unfailing prejudice and exposed a mind steeped in the bigotry and intolerance of the Inquisition.

To come before you implies conviction.

Now in all fairness, do you want a case of this character brought forcibly before you when the defendant feels and believes that you are prejudiced against her?

This time the judge made application to the District Attorney to be taken off the case.

During all these hectic, pre-trial days, she continued to carry her fight to the public. On January 5, 1917, the New York Legislative League debated the issue of birth control before an overflow crowd at the Waldorf-Astoria Hotel. The Women's City Club had to turn away hundreds of women who jammed its birth control meeting at the Park Avenue Hotel. She was guest of honor at another meeting at the Vanderbilt Hotel, where Dr. Charles H. Lyttle of Brooklyn, a Unitarian minister, proclaimed, "Mrs. Sanger deserves the aggressive support of those who regard the present law as the product of unscientific social theories two hundred or more years out of date . . ."

A few days later when the Philosophic Society of Paterson, New Jersey, invited her to speak at its next Sunday meeting, Police Chief Bimson announced he would halt the meeting and "Mayor Amos H. Radcliff," reported the New York *Evening Telegram*, "said he would back up any action taken by his police officials." She fought back instantly. It was always such blatant demonstrations of injustice that roused her to fury. "If Paterson is in the United States," she cried, "I have a right to speak there. If the authorities have arbitrary powers as in Russia or backward Spain, the inhabitants should haul down the American flag." The Mayor relented and allowed the meeting, which by now had attracted such interest it had to be shifted to the larger Institute Hall.

The Brownsville trial, after numerous postponements, finally opened on January 8, 1917. In spite of Mrs. Sanger's insistence that they be tried together, Ethel's case was called first. In addition to members of the Committee of 100, who came to court almost daily, the Brownsville women had sent a large delegation. "Disorder in the form of violent handclapping by the women present, of whom there were nearly a hundred, interrupted the proceedings at one time," reported the New York *Times.*

Ethel freely admitted that she had described birth control methods but scorned the District Attorney's sensational charges that the ten-cent registration made the clinic a "money-making" affair and that "the clinic was intended to do away with the Jews." The testimony of the defense's most important witness, Dr. Morris H. Kahn, physician at Bloomingdale's Department Store, was ruled out as "irrelevant, incompetent, and immaterial." Goldstein was allowed only fifteen minutes for his arguments on the unconstitutionality of Section 1142. "The whole purpose of the law," he asserted, "was to promote a larger population. But what if we had a similar law for fining a bachelor over thirty who had the means to support a wife and family and yet did not marry? Would this clearly not be an infringement of his constitutional rights to life and liberty? What if we had a law that fined all childless married couples unless they could prove they had not consciously avoided having children? Would not this also be the same sort of infringement of personal liberty as this law which forbids people the choice of how many children they will have and when?"

But the judge ruled that Section 1142 must be held constitutional on precedent and declared Ethel guilty. On January 22, she was sentenced to thirty days in the workhouse on Blackwell's Island in the East River. Impulsively she announced what the New York *American* called her "proclamation of defiance."

1. *I shall not touch a morsel of food while in jail.*
2. *I shall not touch anything they ask me to drink.*
3. *I shall not do one article of work.*

She announced that she had made her will and arranged for the disposition of her two children. "To jail and to death," cried Mrs. Byrne as she said good-by to Margaret Sanger in a melodramatic farewell, reported by the *World.* Then she added to newspapermen, "I made up my mind last night to die for the cause. I ate a farewell dinner of turkey and plenty of ice cream. I shall go on a hunger strike. I shall die, if need be, for my sex!"

Ethel spent the first night at Tombs prison while Goldstein worked frantically to get a writ of habeas corpus which would suspend sentence pending the appeal. She was returned the next morning to the Federal District Court of Brooklyn. In the courtroom, she insisted she was going to carry through the hunger strike and whispered to Margaret, "I haven't had a thing to eat yet."

Margaret Sanger, too, favored a hunger strike if it would capture the country's headlines and rouse women everywhere behind the movement. But with the United States plunging toward involvement in the European war, it seemed doubtful that a thirty-day sentence would stir enough national indignation to make a strike effective. "Once you start the strike," she warned, "you'll have to stay with it to the end."

Ethel was ready. A half hour later when the judge refused to issue a writ of habeas corpus and remanded her to Blackwell's Island, she defiantly told reporters she would carry through her strike to death if necessary. In a final act of rebellion, she spent the whole trip to jail giving a lecture on contraception to the other women prisoners in the patrol wagon.

On her arrival, the warden's wife came to the admitting office to look over the new prisoners. A motherly woman with a heavy Irish brogue, she immediately selected Ethel for what was considered a prize job—waiting on tables and acting as chambermaid in the warden's quarters. Ethel refused the job and announced her intention of neither eating nor drinking. During the next twenty-four hours, the old woman pleaded, coaxed, and prayed in an effort to change Ethel's mind. She was terrified Ethel might die in the workhouse. As a final temptation, she sent the odor of bacon and eggs drifting into Ethel's cell. "I'll get you the food secretly," she urged. "Nobody'll know you've taken a bite."

"I'd know," Ethel replied.

Commissioner of Correction Burdette C. Lewis scoffed at the hunger strike. "Others have threatened strikes," he stated. "It means nothing."

But Margaret Sanger knew there was a grain of steel under Ethel's quiet, diffident air. Schooled by long training as a professional nurse, Ethel could resist forcible feeding unless extreme strength was used against her. "Knowing her as well as I did," Mrs.

Sanger wrote later, "I realized that my sister would never give in."

Within a few days, Ethel's hunger strike was competing with the war news from Europe for page one headlines. On January 26, 1917, the right-hand columns of the first page of the New York *Times* announced: "Tisza Hints of New Teuton Move for Peace with 'Acceptable' Terms." The column next to it was headlined: "Mrs. Byrne Weaker, Still Fasts in Cell." The United Press story of the same day reported that "as Mrs. Byrne launched into the fifth day of her hunger strike today, it was apparent that the pale little advocate of birth control is rapidly drawing towards the climax of her struggle against imprisonment."

The case soon dominated editorial and letter columns across the country. "It will be hard to make the youth of 1967 believe that in 1917 a woman was imprisoned for doing what Mrs. Byrne did," wrote Franklin P. Adams in his New York *Tribune* column. In a letter to the St. Paul, Minnesota, *Dispatch*, Dr. Charles T. Miller stated: "The humiliation and righteous indignation felt by every American who has a drop of red blood in his body after reading about Mrs. Byrne cannot be expressed in words."

The opposition comment was equally forceful. "Is there no limit to the mischief which idle women, inspired and abetted by masculine cranks, can work to modern society?" demanded the Milwaukee *Free Press*. In what could easily rank as one of the worst forecasts of the century, the San Jose, California, *Mercury* predicted: "A few more arrests and the propaganda of birth control will vanish as quickly as it appeared . . ."

Commissioner Lewis now barred Mrs. Sanger and all reporters from the workhouse and allowed Ethel's attorney only one visit a day. "I have no patience with Mrs. Byrne's efforts to get advertising for her cause," he snapped, "and I won't encourage such a campaign by issuing bulletins on the progress of her hunger strike." But reporters had their special techniques of getting news from inside the prison. On January 28, next to its front-page story, "Peace by Sword, Kaiser Repeats," the *Times* announced: "Mrs. Byrne Now Being Fed by Force." Commissioner Lewis had finally taken the last brutal step. After Ethel had gone 103 hours without food or water, he established a precedent in American prison annals by ordering her forcibly fed—the first woman in the country to suffer such treatment.

The feeding was accomplished by rolling Ethel into a blanket to limit her struggles and then pouring a mixture of milk, eggs, and brandy through a small tube in her throat. Ethel was already dangerously weakened by over five days without food and water, and Mrs. Sanger knew that the shock of forced feeding might endanger Ethel's life. "Mrs. Sanger said at noon," reported the *Times* on January 28, "that she had received reliable information from Blackwell's Island that her sister was in serious condition." Later she wrote: "Nothing but brutality could have reduced her fiery spirit to acquiescence. I was desperate, torn between admiration for what she was doing and misery over what I feared might be the result."

Mrs. Pinchot and the Committee of 100, however, publicly stated that Ethel's life was "too valuable to the cause" to be wasted and sent her a telegram begging her to abandon the hunger strike. The move only confused Ethel because she thought Margaret had had a part in it. "It makes little difference whether I starve or not," she told Goldstein that night, "as long as this outrageous arrest calls attention to the archaic laws which would prevent our telling the truth about the facts of life."

Meanwhile, Mrs. Sanger and the Committee of 100 were using every public channel to induce the prison authorities to abandon the use of force. A delegation of the committee went to Washington on January 27 to talk to influential Congressmen. "Of a dozen members questioned," said the United Press in a cryptic résumé, "all but one reduced his voice to a whisper when discussing birth control. . . ." Then the committee announced a giant rally in Carnegie Hall for January 29, with Helen Todd as chairman and Mrs. Sanger, Reverend John Haynes Holmes, and Dr. Mary Halton as speakers. The city was covered with announcements, the hall was jammed. Twenty of the Brownsville mothers, who had been caught in the police raid, were given the place of honor on the platform. A hundred students from Barnard College had purchased a block of seats in the orchestra. Such prominent names as Isadora Duncan, Rupert Hughes, and Mr. and Mrs. John Sloan took boxes.

Margaret Sanger arrived at Carnegie Hall after an agonizing day. Her own trial was to open tomorrow in the Federal District Court in Brooklyn and she had just heard from her informants in the workhouse that Ethel's condition had grown critical. Her vision had been affected and her heart was beginning to miss beats due to lack of liquid. "I know she was unconscious for twenty-four hours," Mrs. Sanger was quoted in a story in the Baltimore *Sun*. "She was expectorating blood from the injured membranes of her throat and nose. This meeting tonight may become a memorial instead of a testimonial meeting."

When Margaret Sanger walked on the stage at Carnegie Hall, the audience raised its voice in one great shout. "I come to you tonight from a crowded courtroom, from a vortex of persecution," the *Times* quoted her the next morning. "I come not from the stake at Salem, where women were once burned for blasphemy, but from the shadow of Blackwell's Island, where women are tortured for obscenity."

"I never saw another meeting like that," said Reverend Holmes. "It had the spirit of the abolition days. She took the audience and lifted it up. She had dignity. She had the dramatic air of a person in danger. And she had power. You can tell in five minutes whether a person is an actor or has the real secret of power. She had it—the power of a saint combined with the mind of a statesman. I realized that night she was one of the great women of our time."

The next day she had to be in court at her own trial, but late that afternoon a reporter from the *World* told her he had managed a secret interview with Ethel and that her condition was quickly deteriorating.

She decided to act immediately. With Jessie Ashley and Mrs. Pinchot, who was a friend of Governor Charles S. Whitman and had arranged an appointment, she took the next train to Albany. The Governor, a fair and intelligent executive, listened to their arguments for birth control and promised to appoint an investigatory commission. Then Miss Ashley described the brutal use of force against Ethel on Blackwell's Island. The Governor was sympathetic. "I, personally, do not," he stated, "and I feel sure that the people of this state do not want to see this woman suffer in prison." But he added this provision to any move for clemency: "I would be faithless to my trust if I granted a pardon without a stipulation that she would not go right out and violate the law again."

Mrs. Pinchot wanted the pardon accepted on these conditions. But Margaret Sanger still refused. She could not promise to make her sister abandon the movement for which she had been willing to give her life. Ethel would have to be consulted first. Would the Governor give her a pass to visit Ethel in the workhouse? He agreed and wrote out the pass.

Every minute counted now. They rushed back to New York. Mr. and Mrs. Pinchot drove her to Blackwell's Island in their car. It was a stinging, cold day, and the trip on the ferry seemed endless. But when they reached the prison gate, the Governor's pass and the name Pinchot brought Margaret to Ethel's cell in a matter of minutes. For a moment, she could hardly recognize her sister. She was lying on her cot, motionless, breathing haltingly, not even stirring at the first sound of her name.

"Her appearance shocked and horrified me," she wrote later. "She had grown thin and emaciated. Her eyes were sunken and her tongue swollen. She could not see me. She recognized my voice and asked me to come closer. There was a rash on her face, and when she tried to speak her voice was muffled, a mere whisper. Her mind was already confused.

"'I want to go away,' she kept repeating. 'I must go away.'

"I realized that the look of death was creeping into her glazed eyes. It was useless of me to discuss the question of pardon with a dying woman; I had to make up my mind and assume responsibility for her conduct in the future."

She hurried back to New York and telegraphed Governor Whitman. She told him that Mrs. Byrne was too ill to accept the conditions of the pardon. She would promise on her sister's behalf that Ethel would halt all work for the birth control clinic while the case was being appealed through the courts. It was an agonizing decision for Mrs. Sanger—taking into her hands a decision so momentous to one she loved. Later Ethel might disagree with everything Margaret had done, might even hate her for it. "There was no other course," Margaret Sanger wrote. "Her life was what mattered to me, regardless of her future activities.

"If she had been kept another day in the workhouse," she told reporters later, "it would have meant her death."

The Governor was actually on his way to New York when she sent the telegram. An hour later, she and the Pinchots called on him at his hotel room, where he signed the pardon. They went back to Blackwell's Island immediately. After waiting half an hour, they were told Mrs. Byrne was on her way out. Margaret insisted on going down the long corridor to meet her.

"Along the corridor she came, held on both sides by two burly attendants, the matron following with her wraps," Margaret Sanger described it later. "The martyr's head was falling from side to side, and I could see from the pallor of her face, especially her nose and mouth, that she had already fainted.

"I called out to the matron that she was too ill to walk. But orders had been given and were being obeyed.

"I called Mrs. Pinchot's attention to my sister's condition.

"Without hesitation, Mrs. Pinchot imperiously clapped her hands and in a voice of command insisted that they lay her down on the floor and bring a stretcher. The result was like magic. The word of command from this quarter was not to be ignored.

"A stretcher was brought, Mrs. Pinchot took her own warm fur coat and wrapped it around Mrs. Byrne, and she was carried from the prison to the ferryboat, from which an ambulance, previously engaged, carried her to my own apartment."

"Mrs. Sanger has been sitting up with her all night, and we do not know yet whether she has a chance to recover," J. J. Goldstein told the *World* the next day. It would be two weeks before Ethel Byrne was out of danger—but more than a year before she regained her health.

Her hunger strike gave the intensity of physical renunciation to the birth control movement. The suffragettes of England had never quailed before pain and violence. But in America, Ethel Byrne was a phenomenon. Here it was something new for a woman—and a beautiful and educated woman at that—to risk death willingly for the sake of social reform.

CHAPTER 11

Margaret Sanger's trial opened January 29, 1917, in the same bare, antiquated upstairs Brooklyn court in which Ethel had appeared. A contingent of at least fifty mothers from Brownsville crowded the courtroom. Many held children on their laps and carried extra diapers and bags of food. Mingled with them was the smartly dressed delegation from the Committee of 100, who made the trial, according to a slightly cynical report in the Bay City, Michigan, *Times-Tribune* "more suggestive of a '400' social event than a criminal prosecution."

The New York *Tribune* reporter painted an even more elaborate description. "American beauties in the defendant's arms, society and club women in the front rows of seats, and limousines waiting outside made the trial take on the color of a reception with Mrs. Sanger as the guest of honor. She looked the part, rather than that of a law-breaker, as she sat there, a demure, rather shy-looking young woman. . . ." Turning his attention to the Brownsville mothers, he noted that "most of them were hungry because there was no kosher food to be obtained in the neighborhood." This fact did not deter such stalwart supporters of the movement as Mrs. Rose Halperin of 375 Bedford Street, who, the *Times* reported, came to court with all six of her children.

Fania Mindell faced the court first. "A slip of a woman with a pale and delicate face," the Brooklyn *Eagle* called her. She was in poor health and Mrs. Sanger instructed Goldstein to get her off as easily as possible. Fania was charged with the sale of *What Every Girl Should Know,* and the issue was simply to determine whether this was an "indecent" book. The judges found her guilty and gave her a fifty-dollar fine—a decision that was eventually reversed on appeal.

Jonah J. Goldstein was determined to get Margaret Sanger off with a suspended sentence. To his legal mind, freedom meant victory. The harrowing effect of the hunger strike on Ethel's health convinced him that if Mrs. Sanger followed the same tactic her tuberculosis-weakened body could never stand the ordeal. But she told him flatly, "Not one word about my health at the trial!"

Goldstein also believed that the sympathy aroused in the press over the brutality of Ethel's treatment and the Governor's statement that he considered her punishment overharsh would make the judges lean over backward to avoid a similar sentence for Margaret.

But she was firm. "No compromise," she told him. She had opened the Brownsville clinic specifically to force the courts to broaden their interpretation of the law. "I am right. I must be right," she insisted.

"But, Margaret," he pleaded, meeting her before the trial on the courthouse steps, "if you don't give a little, they'll have to convict you. They have no other choice."

"No compromise," she stated with finality.

Five hundred years before, the prosecutor of Joan of Arc in Bernard Shaw's version of the trial scene protests: "It is always the same. She is always right, and we are always wrong."

Analyzing Margaret Sanger's decision recently, Judge Goldstein confirmed the fact that like Joan's, his client's insight went far beyond the facts. "Certainly she was strong-willed," he said. "Once she set her mind, you couldn't dynamite it. From the legal point of view, she was wrong. But from the long-range point of view, she was right, unassailably right."

So he faced the court, handicapped but still with hope. There was a panel of three judges: John J. Freschi, Italian; Moses Herrmann, Jewish; and George J. O'Keefe, Irish. Judge Freschi, who presided, was the most encouraging factor. He was young and had an open and exploring mind. Goldstein expected little of old Judge Herrmann except that his Jewish origin might make him more sensitive to new ideas. They had no illusions about Judge O'Keefe.

The vehemence with which the District Attorney pressed his charges amazed Mrs. Sanger. He had so little to prove. The last thing in her mind was to deny giving birth control information at the clinic. Yet the District Attorney had subpoenaed thirty Brownsville mothers to testify against her. One after another he called them to the witness stand to corroborate the fact that she had given this information. They smiled at Mrs. Sanger reassuringly, confident that their praise was helping her case, when actually each word tightened the web of evidence around her.

"Why did you go to the clinic at 46 Amboy Street?" the District Attorney would ask each mother.

"To have her stop the babies."

"Did you get this information?"

"Yah, yah, dank you. It wass gut, too."

"Enough," barked the District Attorney, and called the next witness.

Goldstein thought he saw a way to turn the testimony to his client's advantage. He called the mothers back on the stand. How many children did they have? "Eight and three that didn't live," said one. Seven living, two dead; nine living, one dead—the answers all fit the same pattern.

How many miscarriages had they suffered? How much illness? How much did their husbands earn? The replies made up a pitiful record of tortured lives. When he came to the woman who had lost three of her eight children, she replied that her husband earned ten dollars a week—"when he works." He was often sick. He had to lay off one or two weeks every month.

At this point, Judge Freschi slammed his fist on the bench and exclaimed, "I can't stand this any longer!" The court was adjourned for the day.

But it was only a temporary victory, only window dressing that could not cover the central issue of the trial, which was Mrs. Sanger's admitted guilt under the existing interpretation of the law. Brilliant, resourceful, determined to get her off despite her refusal to compromise, Goldstein saw that his one hope was to prove to the court that his intention to appeal the case right up to the Supreme Court made a heavy punishment at this time unnecessary.

His argument boiled down to this: I am convinced we can get a new interpretation of the law in a higher court. So why inflict punishment now?

The Court replied: Why should we let Mrs. Sanger off now so that while the case is being appealed she can go right out, open another clinic, and continue to violate the law?

The argument seemed interminable to Mrs. Sanger. She had almost dozed off in her seat when something in Goldstein's words caught her attention. He had practically convinced the judges to agree to clemency. But on what terms? She sat up. What was he saying? Was he promising to make her "be good," to forget the dream of birth control clinics?

Trying to act as a buffer during this debate, Goldstein had placed himself between his client's chair and the Bench. She tried to peer around him and catch the judge's eye. Each time he shifted from side to side to obscure her motions. She tugged on the back of his coat, but he pretended not to notice. This dodging game continued for three or four minutes, until one of the judges finally broke in. "Your client wishes to say something, Counselor." She would be silenced no longer. Judge Freschi ordered her to take the stand. Margaret Sanger took the stand, and she and the Court then engaged in twenty minutes of caustic, and often strained debate.

THE COURT: You have been in court during the time that your counsel made the statement that pending the prosecution of appeal neither you nor those affiliated with you in this so-called movement will violate the law; that is the promise that your counsel makes for you. Now, the Court is considering extreme clemency in your case. . . . Now, do you personally make that promise?

MRS. SANGER: Pending the appeal.

THE COURT: It must be without any qualifications whatsoever, as stated by the presiding judge.

MRS. SANGER: I'd like to have it understood by the gentlemen of the court that the offer of leniency is very kind and I appreciate it very much. With me it is not a question of personal imprisonment or personal disadvantage. I am today and have always been more concerned with changing the law and the sweeping away of the law, regardless of what I have to undergo to have it done.

THE COURT: Since you are of that mind, am I to infer that you intend to go on in this manner, violating the law, irrespective of the consequences?

MRS. SANGER: I haven't said that. I said I am perfectly willing not to violate Section 1142—pending the appeal.

THE COURT: The appeal has nothing to do with it. Either you do or you don't.

Obviously angry, the judges now directed their attack at Goldstein.

THE COURT: What is the use of beating around the bush! . . . This law was not made by us . . . We are simply here to judge the case. We harbor no feelings against Mrs. Sanger. We have nothing to do with her beliefs except in so far as she carries those beliefs into practice and violates the law . . . We ask her, openly and above board, will you publicly declare that you will respect the law and not violate it? And then we get an answer with a qualification. Now, what can the prisoner at the bar for sentence expect, after the Court is inclined to be merciful and do all we can for her? I don't know that a prisoner under such circumstances is entitled to very much consideration after all . . .

Goldstein then tried to explain that Mrs. Sanger's course of action depended on so many variable factors—the action of Governor Whitman's investigatory commission, a possible change in the law by the state legislature—that she could make no promises binding her for years to come. But Judge Freschi would not hear these evasions and banged his fist on the desk. "All we are concerned about is this statute," he exclaimed, "and as long as it remains the law, will this woman promise here and now unqualifiedly to respect it and obey it!" He turned toward the defendant. "Now, is it yes or no? What is your answer, Mrs. Sanger? Is it yes or no?"

This was the climax of all these days, the decisive moment of the trial. Margaret Sanger turned slowly and faced the judges. "She looked so small and frail it seemed impossible she could stand against the wrath of the Court," Juliet Rublee described this moment many years later. "She was risking a long prison sentence, a five-thousand-dollar fine when she didn't have a penny in the bank. The judge had reeled off a long list of her offenses, and then in his ringing voice, demanded, 'What is your answer, Mrs. Sanger? Is it yes or no?' I was sitting in the first row, and I could see her body stiffen and the muscles in her face grow so tight they seemed to be pressing out of her skin. There was a terrible silence. The whole courtroom seemed to hold its breath. Then she spoke, just one sentence in that quiet, brave little voice: 'I cannot promise to obey a law I do not respect.'

"The tension burst. Every woman in the room began to shout and clap. The judge pounded his gavel for silence. When order was restored, he announced, 'The judgment of the Court is that you be confined to the workhouse for thirty days.' A woman's voice from a far corner of the court cried, 'Shame!' Then it was over."

Margaret Sanger waited quietly in her seat while Goldstein attended to the final legal formalities. "I was not surprised at the conviction," she wrote later. "It was expected. I was relieved at the sentence of thirty days. This would not need a hunger strike." Activated always by policy, not by blind impulses, she realized immediately the foolishness of trying to turn a short prison sentence into a demonstration against the law. Ethel's hunger strike had already stirred the country. But only the day before the *Times* had announced in front-page headlines: RELATIONS WITH GERMANY ARE BROKEN OFF. Another strike now would simply be buried in the back pages of the paper. It would be a useless expenditure of her health and strength which could far better serve the movement a month from now if they were kept intact than if she emerged broken and exhausted from prison.

A few minutes later she was led into the anteroom for fingerprinting with other prisoners from the day's session. Again she rebelled. Why should she allow herself to be fingerprinted and admit that running a birth control clinic put her in the category of common criminals? No fingerprints, she told the police clerk. He appealed to the judges, but they were already wearied by one struggle with her and said the fingerprinting was out of their jurisdiction. So the attendants led her into the courtyard and placed her in a patrol wagon with eight or nine other women, and they were driven to the Raymond Street jail. There a huge, thin-lipped police matron told them to get ready for the medical examination.

Mrs. Sanger did not move. "You hear me?" the matron snapped. "Get ready for the examination."

But again she had decided that every act which put her defiance of the birth control law on the same level with the pickpocket or prostitute must be resisted to the end.

The matron left the room, promising to return with two or three other attendants, ready to force her into submission. But again Mrs. Sanger's determined rebellion changed the minds of the authorities. "You won't have to bother with the examination," the matron came back to tell her. They took her upstairs, locked her in a cell, and left her for the night.

The next day she was taken by van to the Queens County penitentiary in Long Island City. Warden Joseph McCann, a young Irishman who had risen from the police ranks, met her. In her diary of that month under the date of February 7, she noted: "The warden . . . met me, asked me about lunch, and hoped I was not going on a hunger strike, to which I said no:—not unless I was forced on one from bad food. Introduced a very motherly, matronly woman to me, Mrs. Sullivan, and sent up some lunch. Put me in Cell 210, where a woman named Josephine Blank is also near by in same corridor."

Warden McCann later questioned her for the prison record forms. When he came to religion, she replied "humanity." Obviously startled, he rephrased the question. "Well, what church do you attend?"

"None," she replied. Ninety-eight per cent of the inmates, she found later, had been reared as Catholics. The warden could hardly believe the existence of such divergence from the normal. At the end of the questioning, he ordered that her fingerprints be taken. Again she refused.

Margaret Sanger's diary for the second day reads: "Cells open at 7 A.M. but bells ring at 8 o'clock. Breakfast—oatmeal with salt and milk and coffee, two slices of bread (saltpeter said to make it taste so queer).

"Clean cells—a walk in the air. Talked with little colored girl, Lisa, who knew of Mrs. Sanger and called out, 'You'se eats, don't you?' in reference to Mrs. Byrne's hunger strike.

"Dinner of stew and bread. . . . Supper of tea, bread and stewed peaches.

"Third day: Women out in yard look pathetically around the ground to see if the men prisoners have left stubs of cigarettes around. Tragic to see human beings forced to so low a level—digging into the frozen ground with fingers for stubs."

The matron took a nap after lunch and the prisoners could usually count on her not being back until three or four. "This gave them the opportunity," Margaret Sanger wrote later, "to dry their shreds of tobacco under the radiator, then wrap them in toilet paper ready for smoking. At night when all were locked in, they struck the steel ribs from their corsets against the stone floors, and thus ignited pieces of cotton to give them lights. I could see tiny glowing points in the darkness as they puffed away greedily."

Three hundred women and an equal number of men were held in the penitentiary. They ranged from dope fiends, pickpockets, embezzlers, prostitutes, smugglers, and keepers of brothels to "Tiffany" or high-class thieves and a few "transatlantic fliers," who took part in the big hauls from Paris or London. Many of the women, Margaret Sanger found, were mothers. A few kept their children in fine schools and went to any length to hide their prison records from their families.

"The resentment engendered in these caged women," she wrote later, "was like a strong glowing flame, of a depth that I had scarcely believed possible."

What could she do for these women? She was convinced that these poor, twisted lives—the dope addicts, the prostitutes, the shoplifters—were mainly the products of huge families, where children were forced into a desperate struggle for survival almost from infancy. She determined to study the relationship between the size of families and their prison offenses, and asked Warden McCann if she could see the records. This was against the rules, but he agreed to give her the statistics himself, warning her she would find them disappointing. How many brothers and sisters does Marie have, she asked? None. And Rose? A brother, but he's dead. And Florence? A sister in Italy. Case after case turned out the same—each inmate seemed to be the only child or the only surviving member of the family.

But as soon as she had been in prison a week and gained the confidence of the inmates, she found that her original thesis was correct. It was an unwritten law that all prisoners should keep their families out of their problems. Every inmate, without exception, had lied to the police when she stated she was an only child. In her own corridor, Mrs. Sanger took an informal poll and found that of thirty-seven women, each of them averaged seven brothers and sisters in their families.

Why not give a birth control lecture right in the penitentiary? Most of the women were delighted with the idea, so Mrs. Sanger asked the matron if she could go into other corridors during the hour when the matron was having her dinner.

"Go on with you," laughed the matron. "They know bad enough already." But she persisted and got her way. A lecture was held and repeated almost every day after that.

To her amazement, Margaret Sanger found that at least a dozen inmates of her corridor could neither read nor write. She started to give them lessons and wrote letters for them to friends and relatives. Because of her health, she was not forced to operate the machines in the prison workshop, and could spend at least half a day on this teaching and her own reading and writing. Her correspondence was voluminous. With leaders like Eugene Debs, now fighting to rally the working classes against American involvement in the European war, she exchanged regular letters. On February 14, 1917, he wrote her in prison: "You and your sister and comrades are making a brave fight against the wolves of the system. You are being tried in every fibre but you have in you the stuff that stands and you are bound to win." On February 25, he wrote: "You are a brave and noble comrade, and when I think of you caged like a beast, all my blood boils with bitter indignation . . ." Margaret Sanger had already divorced herself from organized socialism but still stood firmly with Debs against a war she considered purely a clash of imperialistic rivalries.

"Oh for a million women rebels," Debs wrote in May 1918, in one of his last tributes to her, "to catch the clarion cry of Margaret Sanger and proclaim the glad tidings of woman's coming freedom throughout the world."

Of all the inmates of the penitentiary, the most aloof and puzzling was the "Duchess." She was a tall, stately woman with white hair and a sensitive, chiseled face that was obviously out of place in these surroundings. She had been in jail for nine months, but never mixed with the other women. It was at least two weeks before Mrs. Sanger could gain her confidence. Bit by bit the Duchess told her story. She had been a teacher for fifteen years before giving up her job to marry a retired minister living on a small pension. He drew constantly on his life insurance, and when he died suddenly, she was left almost penniless. Because of her age and the years since she had taught, she could find no teaching job. She moved from hotel to hotel, so poor that she often had to leave without paying her bill. Eventually she was caught and given a one-to-three-year sentence.

Margaret Sanger saw immediately that the only way to awaken this sensitive, brooding woman, who was convinced that prison had ended her life, was to restore her usefulness in the one way she knew best—teaching. She wrote J. J. Goldstein and had him secure a set of lower-grade textbooks from a friend at the Henry Holt Company. She gave them to the Duchess and put her to work teaching the illiterate girls in the penitentiary.

Months later when the Duchess was released from jail, Mrs. Sanger found her an opening as a hostess at an Adirondacks summer resort. The Duchess was afraid to tell the manager of her prison record. "You've got to tell him," Mrs. Sanger insisted. She had the manager come to her New York office and meet the Duchess. He was impressed with her poise and fine looks, and when he learned how she had taught the prison women, he hired her despite her record. The Duchess made an outstanding hostess. Near the end of the summer, she met a rich widower, vacationing there, and married him. The last Mrs. Sanger heard from her was a letter written on their honeymoon in Europe—spent, appropriately enough, cruising on the widower's yacht.

The day of Margaret Sanger's release was March 6, 1917. She had been treated with reasonable decency almost to the end. "But those last two hours," she wrote later, "were horrible. An attempt was made again, just before I left jail, to take my fingerprints. This was, I felt, an outrageous gesture. I resisted. It was time the authorities learned to discriminate between political prisoners and cutthroats. Why should I submit to having a record of my fingerprints filed away with those of thieves and narcotics? I had been uncomplaining through the thirty days, but I made up my mind to fight this needless assertion of authority even if it meant postponing my release.

". . . It was a bitter-cold day, and outside in the courtyard my friends were waiting for me. I knew they were there, and I longed to see them, but even in order to join them, I would not give in to the demands of Warden Joseph McCann. At first we argued; then he turned me over to the two keepers, who tried to force my fingers down on the printed pad. One of them held me while the others struggled with my arms, but I managed each time to keep my finger tips from touching the pad.

"I do not know from what source I drew my physical strength, for certainly these men tried from eight until ten o'clock that morning to make me submit to fingerprinting . . . My arms were bruised and I was weak from exhaustion when an officer telephoned from the department headquarters, where my attorney had protested against the delay, ordering that I be released without the usual fingerprinting ceremony.

"And then I was free! No other experience in my life has been more thrilling than that release. Through the big metal doorway of the Queens County penitentiary I stepped on that grey day, and the tingling air of outdoors rushed against my face. In front of me stood my attorney, my friends and co-workers, their voices lifted in the martial strains of the 'Marseillaise,' led by Kitty Marion, the veteran of suffragettes. Behind them, at the windows of an upper floor, were the faces of newly made friends, the women with whom I had spent the month, and they too were singing for me.

". . . Something still chokes me as I go through it in retrospect and hear the song again: 'Ye sons of freedom, wake to Glory!' All the beauty and tragedy and hope of life's struggle seemed crammed in that moment of my life."

CHAPTER 12

Margaret Sanger was hardly out of jail before she was in action again on a dozen fronts. A dinner had been planned by her followers at the Delmonico Hotel to celebrate her release. Despite the fact that contracts had been signed—and this was typical of the under-handed opposition the movement constantly faced—the hotel sud-denly announced that its standing in the "debutante set" necessitated the cancellation of this event. Her associates despaired of finding another hotel. Mrs. Sanger not only found one, but made the Del-monico look ridiculous by signing the far more aristocratic Hotel Plaza.

Again at Monticello, New York, when the city fathers tried to stop a meeting by passing a resolution against it, she made the long automobile trip to Kingston and sat on Judge Hasbrouck's steps until he returned home at midnight. The judge was so impressed by her arguments for birth control and this act of determination that he issued an injunction against the Monticello resolution, allowing her to go on with her scheduled speech.

Later, at Hagerstown, Maryland, where a group of women had invited her to speak, she was refused a meeting hall by every owner in town. She finally found an empty and dilapidated dance hall and convinced the local undertaker to rent her a few hundred chairs.

She was always at her best in the midst of battle. She loved its thunder. She was proud to stand forth boldly and tell the world— here is a woman who can crush the bigotry and prejudice of the past and build a new freedom for her sex.

Ellis understood her well. "I know you are not happy," he once wrote, "unless you are doing something daring—as smashing laws . . ." When Hugh De Selincourt, a mutual friend, referred to her as that "shining and gentle woman," Ellis commented slyly, "I don't know if he is aware that the gentle woman has sometimes to be held back from deeds of violence by men in khaki!"

The principal antagonist in most of her struggles was the law. Against it she cried out her defiance. "No law is too sacred to break," she wrote in a February 1917 editorial in the *Birth Control Review.* "Throughout all ages the beacon lights of human progress have been lit by the lawbreaker." As proof, she listed such select company as Moses, Christ ("his leading followers practised their religion in defiance of the law of their time"), Washington, and in more recent times John Brown, Thoreau, and William Lloyd Garrison ("whose sturdy refusal to respect an inhuman law helped to emancipate a race").

In prison, she had planned a long-range birth control campaign of agitation, education, organization, and legislation. Most of her previous battles came under the heading of agitation. Now she saw the necessity of educating a mass audience of women in the basic concepts of birth control. She hit on the technique—then certainly novel for a revolutionary cause—of producing an inexpensive motion picture, called, *The Hand That Rocks the Cradle.* With Mrs. Sanger herself in the leading role, it told the simple story of her early struggle among the women of the Lower East Side. But the authorities had only to learn that the words birth control were to be mentioned on the city's screens and they withdrew the picture's permit on May 7, the day of the opening. Newspaper reviewers who saw the preview considered the decision absurd, the *Tribune* reviewer stating that "the plot is clean and the performance unobjectionable." She fought the decision through the courts, and won the first round when Judge Nathan Bijur issued an injunction against this license revocation. But the higher courts sustained the revocation, and her debut as a professional actress suffered a premature demise.

Far more significant, however, was the founding in February 1917 of the *Birth Control Review*—the magazine which was to be the movement's principal voice for the next twenty-three years. Contrasted with the explosiveness of the earlier *Woman Rebel,* the *Review* illustrated how far the movement had developed along scientific lines. In its pages, Margaret Sanger now collected the most advanced thinking on sociological, economic, and population problems and featured such authorities as H. G. Wells, Havelock Ellis, and Professors Henry Pratt Fairchild of New York University and E. M. East of Harvard.

The *Review* soon had over three thousand subscribers. But this money did not cover expenses, and it was a struggle to keep the magazine alive from month to month. In addition, she was writing a book, the *Case for Birth Control*—a compendium of all favorable evidence which would support Goldstein's appeal from the Brownsville clinic decision as he carried it through the courts. She was so hard-pressed for money for the printer that she wrote Juliet Rublee on July 13, 1917, "I may soon have to take up my bag and return to private practice again." On August 9, she wrote Mrs. Rublee: "The printing man was so hard about the bill that I borrowed $300 from my two sisters and paid him."

All this year and next, she was constantly hounded by finances and stayed borrowed to the hilt. She would never take a salary from the movement itself, insisting that the small contributions which came in from all over the country must go to the *Review* and office expenses. She supported herself through her own lecture fees and by the returns from her magazine articles, and later her books. Her clothing budget was so minuscule on these lecture trips that friends in various cities, where she appeared before distinguished audiences, often made her wear one of their dresses for the evening and then gently insisted that she keep them. Self-pity was the last thing Margaret Sanger ever practiced, but she had to admit in a letter to Mrs. Rublee in December that it had been "a very hard year."

Juliet Rublee soon became one of the financial bulwarks of the *Review*. "How good you are!" Margaret Sanger wrote her on October 10 after receiving a generous check. But on December 31, 1917, she had to write: "The *Review* is out again. The January issue is very good, I think . . . but my deposit for this week was only fourteen dollars!!!" It was at this point that she finally faced the necessity of a permanent organization to finance the magazine, and the New York Woman's Publishing Corporation was organized. She decided to sell shares—"Say 1000 shares at ten dollars each," she wrote Mrs. Rublee, "which would place the *Review* on its feet and keep it going for two years and perhaps for three."

Through this incorporation, new associates—mainly women of money and position—were brought into the movement and became its permanent backbone. Among them were Frances Ackerman and Anne Kennedy. Mrs. Ackerman—though her family was steeped in the orthodoxy of church, Wall Street, and politics—had a warm and sensitive social conscience and served as the devoted treasurer of the movement for eleven years until her death. Mrs. Kennedy, cheerful and motherly, concentrated on circulation and fund raising, and later was to help organize many of the international birth control conferences.

Margaret Sanger was working at a pitch of nervous exaltation. Almost every day she was up at five and sat in bed, reading the hundreds of letters she had taken from the office the night before, making notes on each so that her secretary, Anna Lifschiz, could answer them during the day. Anna, a slight, dark-haired girl, had come to her directly from high school. One of a family of seven children, she insisted on working for a minute salary. Often she waited weeks for that—and even contributed stamps, string, and paste from her own pocket without complaint. Anna's mother used to make cakes and wine for Mrs. Sanger, and when Anna brought them, she always said, "My mother prays for your health, your happiness, and that you will keep well."

"I just kept going night and day," Margaret Sanger wrote later, "visualizing every act, every step, *believing, knowing* that I was working in accord with a universal law of evolution—a moral evolution, perhaps, but evolution just the same. This belief, faith—call it what you will—gave me a feeling of tremendous power. It seemed at times to open locked doors. It attracted the right people; it gave me the physical strength to dictate hundreds of letters through one, ill-paid secretary, to interview dozens of people each day, to write articles, to write and deliver lectures, debates;—in spite of a daily temperature, low but constant, and a decreasing bank account."

Her own personal problems were pushed into the background. She had taken the most inexpensive apartment possible—a forty-dollar-a-month studio in the old Chelsea area on Fourteenth Street between Eighth and Ninth avenues. The house might once have been called "Bohemian." But it had passed from that stage to outright decay. On one visit, Anna Lifschiz was startled to find a dead mouse on the stairs. Another visitor, Ulrick Thompson, described his first visit in a letter. "The stairs were dark and the treads nearly worn through; the walls were cracked and dingy. On the second floor back, I found the name, 'Mrs. Margaret Sanger.' I knocked and was bidden enter. The room was rather bare—an old carpet on the floor, old furniture, a very small fire on the grate, a table piled with books and papers."

Margaret Sanger dressed up the studio as much as possible—draped the windows in the rear with light yellow curtains so that when the sun touched them the room seemed to leap with flame. It was a useful illusion since the only heat came from the small grate. Not that it mattered terribly. She was almost never home except in the early morning and late evening. For her, the apartment came to symbolize the ultimate loneliness. She would return after a lecture trip and find the book lying open on the table, the glove on the floor—just as she had left them a few hours or a few days ago—all testament to the isolation of her personal life.

Since 1914, she had made her separation from Sanger irrevocable and never allowed anyone to ta':e his place. For a few years, it is true, she kept some personal life apart from the movement. On her 1916 trip, for instance, she met Herbert Simonds at a summer resort near Spokane, Washington. Simonds often took her dancing at the local casino. "She was a magnificent dancer," he recalled. "She was always teaching me new steps. Even in this, she wanted to be daringly original. 'Why dance like everyone else?' she would ask. 'Do something different.' "

In many minds, particularly among the bigots, birth control then was somehow linked with "Bohemianism," and even as late as 1924 the New York *Daily News* described her as "Mrs. Sanger, who for years was a member of the advanced school of Greenwich Village philosophers . . ." Her early assertions in the *Woman Rebel* that a woman must be "absolute mistress of her own body" with the "absolute right to dispose of herself, to withhold herself" left her open to this type of innuendo.

But after 1917, the men who surrounded Margaret were always part of the birth control movement—though many eventually threw themselves at her feet. "I want you to know that those two weeks in July [1918] in which we worked on the notes of the book [*Woman and the New Race*]," wrote Billy Williams, "were the happiest, the most inspiring I have ever known. . . . I have loved you beyond my power to understand it; it has gone to depths of my nature that I did not know to exist."

("He may have thought he loved *me*," Margaret Sanger explained twenty-five years later in a note about her admirers, "but I knew what it was he loved—not the physical me but that which emerged from the me and touched the same quality in him.")

Williams, who had resigned as managing editor of the Kansas City *Post* to plunge into the exuberant tide of New York radicalism, was ill that summer. Since Margaret Sanger was working in New

York, she invited him to stay with Stuart, Grant, and her father at the Cape Cod cottage to recuperate. Each night after the boys had gone to bed—"How I love you for the beautiful way you love those boys!"—he wrote with great intensity to his "brave, golden girl." "Never have you been more beautiful to me," one letter went, "than when I have succeeded in expressing to you something of what I feel and have seen, an indescribable, soft, glorious light in your beloved face." Again he wrote: "It's moonlight in Truro, love of my heart, moonlight and I have a close sense of you."

But through these years she insisted on her freedom. The movement came first; she made sure her admirers realized that. "I was hard on men," she wrote later. "I didn't have time to waste on people unless they would do something to help forward the movement. It sounds rough, but it had sense to it."

While she was in Europe in the summer of 1920 investigating a new contraceptive, Williams took dangerously ill. Hospitalized at St. Luke's, he had long periods of delirium. "Emerging today from three months' mental darkness," he wrote her on September 27, 1920. "First sure thought of our work together . . ."

Dr. Mary Halton, who was attending him, wired Margaret in London that Williams was dying. She immediately cabled the hospital: "Billy please make strenuous effort recover . . . Will nurse you back to health." The next day, October 17, however, he was dead, ironically enough two days before death also came in Russia to her friend John Reed.

2

Of all personal problems at this time, the children weighed most heavily on her mind. When she came home at night, it was their laughter she missed. Stuart and Grant were hours away, first at a small school in Ronkonkoma, Long Island, later at Peddie in New Jersey.

Keeping the children at country schools was a compromise she disliked. But the choice had been forced on her. Part of her own family life had to be sacrificed for the enormous demands of a movement that involved countless other mothers and children. The cynics who misunderstood birth control often claimed that Margaret Sanger harbored some deep psychological antagonism against having children. Of all personal attacks, this hurt her most. For the fundamental fact of birth control was that it gave women the freedom to bear only those children who would be completely wanted and loved. Leighton Rollins has called this "the central issue, the imperative need of endowing children with care and love before they enter the world."

What if she had kept the boys at home with her? She could only have seen them a few minutes before bedtime. It was better this way —to have them at country schools under expert teachers where she could visit them on week ends. Furthermore, they needed this stability and discipline. They had still not adapted themselves to the unique and unsettled role of a crusader's sons.

There was the time not long after Margaret Sanger's release from Queens County penitentiary when Grant came home with two slightly blackened eyes. His mother asked why he had been fighting, but he refused to tell. "I'd like to know," she insisted.

"Well, this boy said that my mother'd been in jail."

"What did you do?"

"I hit him and he hit me back. Then another fellow said, 'My mother says your mother went to jail too.' "

Grant had replied, "That wasn't my mother. That was another Margaret Sanger."

"How could you say that?" she asked. "You know that wasn't true."

"Mother," he replied profoundly, "you could never make those fellows understand."

Her separation from the boys often became so painful that on a few minutes' notice she would catch a train for New Jersey or Long Island. "After the first excitement of greeting passed," she wrote later, "they would scamper off to play, quite indifferent to the loving anxiety which brought so unexpectedly to school the busy, over-wrought mother."

These schools were a further drain on her meager finances. But William Sanger, as well as her sisters, Nan and Mary, contributed to the tuition, and Stuart was now old enough to earn part of his way at Peddie. His uncle, Bob Higgins, had been sent to Peddie before him by Nan and Mary, and had made the all-state football team. The Higgins' girls always saw to it that the younger brothers got more advantages in life than the family economic status warranted. Margaret inherited this tradition and enlarged it. Then and later, she always insisted on the best possible education for her sons.

For years, she clung to the dream of being able to spend the summers with them. As far back as 1912, the Sangers had vacationed at Provincetown. When the flood of New York artists and actors over-ran that village, a few of her old friends like John Reed moved to Truro. Seeking a sanctuary between constant foreign assignments for *Metropolitan Magazine,* Reed bought a small house overlooking the Pamet River, which wound silvery and snake-like toward the ocean. An old sea captain had built it, a snug, warm house whose timbers he had brought from the Carolinas and fastened together with wooden pegs. But when Reed was abruptly sent to Russia to cover the Revolution, he sold Margaret the house for a down payment of a thousand dollars—an unexpected windfall of hers from four Chicago lectures.

In the next few years, she was to snatch many week ends of glorious isolation there with the children—but never the whole weeks and months she had planned.

3

Strangely enough, although a score of birth control leagues had opened offices around the country, Margaret Sanger had never had an office of her own until 1917, when she took two small rooms at 104 Fifth Avenue with Dr. Frederick Blossom. On the door in black letters were the words "Birth Control." Inside was an efficient-look-ing collection of desks, steel files, and card indexes. Piled on tables and in corners were the thousands of letters from mothers that had deluged her for the last year.

"The little room is the joy of my life—women coming from all over," she wrote Juliet Rublee on December 4, 1917. "I'm feeling like a mother to the world these days. All kinds of questions and problems to be solved, and men and women seem to think by coming and looking at me—all will be right."

She transmitted to everyone around her some part of her inex-haustible energy. "It was like a religious crusade," Anna Lifschiz recalled. "The office was bedlam—volunteers rushing in and out, perfect strangers just dropping in and sitting in the waiting room, watching. Through it all she moved, serenely confident, giving us all some added strength that would make us work thirteen hours that day when we were sure we couldn't last ten."

Of all the new recruits that she brought into the movement that year, none had such a cyclonic impact as Kitty Marion. Kitty never revealed her real name. Born in Germany, she had run away from home as a girl, worked in the English music halls, and then, roused by Mrs. Pankhurst's fight for woman suffrage, had joined the movement and become one of its most fiery advocates. She was jailed seven times, endured four hunger strikes and 232 compulsory feedings. Even in jail, she fought—chewing holes in the mattress, setting fire to her cell, and once escaping from a nursing home to which the police had confined her. She was even alleged to have thrown a bag of flour at the Prime Minister. To this charge, she retorted, "It's a lie! I never threw anything as soft as flour in my life."

Kitty, who came to the United States at the start of the war when Mrs. Pankhurst feared her German birth might bring internment, supplied the birth control movement with a vigorous aggressiveness and a new technique—the sale of the *Review* on street corners. Day after day she stood at Times Square or at the corners opposite Grand Central Terminal and Macy's until her stoutish, towheaded figure and bright blue eyes became a familiar landmark.

To sell the *Review* (she often sold over a thousand copies a month), Kitty suffered every form of abuse. Irate old ladies would shake their umbrellas at her. Boys would pelt her with tomatoes. But above all, she was the principal target of the police. Almost every Irish cop, seeing the words "birth control," automatically hauled her off to the station house—although J. J. Goldstein continually demanded that the Police Commissioner instruct his force as to the limits of their authority. Once Charles Bamberger of the Society for the Prevention of Vice, who, masquerading as "Mr. Heller," had also trapped William Sanger, secured her arrest by pleading for information for his sick wife. She got thirty days in jail this time. But even then, a note from Agnes Smedley, arrested with her, tells how the indomitable Kitty "is turning the place (Tombs prison) into a birth control branch. And she has held a meeting!"

Dr. Blossom, who had actually arranged for the 104 Fifth Avenue office, brought the movement the advantage of its first professional organizer. Blossom, who had met Margaret Sanger in Cleveland during her 1916 tour, had been so impressed by the importance of birth control that he immediately offered to leave his work among Cleveland charities and give six months toward building the *Review* and the New York league. His attributes were many—not only a rich wife, which made him financially independent, but long experience in raising money from the wealthy and drawing a devoted circle of volunteer workers around him. His gay, laughing charm, enhanced by well-cut features, a strong chin, and slightly graying hair, fitted perfectly into his new role. He was, moreover, a tireless worker, rarely taking more than an apple for lunch and a sandwich for dinner and staying at the office until late evening.

Blossom worked out an efficient system for answering Mrs. Sanger's mail. Almost all inquiries, he found, fitted one of a dozen categories. He developed form letters for each category and trained his volunteers to analyze and answer each letter so quickly that in a few months the huge stacks began to dwindle. He took over all routine organization—the direction of mass rallies like those in Carnegie Hall, the advance preparation for introducing new birth control bills in Albany, and the leadership of the New York State Birth Control League, formed mainly among a Socialist membership which elected him president.

That Blossom had taken over this complex web of organizational detail delighted Margaret Sanger. She hated the petty wrangling of business meetings and committees. She had no hunger for titles. In fact, at this point, outside of being managing editor of the *Review,* she held no official office either in the state or national league.

The sudden and explosive breach between them in May 1917 was the product of Blossom's personal ambitions. Having become a Socialist only a few years before, he now saw through birth control, with its still predominantly Socialist or radical base, the opportunity for him to become a nationally important figure in radical circles.

Blossom's major error was that he badly misjudged Margaret Sanger's strength in thinking he could seize the leadership from her. He considered her purely an inspirational woman on horseback who had roused the country with her daring and often oversensationalized tactics. He failed to see that in touching the needs and hearts of mothers everywhere, she had actually become the protagonist of motherhood. Her leadership did not need the sanction of official title. It was an all-consuming flame—intangible as spirit yet based on the most fundamental scientific principles—that could no more be supplanted than Gandhi could have been supplanted as the spiritual symbol for millions of Indians.

Ironically enough, the immediate break came over a side issue, Mrs. Sanger's editorial opposing the country's entry into war which she had written for the June 1917 *Review.* Blossom, an ardent Francophile, considered her stand as wrong as if she had supported Germany. But she was neither pro-Allied nor pro-German. She was simply a devout pacifist for whom birth control and the population question so dominated her whole thinking that anything else, whether economics, politics, or Prussian militarism, became insignificant. She opposed the war as a pacifist, as a population expert who saw Germany's sudden increase from a 40 to 70 million population the sole reason for its drive for expansion, and most of all as a mother. Was not the very basis of birth control to free woman from those national laws which caused her slavery? A woman's instincts, she cried in her editorial, "are essentially creative, not destructive . . . [Women] must deny the right of the State or Kingdom hereafter to make her a victim of unwilling motherhood and the handmaiden of militarism."

Blossom brought the conflict into open warfare when Mrs. Sanger arrived at 104 Fifth Avenue one May morning to find that he had stripped the office of every piece of furniture, file, business record, and voucher. Nothing remained but the telephone sitting on a lonely packing box.

Mrs. Sanger and Anna Lifschiz immediately rushed over to Third Avenue to refurnish the office with a few dilapidated pieces of secondhand furniture. Then she brought charges against Blossom—her attorney, J. J. Goldstein, even seeking the intervention of the District Attorney. Blossom, in turn, appealed his case to a special investigating committee of the Socialist party. The charges and countercharges involved a complex, heated, and highly confused postscript to what might have been a valuable partnership. It was four years before the Socialists rendered a final report. Mrs. Sanger was upheld; Blossom severely condemned.

With the tumult of the Blossom affair, the seemingly endless struggle to keep the *Review* alive, to pay bills for the printer and the office, to maintain an expanding organization and answer often hundreds of letters a day with an ill-paid secretary and a few volunteers, it is little wonder that at a low point on December 4 Margaret Sanger could write Juliet Rublee: "Were it not for your friendly spirit, I am afraid I should have run away this week to some cave and spent the rest of my life in laughing at the world."

Then on January 8, 1918, came a momentous turning point. Goldstein had been fighting the Brownsville clinic conviction under Section 1142 and had lost the first round in the Appellate Division. Now in the Court of Appeals, the highest appeals court in the state, Judge Frederick E. Crane rendered the final decision. He sustained Mrs.

Sanger's conviction—but with an opinion so broad that it actually gave her many of the objectives for which she had been fighting.

What Judge Crane did was to affirm the constitutionality of Section 1142, which prohibited birth control information—yet at the same time, writing an interpretation that vastly enlarged the scope of Section 1145. This section said that physicians could give advice to prevent or cure disease. Always before this had been held to mean only syphilis and gonorrhea. But in Judge Crane's liberal interpretation, "disease" was now to include everything in the definition of Webster's International Dictionary—"an alteration in the state of the body, or of some of its organs, interrupting or disturbing the performance of the vital functions, and causing or threatening pain or sickness; illness; sickness; disorder."

Section 1145, according to Judge Crane, protected the physician who gave birth control advice to a married person for her health.

Margaret Sanger was jubilant. At last, the sword over every doctor's head—the fear of violating Section 1142 and the possibility of losing his license—had been legally removed. Even the druggist, acting on the doctor's order, was protected. She had steadfastly insisted that contraceptive information and techniques must be under medical supervision. The Crane decision confirmed the accuracy of her vision. The Brownsville clinic, opened as a test case to prepare the way for hundreds of later clinics, had brought a resounding legal victory.

CHAPTER 13

In 1915, just after the start of the war, Havelock Ellis had told Margaret Sanger about a new chemical contraceptive, a jelly made in Germany, which he considered a decisive advance over the antiquated methods described in *Family Limitation*. Ellis no longer knew the chemical's name or what firm manufactured it. All he could do was refer her to a few Berlin doctors who might send her in the right direction. It seemed like a ridiculous gamble—"my search for the Holy Grail," she jokingly called it. But she had pushed relentlessly toward her goal of setting the movement on a completely scientific basis, first in the sociological and economic scope of the *Review,* then with the Brownsville clinic and the Crane decision. Now if she was to seek the support of the medical profession, it was essential that birth control be correlated with the latest and most accurate technique—even if she had to search through the chaos of postwar Germany to find it.

Before she left for Europe, however, she made two shorter trips —the first to Coronado, California, to work on the book which would crystallize her whole philosophy of birth control. With the advance payment from the publisher, she rented an inexpensive cottage on the beach for three months, and taking Grant with her, settled down to finish *Woman and the New Race.*

Woman was an amazing book—breathless and soaring, exploding with all her unique and passionate intensity. It was the cry of a feminist. It was a fierce demand for woman's new role in the world— and in this respect, it was the rightful heir to Mary Wollstonecraft's *Vindication of the Rights of Woman* of a hundred and twenty-five years before.

But the book's strength and originality was that it went far beyond the previous feminist platform—political, economic, and social. For the first time, Margaret Sanger united the feminine rebellion with the biological revolution of Huxley and Darwin and crossed the scientific frontiers of H. G. Wells and the psychological frontiers of Freud and Ellis.

The most vital factor of a woman's existence, she said, was her power to reproduce the race. In psychosexual terms, this made "love . . . the greatest force of the universe." On the biological level, it gave women control of the race, its numbers, and quality.

Women, however, had never been mistresses of their own bodies until birth control freed them from "biological slavery." It put in each woman's hands the ultimate freedom—the right to decide when and how many children she would bring into the world.

This meant personal emancipation on the psychological level. For she believed strongly that "the need of women's lives is not repression, but the greatest possible expression and fulfillment of their desires upon the highest possible plane."

But birth control also gave women the scientific means to mold the race on a gigantic scale. She saw that if women used birth control, not just as individuals but working together for the total welfare of the state, they held a power far greater than that of kings or prime ministers. A penetrating vision! It would be almost a generation before governments like India faced the fact that their national survival depended on birth control!

The book is a testament to motherhood and "the feminine spirit." Again and again she demands a casting off of the old world, with its masculine prejudices and limitations. A woman's "mission is not to enhance the masculine spirit, but to express the feminine; hers is not to preserve a man-made world, but to create a human world by the infusion of the feminine element into all its activities." She envisioned not only a new and cleansing morality but a eugenic and scientific control of the race. "The race is but the amplification of its mother body . . ." The standards of reproduction must be changed; they must no longer be the demands of militarists for troops, of factory owners for an endless labor supply. The only standard must be beauty and love. "When motherhood becomes the fruit of a deep yearning, not the result of ignorance or accident, its children will become the foundation of a new race."

Sometimes brash and farfetched in its language, often overobsessed with the role of women, the book was still a major landmark in feminist literature. Although she finished the rough draft at

Coronado, working a furious pace, she rewrote much of it during the next twelve months. *Woman and the New Race,* published in 1920, became the bible of the movement, selling 250,000 copies in one year in the United States and many thousands more abroad.

2

Margaret Sanger's second trip was an invasion of that most conservative bulwark of the country—the South. In the first birth control meeting ever held below the Mason-Dixon Line, she addressed a mixed audience of more than eight hundred people on Sunday, November 2, 1919, in an Elizabeth City, North Carolina, theater. "It was a timid audience at first," reported the Elizabeth City *Independent,* "an audience that seemed to fear being shocked." Many of the local farmers had come from great distances. It had rained all day before the meeting. The atmosphere in the theater was taut.

"But Mrs. Sanger's charming personality put the audience at ease at once and she carried it with her for an hour and a half," continued the front-page story. "Mrs. Sanger is an unusual woman, a feminist who has endured years of misunderstanding without getting soured. Through all of her harsh experiences, she has emerged still fresh, sweet, modest and radiant with human kindness and genuine goodwill. Only such a personality could have discussed the delicate subject of birth control before a mixed audience in a small southern town."

At the conclusion of the lecture, so many women crowded around the platform, asking specific questions on contraception, that Mrs. Sanger asked the men to leave the theater and turned the end of the meeting into a discussion of techniques. "Mrs. Sanger told the women what they wanted to know," concluded the *Independent's* reporter, somewhat dazzled by the enthusiasm of the reception. "A more astounding, a more revolutionary thing probably never occurred in the staid, conservative old state of North Carolina." What the reporter did not know was that the trip was soon to open up the whole South to the birth control movement.

3

Sailing for England in the spring, Margaret Sanger crossed the Channel to Holland by boat and then took the train to Germany. Berlin in 1920 was a dead, broken city. The streets were silent. There was almost no traffic. Pedestrians moved stolidly; they seemed

to have forgotten how to smile. Instead of displaying food or clothing, the shop windows were decorated with streamers of colored
paper. Money meant nothing; food everything. Fresh vegetables
were so scarce that when old peasant women came in from the
country with bags of potatoes on their backs they were sold out
fifteen minutes after reaching the market place. For months, many
people had nothing but turnips—turnip soup, turnips raw, turnips
mashed, turnip salad, even turnip coffee. "Ordinarily I could go
without eating if I had plenty of water," Mrs. Sanger recalled
later, "but in Berlin I found myself haunting grocery stores like a
hungry animal . . ."

The condition of the women horrified her. The best food was
given to the men, the wage earners. "Women . . . had to go without or subsist on what they could scrape together," she noted.
"They nursed their babies beyond two years to supply milk . . . I
heard countless stories from mothers who had been tortured by
watching their children slowly starve to death—pinched faces growing paler, eyes more listless, heads drooping lower day by day until
finally they did not even ask for food. You saw a tiny thing playing
on the street suddenly run to a tree or fence and lean against it
while he coughed and had a hemorrhage."

German statistics showed that during four years of the war over
51 per cent of the women had remained barren. Was this the result
of malnutrition?

This question Margaret Sanger put eagerly to the gynecologists
and pediatricians to whom she had letters of introduction. She
sounded out their opinions, then carefully steered the conversation
toward birth control. At this point, the doctor would usually rise
brusquely from his chair, demanding, "Why should a nurse take an
interest in such things?" She tried to explain how she had led the
birth control movement in her country. "Nein, nein," he would shout.
"Not in Germany. In Germany it is abortions, not birth control. With
abortions, it is all in our hands. The women must come to us. Never
will Germany give control of its population to women! Never will we
let women control the race!"

Here in this nation where woman's role had always been subservient to man's, Margaret Sanger saw the ultimate battleground of
woman's struggle for freedom. The doctor's words were so ironically
perfect—"in our hands!" Here was the essence of everything she
fought—the gross conception that a woman was nothing more than

breeding stock for the authoritarian male who sat in judgment over the race, nothing more than an instrument for the use of militarists and the state.

She would leave the office shaking with anger. But she went on to the next appointment, always hoping that she would find some small clue. One gynecologist sharply demanded where she had come from.

"New York," she told him.

"Are you sure you are not from France or Belgium?"

"Certainly not."

"Nobody who has the welfare of Germany at heart could favor contraception over abortions," he roared. "Only enemies of Germany could come here to give such information to our women."

At the office of Dr. Magnus Hirschfeld, renowned director of the Institute for the Study of Sex Knowledge, she found her first clue. Dr. Hirschfeld thought he knew the name of a Dresden firm which might be manufacturing the chemical. She took the train to Dresden, but at the factory they only shook their heads. No, it must be that firm in Munich. Another dead end—except in Munich they were sure that the formula was being manufactured by two chemists, a father and son, at Friedrichshafen on Lake Constance.

She went to Friedrichshafen. A small, poorly dressed man—his coat patched, his hair at least ten days overgrown—met her at the station. In his hand, he held a bunch of wild flowers wrapped in newspaper, his quaint welcome to his city.

She could not ask her questions fast enough. Was he making the chemical jelly? Yes, he and his father and brothers had a small factory with a half dozen employees. Could she go to the factory? No, no, they should talk. They should sit and have a coffee first.

He kept her talking for two hours while she fretted impatiently. "Now we will see the factory," she said. Not yet, not yet. He was afraid she would steal the formula, she finally realized. The family allowed no visitors near the factory. But he had a sister living in New York who was now in business as the firm's agent, and Mrs. Sanger could buy the jelly from her. They discussed amount and price, and she signed an agreement.

She refused to leave Friedrichshafen, however, until she had secured enough samples so that the formula could be tested in New York. It was not, she eventually found, the magic solution to the problem of an efficient chemical contraceptive. It turned out to be expensive and difficult to import into the United States. But it was the first important step toward her goal. The formula, later analyzed and improved by American chemists, became the basis of many new chemicals eventually used in clinics throughout the United States.

Even this climax to her search could not dispel the mood of depression that had settled over her with each day in Germany. This degradation of the feminine spirit—women in the fields, reduced to the state of animals, pulling plows in place of draft horses; the sickly children—"God, what pinched, empty little faces!" she wrote—all combined to reduce her to a state of actual physical illness.

Here was the old pattern again—the beauty and dignity of life stamped out by the remorseless havoc of war and new attempts to build up the birth rate of Germany. Population and war! The combination was inescapable. Every fiber of her being cried out against this senseless repetition of the cycle that had just carried Germany to one disaster.

Back in England, she stayed in her hotel room. Her hacking cough left her exhausted. She struggled to emerge from her depression by catering to the simplest of feminine needs—color. She went to a draper's, bought yards of colored materials, bright yellows, oranges, and reds, and sat all day fashioning new dresses. Ellis, who had rushed to welcome her after five years of separation, wanted her to leave immediately for a vacation in Ireland. But she put him off. As soon as she had the strength to spend a few hours away from her hotel, she shook off the last haunting memories of Germany by the one method that always lifted her to new heights—action!

Dr. Alice Vickery arranged for her to give a series of thirty lectures to the wives of workers who belonged to the Women's Cooperative Guild. Each day she went to a different district of London. At the dockyards area of Rotherhithe, one of London's worst slums, she and Dr. Anne Martin held a demonstration of contraceptive techniques, probably the first informal clinic of this kind in England. "A good lecture yesterday afternoon to working women," she wrote Juliet Rublee on May 29. "Another June 2, 3, 5, 9, 25, 28th and every day to July 15th."

Then she was making contact with a number of important English men and women who were now supporting birth control. She had met Clinton Chance, a wealthy manufacturer. Always uppermost in her mind was the dream of a new birth control clinic, this time to be sponsored by the medical profession. She had discussed the idea with him, and he and Mrs. Chance had invited her to their home for the week end. "He is to retire and devote all his wealth and time on birth control," she wrote Mrs. Rublee on July 7. "It is the only cause he believes in doing anything for . . . If Mr. Chance will support the clinic for a year, so I can feel it worthwhile, I will engage a nurse and a clinical worker, get rooms and supplies. . . ."

The English attitude on birth control had improved remarkably since the war. Marie Stopes' book, *Married Love*, for which Mrs. Sanger had found an American publisher, had run up huge sales in England and made a deep impact on the educated classes. Among birth control's staunchest supporters were two leading physicians and two churchmen—Sir James Barr, ex-president of the British Medical Association, Dr. C. Killick Millard, Health Officer of Leicester, the Bishop of Birmingham and Dean Inge of St. Paul's. The majority of medical men and Anglican clergymen still opposed it. But Harold Cox, former M.P. and now editor of the *Edinburgh Review*, rebuked them sharply in a speech by pointing out that the birth rate among these two groups was just about the lowest in the country.

Already planning an international conference in New York, Mrs. Sanger saw the importance of recruiting international names. She made her way effortlessly into the best London drawing rooms. "I had a most enchanting time with Lord Greenborough yesterday," she wrote Mrs. Rublee on May 29. "I felt like Grant when I took him over the U.S.A. border into Mexico. He looked up at the sky and all around, and then said: 'Is it really Mexico, mother? Why, the sky is just the same.' The simplicity and ease of Lord Greenborough was a treat."

She met Harold Cox, Dean Inge, the "gloomy dean" who had become one of birth control's most vociferous supporters, and J. O. P. Bland, Britain's foremost writer on the Far East. The driving force of her convictions made such an impression on Bland that he wrote her: "You have stirred up a wind in the valley of dry bones, and we need more of it and of you."

Guy Aldred, whom she met during her 1914 exile, arranged a speaking tour of Scotland. It was July when she left for the North and plunged eagerly into the lush countryside of the Scottish summer—"bluebells so thick in spots that the ground was azure, long twilights when the lavender heather faded the hills into purple," she described it.

But all this beauty was quickly shattered by the misery of the working-class mothers at her meetings. "Meetings here overcrowded," she wrote Mrs. Rublee on July 7. "Oh, Juliet, *never* was there such a cause. Poor, pale-faced, wretched wives. Men beat them. They cringe before their blows, but pick up the baby, dirty and unkempt, and return to serve him."

Always it was such degradation of the feminine spirit that touched the deepest springs of her feelings and drove her forward with a new and even more frantic urgency. Speak, speak, write, teach! At such moments, she felt she had to convert the whole countryside to birth control overnight, before these mothers collapsed from the weight of their own misery.

On July 4, she addressed a mass meeting of shipyard workers on Glasgow Green. It was an impressive turnout—nearly two thousand workers standing in the bright sun to hear a problem discussed that would have brought only laughter and scorn a few years back. "What a sight it was!" she exulted later. "Nearly two thousand men in caps, baggy trousers and working togs, standing close together, eager to catch every word. What silence, what interest, what an intelligent attitude, demonstrated as by no other group equally large anywhere!" The men seemed hypnotized by the earnestness of that cool silvery voice on the sticky afternoon air. "She grips ye," one worker told Aldred later.

That evening she spoke at a Socialist meeting. The hall was jammed, and even the women, who rarely attended, joined actively in the discussion. One old-time Socialist said he had been attending these Sunday-night meetings for years but had never before been able to get his wife to come. "The women have practically crowded the men out of the hall," he announced.

She spoke at a small, ragged town near Dunfermline, where Andrew Carnegie had been born. Arriving at the railroad station in a driving rain, she had neither raincoat nor umbrella, and the station did not boast a single taxi. She trudged through the storm and was soaking wet when she reached the cottage of her hostess. A hurry call was immediately sent to all neighbors for an extra skirt and pair of shoes—but in that town of five thousand people no one had an extra skirt and only a determined search turned up a pair of Sunday shoes.

With no inn for miles around, Margaret Sanger slept that night after her speech in the one bed in her hostess's cottage. But she knew that the village had given her its best, for only a few months before Sylvia Pankhurst, the suffrage leader, had stayed there.

"Oh, I am busy and tired," she wrote home. "Things are hard here—
terribly hard. Try to move that mountain before you with a shovel,
and you have an idea what it is here—but it is moving."

4

She returned to London. Ellis kept writing her, "The summer is
all slipping away and there has scarcely been a chance to carry out
any cherished plans for us." She was suddenly surrounded with admirers, H. G. Wells, Hugh De Selincourt, Harold Child, E. S. P.
Haynes, a lawyer and friend of Wells—all eager to weave bright
dreams around her. Why shouldn't she take them? She had shunned
entanglements for years and never divorced Sanger—maintaining
the formality of marriage as a protection. But before leaving for
England she had at last instituted divorce proceedings and the final
decree was due in October.

With Ellis, she spent a week in Ireland, wandering from town to
town by train, tram, car, and even jaunting car, sitting back to back
with him as they bounced from Glengariff to Killarney. They
climbed over the countryside, explored the towns where Margaret
believed her mother's family, the Purcells and Fitzgeralds, had
lived, and talked for long hours over coffee cups and on midnight
walks. ". . . I shall never, never forget our peaceful and calm Sunday on the terrace at Killarney," he wrote her later. And again: "I
have so many varied and vivid pictures of you, trim and quick, which
often come before me and are always sweet and consoling to see."

Ellis introduced her to his circle of friends at Wantley, Sussex, and
this house became the center of her new world. It was built of
stone, at least four hundred years old, the living room roofed by oak
beams, a large inglenook fireplace dominating the stone-flagged
dining room. A wonderful harmony united house and gardens. Apple
trees, laden with blossoms, flanked one side so close you could touch
the boughs from the windows. Wisteria covered the south and west
gables; delphiniums stretched beyond the dining-room window; and
a lilac walk of dazzling color led toward the main gardens.

Appropriately enough, the house had belonged to Shelley's father.
The spirit of the poet filled the house and shaped the lives of its inhabitants. Its owner, Hugh De Selincourt, a poet and novelist of intense good humor, was an expert on Shelley and Blake; his wife,
Janet, was a musician, with dark braids always bound tight around
her head, the perfume of exotic flowers in her hair. Harold Child,

the dark-haired, classic-faced, second editorial writer of the London *Times* lived there also, and shared in the responsibilities of the house and its expenses. Ellis came whenever they could snatch him away from Brixton, and so did Madame Françoise Cyon, his close friend; but there was no line between inhabitant and visitor. It was a community to which everyone contributed the special elements of beauty on which it existed.

Like Shelley, the Wantley "circle" strove to bring the poetry of dreams into daily life, to lay bare, as Trelawney had said of the poet, "those mysterious feelings and impulses . . . in a form so purified of earthly matter that the most sensitive reader is never shocked."[1]

Life at Wantley was a magnificently plotted game that filled each day with music and reading aloud from their favorite books and midnight walks on the moors. At night, they would sit around the fire, the conversation flowing among them, Janet usually sewing on fine needlepoint. Then someone would call for music, and Janet, a skilled pianist, and her daughter Bridget, with violin or cello, would fill the house with Beethoven and Brahms. Often they would simply sit under the stars, like Shelley before them, "watching the changing and eternal heavens—their gathering thunderstorms, their delicate gossamer clouds and white woolpacks, their sheet-lightning and their nightpiece of moon and stars."[2]

Like the Shelley-Byron circle in Italy a hundred years before, with its complex interweaving of Shelley and Claire Claremont, Byron and Claire, and Mary Shelley and Jefferson Hogg, the Wantley household too had its tangled web. For it was built on love, and love was its main preoccupation. It was something to be shared and enjoyed and became as much a part of their lives as the wild perfume of the garden and the clean air of the moors.

"Wantley," Margaret Sanger recalled many years later, "was not dedicated to love in the sense of sex. It fused friendship and love as a spiritual unit, outlasting sex love. This was its special significance."

Jealousy had no part in it. Janet's beauty touched everything and everyone. Harold Child particularly, then a neighboring doctor, came under its spell. Yet both Child and De Selincourt always helped her pick the bouquet which she delivered daily to this

[1] Edward J. Trelawney, *Last Days of Byron and Shelley* (New York: Philosophical Library, 1952), p. 53.
[2] Edmund Blunden, *Shelley* (Toronto: Collins, 1946), p. 210.

doctor. It was of the very essence of Wantley that love should not
be confined, that it should grow and give strength as it spread, that
its very presence in the household was like a benediction for all
inhabitants. It was only natural that De Selincourt's unbounded
admiration for Ellis should forge a special link between him and
Françoise Cyon, who was living with Ellis. And once Margaret
Sanger came to Wantley, they were all at her feet. She was to bring
the house that special quality of radiant and heroic love that would
become a part of it with the years.

For them, she was the ideal made real, the woman rebel, the
fighter who had challenged the world and yet could express the
poetry of dreams in their moments together. It is no wonder that
she seemed to them the finest expression of Shelley's vision—Shelley, who had started as a crusader, tossing his political leaflets
to the crowd from his balcony, but eventually forced by an antago-
nistic world to confine the poetry of living to the written word.

She had not only fought in the courts and on street corners to
make love the greatest force in the world, she had lived her ideal.
For them, she was love incarnate, "sweetening the air you breathed
in her presence," De Selincourt wrote.

Their letters to her exude the wonder and excitement with which
she touched the Wantley circle. "The whole place breathes your
sweetness," De Selincourt wrote her after her first visit. ". . . Every
nerve of me continues in tumult . . . Ah! the glory of you."

Again he writes: "My whole life has widened out under your
touch . . . I'm like a drunken man—all of a rapture . . . I was aching and beaten and sore. You've given it all back to me in renewed
power and loveliness."

Harold Child described her adoringly in a later letter.

. . . You have the eyes and brow of a saint—your eyes very far
apart and so quietly, unaggressively, immorally brave and candid
and simple with the simplicity of a spirit. And the nose so exquisitely
sensitive—not broad nor yet too fine for emotion . . . and then the
mouth and chin, all compassion and sweetness and yet all resolution
and strength.
. . . A saint's face, a lover's face, a child's face . . .

Margaret Sanger came to Wantley, first for a week end, then for
a week at a time, and in future years, she would return there inevi-
tably, as if all her instincts drew her to this house. Juliet Rublee,

her closest confidante, wrote her at the end of that summer, questioning her attachments and the possibility of marriage. But even Juliet did not understand. It was no more possible than if you could marry the moon—but you could be in love with the moonlight. To those who did not know Wantley, it seemed effervescent and unreal, the quality of this thing. But to Margaret it was the truest reality. Ever since 1917, she had eliminated almost all personal life in America. The bigots would always misinterpret her actions, would call her "Bohemian." Only here in England, now and for much of the rest of her life, she could combine that essential duality of her nature —the woman rebel and the woman in love. She could be the incarnation of that soaring and triumphant woman, that feminine Ariel of Shelley's dreams. She could live as though "to live and love were one."

5

From this house of saints and lovers, Margaret Sanger plunged into the witty, sarcastic, flirtatious, and intensely pragmatic world of H. G. Wells. In July, she spent a week end with Wells and his wife, Catherine, whom everyone knew as Jane, at their estate, Easton Glebe, in Essex. From the glory of his stately red brick Tudor house, with its great lawns and tall, blue cedars, Wells, the novelist whose books had sold millions of copies in almost every country, Wells, the apostle of the new science, Wells, the messiah of rationalism and giant killer of all humanity's ignorances and frailties, spread out his arms to the intellectuals of the realm. Into his home on any normal week end came Arnold Bennett and Bernard Shaw, philosophers like Bertrand Russell, lawyers and economists, professors and preachers—all swept into the enormous week-end ritual, over which the huffing, grunting, and often riotous figure of Wells with his high squeaking voice presided like a joyous schoolboy.

Everything moved at an enormous pace here. Not just the conversation, which was always fast and bright, but the never ending round of games. They played tennis on the lawn. They took long walks in the woods, Wells always striding at the head of the column. After a huge luncheon, there would be cards, music on the phonograph, a sumptuous tea to which the two Wells boys, Frank and "Gyp," then at Cambridge, would attend with a dozen or more of their classmates. Then there was charades, always charades. Jane Wells kept the drawers and closets of the attic stocked with strange

costumes and eccentric props for the guests to explore at the height
of the evening's frenzy and then reappear a few minutes later,
clothed in the wildest fancies of their imaginations.

Wells himself, his rotund body squeezed tight in the tiny car
he called his "Pumpkin," called for Margaret Sanger at Dunmow
station. "He's very fascinating to women . . ." she described him in
a letter home. This was something of an understatement since Wells'
reputation had become public property from the time he had left his
first wife over twenty-five years back and openly flaunted Victorian
morals by going off to live with Jane, whom he later married. Even
the three spinster sisters, in whose London household Mrs. Sanger
was staying, were well aware of these exploits. On her return Mon-
day night, she recorded in her *Autobiography* ". . . in came the
three ladies, hair in braids . . . They had stayed wide-awake to
hear all about my weekend. I told them as much as I could remember . . . When I had finished, the eldest leaned forward and hesi-
tatingly, but loudly whispered, 'Did he try to kiss you?'

" 'What? Who?' I asked.

"She looked a little abashed at this, and another voice explained
apologetically, 'Sister means that Wells has a magnetic influence
over women!' "

Although Wells and Jane had long ago faced the fact that they
were "as unlike as torrent and brook" and that "it was not only sexu-
ally that Catherine could not satisfy Wells" but that "intellectually
his enormous reach and grasp simply, on occasion, bewildered her,"[3]
they had made the compromise and lived together in splendid harmony. "Our alliance was indissoluble," Wells stated in his autobiography. "We had inter-grown and become parts of each other." If
not lover now, Jane was everything else to him—practical housewife,
hostess supreme, business manager of all his financial and publishing affairs, and stout bulwark between him and the outside world.
"The sun would set if anything ever happened to Jane," Wells admitted to Margaret that week end.

Always searching, as if this dream had been denied him in youth,
for those "unimaginable goddesses" now come "to earth in all their
loveliness,"[4] Wells was fascinated by Margaret. Like her, he had
come up from the poor in a state of flaming rebellion. In his books,
he had preached the new rationalism. He had thundered to man-

[3]Vincent Brome, *H. G. Wells* (Toronto: Longmans, 1951), p. 75.
[4]*Ibid.*, pp.123–24.

kind to throw off the shackles of the past and grind prejudice, ignorance, and superstition underfoot. Science was his religion, the new religion which would not only control externals like hunger, but the very social relations between the sexes. In his *Modern Utopia* in 1905, he had cast his thunderbolts at the rigid social code of the Victorian era and demanded that men and women be liberated from medieval enslavement.

But Wells had only preached. Margaret Sanger had shaken the walls of ignorance to their foundations. Wells was fascinated by audacity, and most of all, by women of action. For him, Margaret was the symbol of all that was heroic in the opposite sex.

After the week end, she returned to London and Wells tried hard to see her. The address she had given him, that of the American Express office, blocked him momentarily. In a note to her on black-bordered writing paper of The Reform Club, he complained testily: "This paper is in mourning because I suddenly wanted to ring you up for lunch and couldn't. Six Haymarket isn't an address; it's a letter-drop."

He came to New York the following year, and trying to arrange a meeting with her at the home of a mutual friend (Thomas Lamont), he was again insistent on better treatment. ". . . I'll go there gladly if it really means a sure, sweet access to you," he wrote on December 7, 1921. "But not if it means just tantalizing glimpses."

"I'd like to be somewhere convenient to you . . ." he wrote her again from Washington. "Have you any ideas?" I'm very much at your disposal." Then he asked with finality: "Can't I carry you off somewhere for a day or so?"

Neither Wells—nor anyone else for the time being—was to carry her off though these moments at Wantley and Easton Glebe represented, and would always represent, the major threads of her life. De Selincourt was her link to the Romantic rebellion—the tradition of Shelley and Madame de Staël that love was a divine instinct, the art of loving a positive good.

Through Ellis and Wells, she united the Romanticists with the new psychology and science. Ellis had cleansed love of the dark ignorance of the past. She lived his teaching and raised it to a new and therapeutic wholesomeness. Like Wells, the herald of the scientific revolution, she united the basic instincts of nature with the goal of a planned and eugenic society which would carry men and women to new perfectibility.

All these men would remain an integral part of her life. Yet the paradox was that none of them—De Selincourt, Wells, or Ellis—could hold her. The man she would eventually marry—and that time was closer than she possibly realized—would be as different and remote from Wantley and Easton Glebe as if he had come from another world.

CHAPTER 14

From what she had seen of the misery of postwar Germany, Margaret Sanger issued a blunt warning to the women honoring her return to New York with a dinner at the Commodore Hotel on December 8, 1920. "Birth control," she said, "must save the world from another and more devastating holocaust. . . ."

Would anyone in the United States in these fat, indolent years of prosperity be concerned about Germany's expanding population? Population growth and its relation to war was not taken seriously even in the universities. Only a few professors like E. M. East, Henry Pratt Fairchild, and Warren Thompson conceived and taught it as a science.

A few weeks later, she issued a second warning. In the Far East, Japan's teeming millions, crowded into a handful of islands, she predicted, would one day explode beyond their borders unless birth control was adopted immediately. This time at least the Japanese Government heeded her words. Mrs. Sanger, it suggested, should keep her opinions to herself. Japan wanted nothing of birth control.

At a time when everyone was shouting for the good old days and business as usual, few people made a stand on any issue—and certainly not birth control. Despite Judge Crane's decision, few doctors had committed themselves on contraception. Margaret Sanger realized she would have to force them out of their frightened neutrality. She asked Dr. Mary Halton, always an indomitable supporter, to test the courage of Manhattan's hospitals.

With two women patients, one afflicted with tuberculosis, the other a kidney disease so serious that pregnancy to either would be fatal, Dr. Halton visited all twenty-nine Manhattan hospitals. Would the superintendent or responsible official allow contraceptive advice to save these women's lives? Without exception, all twenty-nine refused.

Margaret Sanger was also using subtler methods to enlist the support of prominent doctors. At least once a week Juliet Rublee would invite a number of obstetricians and pediatricians to her lavish dinners. Determinedly she steered the conversation toward birth control, and before the evening was half over her guests were in the midst of furious debate. At this point, she would telephone Margaret. Wearing a simple black dress (the more radical your ideas, the more conservatively you must dress, Bessie Drysdale had told her), Mrs. Sanger would arrive in the doorway of the living room with Juliet's arm around her. "Now here is the woman who can answer all our questions!" Mrs. Rublee would say.

It was a dramatic entrance that led easily into a short talk on birth control and often won new converts.

In England, the medical profession was far more courageous in its support. Lord Dawson of Penn, court physician to King Edward VII and now to George V, astounded the Lambeth Congress of the Anglican Church by coming out for birth control. "Imagine a young married couple in love with each other," he stated, "being expected to occupy the same room and to abstain for two years. The thing is preposterous . . . Romance and deliberate self-restraint do not, to my mind, rhyme very well."

When newspapers headlined the speech, KING'S PHYSICIAN ASKS CHURCH TO SANCTION BIRTH CONTROL, with the inference that His Majesty was endorsing it, stolid Britishers gaped.

England now also had two birth control clinics—one run by Marie Stopes where instruction was given by a midwife, the other, known as the Walworth Center, directed by Dr. Norman Haire, an Australian gynecologist and a lay group under the sponsorship of Harold Cox, Bessie Drysdale, and the Neo-Malthusians.

Recognizing the necessity of rallying scientific support for birth control from every possible quarter, Margaret Sanger now drew up a detailed questionnaire and sent it to colleges and universities throughout the country. Here was an untouched reservoir of aid! Not just old friends like Professors Ross of Wisconsin and Carver and East of Harvard stood behind her, but a group of new cohorts like Raymond Pearl of Johns Hopkins, Dr. C. C. Little of the Carnegie Institute, and Professor W. F. Wilcox of Cornell.

Her associates had been working hard to win over the women's groups, and on October 15, 1920, came the first impressive victory. Despite the bitter opposition of a Catholic minority, the New York State Federation of Women's Clubs at its annual convention overwhelmingly passed a resolution in favor of birth control.

In the courts, another victory! Fania Mindell's conviction for passing out the book *What Every Girl Should Know* at the Brownsville clinic was reversed by the New York Court of Appeals. The movement was now guaranteed more freedom in its distribution of books and pamphlets. The New York police would have to restrain their free-and-easy arrests of street-corner workers like Kitty Marion.

Margaret Sanger now concentrated on the most frustrating of all objectives—birth control legislation. All through the winter months of 1921, she labored in Albany. First a new and liberalized law had to be drawn. Then she tramped from office to office, interviewing assemblymen and state senators, pleading for their support. She gave speeches, attended women's groups, and held press interviews to make the public understand the purpose of new legislation. The amount of hostility in Albany was so pronounced that it often took her weeks to gain an interview. One Brooklyn assemblyman who first promised to introduce the new bill later wrote: "I am told it would do me an injury I could not overcome for some time." Another refused on the grounds that his support would rouse too much "levity from his associates." She finally found a courageous sponsor, Assemblyman Samuel Rosenman, later a prominent judge and adviser to President Franklin D. Roosevelt, but the bill was defeated.

When one of her younger associates lamented that months of furious energy had been wasted, she reprimanded her gently, "Thousands of mothers who never understood birth control before hear these debates. Every additional mother is a victory."

In Connecticut, where Margaret Sanger now carried the legislative fight, she had two of the movement's staunchest supporters by her side—Mrs. George H. Day, Sr., a grandmother who never missed a birth control board meeting in New York, and Mrs. Thomas Hepburn. Connecticut's law was the most medieval in the country. It was the only state where even "to use a contraceptive" was a criminal act—as if the legislators could station a policeman in every bedroom. The bill went down to defeat, but only after Margaret Sanger had stood up against the Church's representatives in a debate that made headlines throughout the state.

That winter one long-range objective dominated every spare min-

ute of her time—a conference in the fall—the first National Birth
Control Conference ever held in America. To it she would invite
birth control advocates not only from this country but Europe and
Asia. Most important of all, the conference would include a series
of medical demonstrations which would break down the wall of
ignorance surrounding contraceptive techniques and teach hundreds
of doctors the most advanced methods of birth control.

But the strain of this project on top of her exhaustive legislative
campaign, her speaking tours, and the responsibility of editing the
Review and running the office took its toll by spring. Dr. Halton
warned her that a complete rest was essential. The pain of her
tubercular glands had become unbearable, and when Jane Wells
kept writing from London that a doctor she knew had performed
similar operations successfully, Margaret at last agreed to try
surgery.

All her English friends, but particularly Hugh De Selincourt,
demanded that she take a European vacation. ". . . You are more
important than ANY movement," De Selincourt wrote her. "I shall
go on dinning this obvious fact into your lovely ear, and one day
you will believe me if you see yourself clearly enough in the lovely
mirror of your epoch-making work."

. But Margaret Sanger had an even more important reason than
health for making the trip. For the climax of the birth control conference she had planned a mass public meeting, and she needed
speakers whose names would command international respect. Havelock Ellis, H. G. Wells, Harold Cox, or Dean Inge would insure
the success of the conference. But to convince any one of them,
she knew, would take persuasion on the spot. Leaving the highly
efficient Anne Kennedy in charge of arranging the details of the
conference, she booked passage on the *Aquitania* and sailed early
in May.

Harassed as always by a shortage of money, she traveled second
class. "I am borrowed to the hilt," she wrote Juliet Rublee from
shipboard on May 17, "but what difference does it make! I feel
like an object of charity anyway, but my book (a new one she was
working on) will be out in September, and I get an advance on
that."

Mrs. Rublee as always was overgenerous in her support, and later
wrote that she would pay the rent at 104 Fifth Avenue while Mrs.
Sanger was away. But she answered: "Please *don't* send that thirty

dollars for the room. I left my royalty money (from *Woman and the New Race*) to be drawn upon. . . . You have been so dear and generous—heavens, it makes me gulp down tears when I think of it."

She discovered as soon as she boarded ship that instead of the two-passenger cabin she had booked, a strike on other lines had swamped the Cunard Company and she had been moved into an inner cabin with three children and a mother. Her Irish mettle was roused. "I absolutely refused to accept anything but what I had booked for," she wrote home. "The Purser said there was nothing else on board for me. So I decided to sit up and out on deck *all the way across!* I refused with such consistency and politeness that the poor gentleman was disturbed. Finally when he saw that I meant it, he got me room with a woman who had paid for a single cabin."

Even then she had little rest. As soon as they heard of her presence, dozens of passengers came to knock on her door.

By the time she reached London, she was close to exhaustion, and hid herself away in a small hotel. "I've been here a week," she wrote Mrs. Rublee, "and have kept in bed all the time . . . I shall not speak or visit or work or read or write or do anything but devote my time to getting rid of this neck trouble . . . I have seen no one!!! Havelock is ill and away. I'm not strong enough spiritually to meet Hugh yet. He's so vigorous and healthy and pours out upon you such enthusiasm . . . It's too queer for words to be here alone and so lonely I could die. But I'm going to stick it out a little longer."

By the middle of June, however, she had regained enough strength to go to a housewarming at Dr. Drysdale's and spend three quiet days with Ellis at Canterbury.

Margaret Sanger's letters to Juliet Rublee now mention for the first time the name of J. Noah H. Slee. "I had a very nice letter from Mr. S., who is at the Hague," she wrote on June 23. ". . . He asks if I am to be in Paris, and if not he will fly over to London to spend the day. That is the fashion now, to fly over and back in a day."

Mr. Slee was president of the Three-in-One Oil Company, a prosperous businessman, a tall, ruddy-faced, country squire, a pillar of the Episcopal Church and Union League Club in New York. Taken to one of Mrs. Sanger's meetings the previous winter, he had been immediately stricken by two conflicting feelings—his wariness of birth control and his admiration for Margaret. The latter gradually predominated, however, for he began to attend her meetings regularly and then send large bouquets of roses to her office. At this point, Juliet Rublee was obviously impressed by the ardor of his attentions, for Margaret wrote her in the same letter: ". . . Don't worry your blessed, dear head a minute about me and Mr. S., darling girl. . . . I am *not* inclined to marriage. Freedom is too lovely, and I mean to enjoy it for a time."

That Margaret Sanger was constantly pursued in London by a devoted band of admirers is confirmed by a note to her from Ellis. "Nowadays you are such a famous and popular person that scarcely a moment can be permitted to the 'wisest living English.' De Selincourt is most disconsolate, not even having been able to kiss her darling feet for an hour or two (greedy man) because the nurse kept popping in. Heaven knows how many more bleeding hearts are lying in the track of your chariot wheels."

But she had neither the strength nor the time now for those flights into the golden world of the Wantley circle or Easton Glebe. She had seen Wells briefly. He had been forced to turn down her invitation to the conference, but agreed to write the introduction to her new book, *The Pivot of Civilization*. Dean Inge, too, turned down the invitation. And such was Ellis's overpowering shyness that no one, not even Margaret, could persuade him even to attend the conference.

Juliet Rublee now expressed concern over the lack of a prominent speaker, and Margaret replied, "Darling, don't worry over the conference, please, and do not put so much *faith* in personalities. Let us put it into the Spirit of Universal Progress. Let *it* guide and direct and choose our speakers for us. I am going to be guided in the future by this as I was in the early days—making principle work out our problem for us. I always get a truer vision of things when I get away alone. Then strength and decision comes back strong."

A week later Harold Cox, who had been a confidant of King Edward VII, a member of Parliament, and was considered one of England's finest orators, agreed to speak at the conference.

In July, Margaret Sanger went to Switzerland, staying at a small hotel at Zermatt, seven thousand feet up, where she could look directly from her window at the soaring peak of the Matterhorn and hear the soothing roar of mountain streams just outside her room. "I am resting, dear," she wrote Juliet Rublee. "Open air since July 1st, night and day . . . Pain all gone from neck, tissues softened, and really I feel like my old self before you knew me. You blessed woman. Why *will* you worry, Juliet? I will never die doing the work I love." In the same letter, Margaret told her that she was dictating to a secretary a few hours a day and had completed much of the first draft of *The Pivot of Civilization*. The combination of rest and work stimulated her immensely. "I never had greater confidence in the work than now. It is absolutely the only issue which is alive, which is fundamental, and which can save civilization from the wreck which charities and other weak and sentimental agencies have made of society."

In September, she attended a conference on birth control techniques at the Hague and returned to London for the operation. "Imbedded tonsils were removed from the source and recovery was near," she wrote later. "This after twenty-three years of suffering!"

She was still in a nursing home a few days before her ship was to sail. Doctors, nurses, and friends urged her to postpone the trip. But she had to get back to New York to make the final conference arrangements, and as usual, illness was not allowed to stand in her way. Ellis insisted on taking her to Plymouth for the boat. "It was well I went," he wrote De Selincourt, "for she certainly ought to have remained at the nursing home a few days longer. Just before we reached Plymouth, the throat became troublesome and she could not speak. She was quite cheerful over it, and wrote on a scrap of paper: 'You will have to hang a card around my neck and write on it in large letters, SHE IS DUMB.'"

2

Back in New York, Margaret Sanger was now working frantically on the conference which was to open November 11. Although she had always remained suspect of formal organizations ("There was something heavy and ponderous, something lifeless and soulless in the mechanism of those I had known"), she realized that birth control, particularly the conference's medical aspects, needed a responsible group of citizens behind it. The American Birth Control League, therefore, was formed, with Mrs. Pierre Jay, Mrs. Rublee, Robert M. Lovett, and Dr. John Vaughan on its board.

For the climax of the conference, the public meeting at Town Hall on Sunday, Mrs. Sanger had selected as the subject, "Birth Control: Is It Moral?" The meeting was intended not for headlines, but to present a variety of viewpoints from professional leaders like

Harold Cox and Dr. Royal S. Copeland, Health Commissioner of New York. Town Hall had been reserved and paid for three weeks before. The meeting was scheduled for 8:30 P.M., the doors to open at seven o'clock.

Despite the success of the first two days, Margaret Sanger was filled with premonitions all that afternoon. Her brain seemed numb. Always when she was to speak, she could actually visualize the hall and her audience and its reactions ahead of time. Now she could not even think through her speech. Her strong sense of mysticism was particularly troubled by her dream of the night before, a dream in which she struggled to carry a baby up a steep hill. "I came very abruptly to a side hill which became a mountainside of rock and slippery shale," she wrote, "and I had nothing to hold on to to keep me from slipping. The baby kept crying and I tried to comfort it, but I dared not use my right hand, as it seemed to be held up like a balancing rod which kept us both from falling. The wretched dream kept me drowsy all day—always when I dreamed of babies there was some kind of troublesome news not far away."

She dined at seven with Mrs. Rublee and Harold Cox while Mrs. Kennedy went ahead to Town Hall. A little after eight the three of them took a taxi. When they reached Forty-third Street, the taxi slowed to a crawl. Thousands of people jammed the street. "An overflow crowd," Margaret thought to herself. "A wonderful turn-out!"

They had to leave the cab and push their way to the entrance. She was astounded to see two policemen barring the doors. She attempted to go in, but the policemen blocked her with their arms.

"You can't get in this place tonight," one policeman announced brusquely.

"Why not?" she asked.

"There ain't going to be any meeting."

"But who stopped it?" she demanded. "I am one of the speakers. Mr. Cox is another."

"You can't go in," he repeated. "That's all I know about it."

A newspaperman standing near by suggested that Mrs. Sanger telephone Police Commissioner Richard Enright.

She and Mrs. Rublee rushed across the street to a telephone booth and called Police Headquarters. No one would say where the Commissioner was. As far as they knew, no orders to forbid the meeting had been issued.

She was about to call Mayor Hylan when across the street she
saw that the two policemen at the door were allowing a trickle of
people to leave the hall. At the sight of the open door, she hung up
the receiver and pushed her way back through the crowd.

Instinctively she knew she had to take command of the meeting.
Who had stopped it, she still didn't know. The only way to find out
was to get inside. While the two policemen fought to hold back the
outside crowd at the same time as they opened the door to let a
few insiders out, she sprang forward and stooped under one policeman's arm. She was inside the hall!

Most of the audience was milling in the aisles. She rushed to the
footlights. But they were as high as her shoulders and another blue
uniform obstructed the steps leading to the stage. "A tall, handsome
man stood near me," she described it later, "looking vacantly around
and much perplexed. A small messenger boy with a large bouquet
of pink roses also stood near by. As I stood looking up at the stage
and wondering how on earth I could get upon it and call out to the
audience to come back, I was suddenly caught up in the strong
arms of the handsome man beside me and lifted—no, really flung
over the footlights onto the stage. Before I could pick myself up
and recapture my poise the same man grabbed the flowers from the
messenger with the vacant stare, leaped upon the platform with the
quickness and agility of an athlete, and placed the huge bouquet
of roses into my arms . . ."

The man, who turned out to be Dr. Lothrop Stoddard, shouted
to the audience, "Here she is. Here's Mrs. Sanger!"

She stood at the front of the stage, a small figure, ignoring the
chaos around her. She was angry now. "Don't leave," she called to
the audience. "We're going to hold the meeting!"

The hall was in turmoil. People—many of them distinguished
public-health officials from all over the country, lawyers and judges
who had been especially invited—scrambled back to their seats.
Mrs. Sanger knew that the meeting could be legally closed if fire
regulations were breached and urged that the aisles be cleared.
At this point, the *Tribune* estimated that five thousand people were
jammed outside Town Hall. Many succeeded in fighting their way
back inside.

"Then began such a thundering applause, as if it were the only
relief for their angry, indignant, rebellious spirits," she wrote later.
"The fight was on, and every man and woman in that hall was there

beside me to fight to the finish. I felt it in the air, in their voices, as they called out to me to speak."

While she waited for the audience to be seated, Anne Kennedy, who had mounted the stage, described what had happened before Mrs. Sanger's arrival. At eight o'clock, with the hall already half filled, an unidentified man, accompanied by a police captain, had come up to her on the platform and announced, "This meeting must be closed."

"Why?" she demanded.

"An indecent, immoral subject is to be discussed."

"On what authority? Are you from the police?"

The man identified himself as Monsignor Dineen, the Secretary of Archbishop Hayes.

"What right has he to interfere?"

"He has the right." He turned to the police captain with him.

"I'm Captain Donohue of this district," said the officer. "The meeting must be closed."

The New York *Times,* after an all-night check by its determined reporter, corroborated this startling incident in next morning's front-page story. "The police suppression of the birth control meeting at Town Hall Sunday night," it stated, ". . . was brought about at the instance of Archbishop Patrick J. Hayes of this Roman Catholic Archdiocese." What had brought Captain Donohue to the meeting? A telephone call to his desk lieutenant from Police Headquarters, he stated. From whom at Headquarters? He claimed he didn't know. ". . . Captain Donohue did not know why he had been sent to Town Hall until he met the Monsignor there."

After this ultimatum from Monsignor Dineen, Mrs. Kennedy had coolly replied, "We'll write this down, and I'll read it to the audience: 'I, Captain Thomas Donohue of the 26th Precinct at the order of Monsignor Joseph P. Dineen, Secretary to Archbishop Hayes, have ordered the meeting closed.' "

"When I saw this statement," Margaret Sanger wrote later, "I grew hot with indignation. It was one thing to have halls closed by a mistaken or misguided ignorant police captain, but a very different thing to have a high dignitary of the Roman Catholic Church order a meeting closed. I knew the law of the city: I knew the rights of citizens guaranteed under the Constitution . . . At the thought of this official impertinence, this bullying, this arrogant dictatorship, this insolence of a Roman Catholic Archbishop, my resistance, my resolution became set. I would not close the meeting unless I was forced by arrest to do so. I knew our rights were being violated by the police captain. They must go the limit. Unless I stood my ground and got arrested, I could not take my case into the courts."

She had made her decision—a decision of special portent to the birth control movement. Standing in this howling maelstrom, she had grasped the facts instantly. She had taken command. This act of suppression must be fought to the end, must be made a symbol of the determination of all intelligent people to refuse to bow to authoritarian and illegal power when their constitutional rights had been breached.

She stepped to the front of the platform and raised her hand. The audience quieted. "Ladies and gentlemen," she cried, "you have all seen——"

That was as far as she got. Two policemen stepped forward, held her, and ordered her to stop speaking.

"Where's your warrant?" she demanded. "What's the charge?"

The audience burst out in angry catcalls and hisses.

Harold Cox, tall, white-haired, with the distinguished bearing of an elder statesman who had spoken for the British Empire in the halls of Parliament, stepped to the front of the platform. "I have come from across the Atlantic——" he cried. But he got no farther. Another policeman pulled at his arm and led him back to his seat.

Then Miss Mary Winsor, a distinguished suffragist, president of the Pennsylvania Equal Suffrage Association, sprang up to speak. She too was stopped.

The *Times* in next morning's edition described the scene:

The stage was in tumult. Several women began to address the audience, and as fast as one was seized by the police, another began to speak. Mrs. Sanger was still the storm center, and her friends crowded around her and all but swept the policemen off their feet.

"If you would help us," one woman told the audience, "we could remove the police from this platform." There were cries of "Put out the police," but wiser counsel prevailed . . .

Again Margaret Sanger tried to speak and was stopped. Again Miss Winsor and other women stepped forward to take her place, and each time the policemen pulled them back to their seats. At each intervention, the audience roared in protest. An ugly mood of defiance rippled through it. A second squad of reserves had entered the hall and was now trying to force the people in the rear seats to leave.

"People now jumped excitedly on the platform to help me in case of trouble," Margaret Sanger stated later. ". . . I have never been afraid of the police but it was a glorious feeling to see those men behind me with eager, determined faces with jaws set and eyes blazing with indignation."

At the back of the platform, leaning against the wings, stood Monsignor Dineen, giving directions by a nod of his head or a whispered command to the policemen who acted as messengers between him and Captain Donohue. At last, he gave the final command. The captain ordered the policemen flanking Mrs. Sanger to put her under arrest.

Miss Winsor started to speak again and she too was put under arrest.

With policemen holding each of their arms and Captain Donohue leading the way, the two women were led from the hall. No speech had been given! No law had been broken at this legally authorized meeting—except by the policemen who made the arrest! As the women were led into the street, a few people began to sing, "My country, 'tis of thee," and suddenly everyone in the crowd joined in the swelling, ironic chorus of indignation.

Juliet Rublee, following close behind, shouted at one police officer, "I spoke. Why don't you arrest me, too?"

"Come along," he said.

"Scores of automobile owners," reported the *Tribune* in next morning's edition, "volunteered to take Mrs. Sanger and Miss Winsor to the police station, but Captain Donohue insisted they would have to go in the patrol wagon. When the women protested against this indignity, they were marched through the packed streets to the station house. . . ." A cordon of police surrounded them, but the crowd pressed in close, thousands of people, singing, shrieking, hissing at Captain Donohue and other officers. It was one of the wildest parades that New York had ever seen.

At night court, Robert McC. Marsh, a prominent lawyer and son-in-law of Mrs. Delafield, volunteered to defend the women. The magistrate released them on their own recognizance and ordered them to appear in court the next morning.

It was well after midnight, but Mrs. Sanger, Miss Winsor, Harold Cox, and other friends returned to Mrs. Rublee's house. Reporters flocked in. A few who had not been in the hall when the police first stopped the meeting at Monsignor Dineen's order were amazed and dubious that a religious body had dared commit such a flagrant violation of civil rights. The *Times* reporter decided to get verification from the Monsignor himself. After persistent telephoning, he finally reached him at his office at St. Patrick's.

"Yes," said the Monsignor, "I ordered the meeting to be closed."

Early the next morning, after a few hours' sleep, Margaret Sanger appeared in court before Magistrate Joseph E. Corrigan. "How can you stop anything which has not started?" he asked the arresting policeman cryptically. No one answered. Where was Captain Donohue with the charges? They waited an hour. The captain never appeared. Assistant District Attorney Richard Gibbs finally admitted there was no evidence of illegality on which he could draw a complaint. The case was dismissed.

But it was just the beginning of an eruption that was to shake New York for many months to come. Margaret Sanger's determination to carry on the meeting until Monsignor Dineen had openly stepped in and ordered her arrest bared with frightening clarity the extent of the Church's power in New York politics. The city was stunned. Every New York newspaper featured the story in front-page headlines and excoriated Church and police in biting editorials.

From the *Tribune* came this protest:

". . . *The police broke up the meeting without waiting for any expression of opinion which would warrant repression . . . It was arbitrary and Prussian to the last degree . . . If the police deny even the right of assemblage to one group of citizens, what is to stop them from denying it to another group against which they or their advisers have a personal prejudice?"*

The *Post's* editorial warned:

"*If people cannot come together in a perfectly orderly and open way to debate whether or not a matter is moral, then our boasted freedom of speech is a mockery.*"

Said the *World:*

"*The issue Sunday evening was bigger than the right to advocate birth control. It is part of the eternal fight for free speech, free as-*

sembly and democratic government. It is a principle which must always find defenders if democracy is to survive."

Overnight Margaret Sanger had taken the shattered pieces of a disrupted meeting and turned the birth control conference into a general offensive for the right of free speech and free assembly. She called together the executive board of the American Birth Control League. A new meeting was announced, this time for Friday evening. The issue was out in the open now. She had flung out her challenge to the police and the Church, and not only newspapers in the United States but in England and Europe waited expectantly for the next round. From Cambridge University, England, after he had read the story the next day, an illustrious professor, Telou Porter, sent a telegram to birth control headquarters: "Arrest and release greatest victory yet."

It was addressed to "Saint Margaret, New York."

CHAPTER 15

"The Archbishop is delighted and pleased with the action of the police, as I am, because it was no meeting to be held publicly and without restrictions," Monsignor Dineen told the New York *Times* reporter the next day. The statement was enormously significant both for the Catholic Church and the birth control movement. Minor members of the hierarchy had attacked birth control intermittently for the last five years, but this was the first time that an Archbishop had declared open warfare. Margaret Sanger might well have considered it a backhanded compliment. For the Church now recognized that the movement had achieved such strength and drawn so many Catholics to its principles that it must be classed as a serious opponent.

For almost any other public figure the enmity of the Church would have meant certain disaster. Not for Margaret Sanger. Always at her best in a fight, she welcomed the chance to face the Archbishop in the open arena of newspaper headlines and public meetings instead of through undercover boycotts and subtle political pressure, which had previously been the Church's weapons. Here was her old antagonist—that same power which had practically hounded her father out of Corning for his espousal of Henry George and Robert Ingersoll and had made her a heretic in the eyes of her schoolmates. This was the battle she had awaited.

That the Archbishop had struck first—and most unwisely—gave her an advantage that she exploited to the limit. In its zeal to crush the birth control movement in one critical blow, the Church had closed a public meeting, a completely legal meeting, through its special influence in the Police Department. It had openly transgressed that most treasured constitutional principle of free speech and assembly.

Margaret Sanger, therefore, fought back not on the issue of birth control but as the defender of constitutional freedoms. Much of the nation's conservative press, which up to now had considered her a "crackpot" and "fanatic," was suddenly forced to recognize her as a staunch defender of the Constitution. Overnight her strategy brought birth control hundreds of headlines and favorable editorials that years of campaigning had never been able to win.

Further, her announcement that the halted meeting would be held again on the coming Friday immediately put the Church on the defensive. The Archbishop made a stumbling attempt to regain the initiative in the middle of the week when Monsignor Dineen defended the Town Hall raid by saying, "I was shocked and horrified when I saw that children were being admitted to the meeting. I counted no less than four or five within a few minutes," he was quoted in the *Tribune*. Mr. Marsh, Mrs. Sanger's lawyer, deflated this statement by offering factual proof that the four "children" were actually Barnard students—all twenty or older—who had been sent to observe the meeting on assignment from their sociology class.

Since Town Hall was unavailable for the second meeting, the Park Theatre at Columbus Circle was booked for Friday evening. At eight o'clock, the crowd outside was so dense that only a single door could be opened. Fifteen minutes later the theater was packed. Some of the thousands left outside tried to get in by climbing the fire escapes. 4,000 ATTEMPT TO BATTER WAY TO BIRTH TALK, the New York *American's* headline described it. "So great a crowd . . . besieged the theatre," reported the New York *World*, "that the police were nearly torn loose from their blue coats and ash night sticks."

It was a serious audience, not a collection of curiosity seekers. The boxes were filled by distinguished names like Paul Kellogg, Mrs. Dexter Blagden, Mrs. Haggerty Pell, and Mrs. Marshall Field, who came from Chicago to attend. When the London newspapers described "the caravan of fashionable people in distinguished autos," Havelock Ellis could not help chiding Margaret in his next letter about "the fashionable character" of her meetings.

Margaret Sanger had captured the headlines so effectively with her Park Theatre "coup" that Archbishop Hayes himself now made his first public statement on birth control. The main point in his lengthy invective was the advantage to society of large families as demonstrated by John Wesley, who was the fifteenth child, Benjamin Franklin, the fifteenth, and Ignatius Loyola, the eighth son.

Mrs. Sanger countered this argument with her own public statement by going right to the Bible. "Isaac," she pointed out, ". . . was an only child, born after long years of preparation. Samuel, who judged Israel for forty years, was an only child. So was John the Baptist."

Later in his Christmas Pastoral, the Archbishop again returned to the attack—proof birth control had at last reached the point where it demanded major attention in this important message. "Children troop down from heaven because God wills it," the Archbishop proclaimed. "He alone has the right to stay their coming . . . Woe to those who degrade, pervert, or do violence to the law of nature . . ."

"Why then, I wonder, do priests and nuns remain unmarried?" Margaret Sanger commented dryly. "Why then are celibacy and self-control—a most unnatural law of nature—approved and extracted?"

But she was less interested in such religious rhetoric than in the legal, or illegal, connotations of the raid. "I consider my arrest a violation of the first principle of liberty for which America stands, and I shall take this case to the highest courts, if necessary, to preclude the possibility of it ever happening again," she announced to the press. For weeks after the raid, telegrams and letters flooded local newspapers demanding court action for false arrest. The American Civil Liberties Union offered her its legal services. When twenty-eight of the city's leading citizens wrote an open letter to Commissioner Enright demanding Captain Donohue's punishment, the Commissioner was finally forced into action. He ordered Chief Inspector William J. Lahey to make an investigation of the raid.

The investigation, alternately resembling a comic opera and a Spanish inquisition, offered a field day to local reporters, who covered it with irony and exuberance. Neither Captain Donohue nor Monsignor Dineen was called to the first hearing. The only witness of significance was a tall, aristocratic business tycoon named J. Noah H. Slee, the same Mr. Slee who had followed Margaret to London the summer before. A faithful suitor, he had naturally gone with Margaret to the Town Hall meeting and gave a lucid and staunch defense of her actions.

At the next hearing, when for a second time neither Donohue nor Monsignor Dineen was called, it was obvious that Lahey was investigating not the raid but the birth control movement. Seated next to Lahey at the table in the hearing room was a hulking figure in a black alpaca coat, later identified as Assistant Corporation Counsel Martin Dolphin. "His large head, his dull, heavy features with full hanging lips and coarse mouth and jaws loomed before me," Margaret Sanger wrote later. "His eyes were fixed straight on my face, as if he intended to hypnotize me and influence by sheer terror what I had to say."

For over an hour, Lahey battered Mrs. Sanger with questions, not on the Town Hall raid but on the Brownsville clinic arrest of five years before, "until I felt physically bruised, as though parts of my body had been beaten black and blue." Lahey undoubtedly considered himself a master of the strategy of diversion. At one moment, he pointed dramatically at the closed door behind him and produced a witness who gave such inaccurate testimony about the Brownsville raid that Mrs. Sanger told her bluntly she was lying.

But the dramatic climax undoubtedly came when Mrs. George Rublee was called to the witness chair. The mysterious stranger, Martin Dolphin, suddenly took charge of the questioning. "A spirit of evil seemed to exude from him and to surround him," Mrs. Rublee recounted later.

"Did you ever read the law, Section 1142?" Dolphin demanded. Mrs. Rublee, wife of one of the city's most prominent lawyers, said that she had.

"When?"

"Yesterday, with Mr. Marsh," she replied.

"Did you ever read it before?" demanded Dolphin.

"Yes, about five years ago."

"Did you ever talk it over with Mrs. Sanger?"

"I might have."

Dolphin suddenly stood up and pointed accusingly at Mrs. Rublee. "Arrest that woman!" he shouted to Patrolman Thomas J. Murphy, who was sitting near by.

For a few seconds, everyone in the room sat paralyzed. Then Mr. Marsh turned to Dolphin and asked, "On what grounds is Mrs. Rublee arrested?"

"She has violated Section 1142," snapped Dolphin.

"She has read the law—is that a crime?"

There was no answer.

"Who makes the charge against Mrs. Rublee?" asked Mr. Marsh.

Patrolman Murphy looked helplessly at Dolphin and finally mumbled, "I do."

"My brother of the Bar," Marsh asked Dolphin again, "will you give me your name?" Again there was no answer. "At least it is a courtesy between attorneys to know by name with whom we are dealing."

"I am merely a bystander," replied Dolphin.

"Well, Mr. Bystander, will you be specific and say what the charge is that this woman is arrested on?"

Dolphin stood up and advanced threateningly toward Marsh. "Do you want to get into this?" he shouted. "If you do, now is the time to say so." Just as suddenly, he turned on his heels and stalked from the room.

The farce was played to its conclusion at the Elizabeth Street court, to which Patrolman Murphy escorted Mrs. Rublee and Mrs. Sanger—all riding in the chauffeured limousine of Mrs. Dexter Blagden. "What was she selling? Where are the articles?" demanded Magistrate Peter A. Hatting. Murphy admitted with some embarrassment that there were none. Angrily, Hatting gave the police until four that afternoon to produce some evidence. At that point, when neither Dolphin, Lahey, nor any evidence had made an appearance, Hatting dismissed the case.

It was the second major blunder of the Police Department, and the New York press greeted it with obvious relish. The *World's* editorial on December 3 demanded:

What further step can be expected than the arrest of witnesses in that inquiry for purposes of intimidation? And if intimidation was not the purpose in Mrs. Rublee's arrest, let it be known what the purpose was.

Mrs. Rublee, however, was not easily intimidated although, as she told reporters, she had already received a postcard warning "unless I ceased my attacks on Monsignor Dineen and the Roman Catholic Church, I would be killed."

She and Mrs. Sanger invited a score of the most prominent citizens in New York to a protest meeting at the Rublee house that night. The issue had now gone far beyond birth control and approached open domination of the Police Department by the church hierarchy. Such leaders of finance, industry, and law as Henry Morgenthau, Sr., Herbert L. Satterlee, Lewis L. Delafield, Charles C. Burlingame, Samuel H. Ordway, Pierre Jay, Paul M. Warburg,

Charles Strauss, Montgomery Hare, and Paul D. Cravath considered the danger critical enough for an open letter to Mayor Hylan.

The action of the Police Department constitutes such a wilful violation of the right of free speech as to cause grave alarm to the citizens of New York, who have a right to know why such outrages have taken place, what motives and influences are behind them, and whether any conspiracy exists in the Police Department to deny the right of free speech and the equal protection of the law to citizens of New York . . .

The Mayor replied promptly enough by ordering his Commissioner of Accounts, David F. Hirshfield, to make another investigation, or what one newspaper acidly called "an investigation into the previous investigation." After one fruitless hearing on January 24, 1922, Captain Donohue was finally called as a witness on February 17 and proved so amazingly inept that even the Commissioner commented to Emory Buckner, now Margaret Sanger's lawyer, "You don't have to examine any other witnesses to show the intelligence or lack of foresight on the part of this captain."

Why did Captain Donohue go to the Town Hall meeting?

". . . Lieutenant Courtney on duty at the station," the *Times* reported the captain as saying, "had told him that an order had come from Police Headquarters."

From whom at Police Headquarters? As far as the captain knew, it was only the telephone operator.

Whoever made the call from Headquarters was obviously being well protected by the captain. "The violation of the Constitution was committed directly by a little group of the police, evidently inspired by somebody at Police Headquarters," stated the *Herald*. "Whose was the motive behind this inspiration . . . ?"

As the hearings dragged on through February, it became apparent that Commissioner Hirshfield had no intention of pinning direct blame on the real instigator of the raid. "From the Mayor down, city officials were literally 'thumbing the nose' at its taxpayers," Margaret Sanger fumed. "The hierarchy of St. Patrick's Cathedral was smugly complacent, knowing that though somewhat dulled, the tools of a city government were still in their hands."

Despite Hirshfield's gaudily cloaked attempt at bringing those responsible for the raid to justice, not the slightest whisper of blame was attached to Monsignor Dineen. Not one single person in the

Police Department was even punished. Amazingly enough, when the
storm had blown over a few months later, Captain Donohue was
promoted to inspector and then quietly retired.

Even the blatant antics of Martin Dolphin in ordering Mrs.
Rublee's arrest escaped legal retribution. A distinguished panel of
New York lawyers brought charges against him before Judge John
W. Goff. Goff immediately recommended prosecution. When the
charges reached the Court of Appeals, Dolphin's conduct was labeled
"arbitrary and unlawful." But the charges were finally dropped on
the flimsy pretext that he had not been acting in an official capacity
when he ordered Mrs. Rublee's arrest.

The final outcome was that despite two investigations into the
Police Department's raid, no report was ever issued. Three years later
the New York evening *Mail* commented tartly that Commissioner
Hirshfield still "has made no report, and the conclusion he drew
from the evidence placed before him remains a profound mystery
to this day."

But despite the lack of legal retribution, Margaret Sanger easily
emerged victorious in this first open encounter with the Catholic
hierarchy. Not only in New York but throughout the country, she
had gained an overwhelmingly favorable press. The Church's part
in usurping constitutional liberties was widely censored.

Instead of making America an example for the Western world and
quashing its birth control movement early in its development, the
Church here was actually on the defensive. Summarizing its continued defeats in an article in the June 1928 *Review*, Charles V. Drysdale wrote: "In France the adoption of Birth Control commenced
with or soon after the Revolution although the great mass of the
people still remained Roman Catholics . . . It [the Church] has
absolutely failed to check it in Belgium. . . . in spite of being
crowded with priests . . . It appears to be failing even worse in
Roman Catholic Austria . . . There are limits even to the religious
subservience of women, and when they realize that they are still
to be debarred the use of chemical contraceptives and be required
to dissuade their husbands from intercourse when they do not
desire children . . . not even the Pope and all his majesty and
ministers will restrain them."

CHAPTER 16

"The greatest threat to the peace of the world is to be found in the teeming populations of Asia," Margaret Sanger wrote in the January 1922 issue of the *Review*. This was a theme—the direct connection between overpopulation and war—she had been enunciating since 1917. Despite the mounting influence of the militarist clique in the Japanese Government, the younger progressives like Baroness Shidzue Ishimoto were visibly stirred by Margaret Sanger's predictions. Now in the very midst of the Town Hall investigations, one of their leading voices, the publishing house known as the Kaizo group, urged Mrs. Sanger to make a lecture tour of Japan. It was an impressive invitation. Only three others whose ideas rated international attention had been invited—Bertrand Russell, Albert Einstein, and H. G. Wells.

It had been only eight years since Margaret Sanger had spoken out for birth control in the *Woman Rebel*. They had called her then the high priestess of a new gospel of sex knowledge—a "vigorous, constructive, liberated morality." In those years, the movement had been based on the emotional needs of women, particularly working women, searching for some escape from the slavery of excessive childbearing. But she had carried the movement into new scientific channels—clinics, doctors, better techniques of contraception. Now with this trip to Japan, she would, in one dramatic step, broaden the impact of birth control so that it would become the key to the population problem of whole nations.

Here was the very essence of her genius, that simplicity and directness of mind which could formulate this new vision and then immediately set forth to turn it into a practical program for Japan and the rest of the world. H. G. Wells was one of the first to appreciate the "extraordinary breadth of outlook and the real scientific quality of her mind." For birth control, the perfect biological tool by which human beings could harness the blind instincts of nature, could shape not just the happiness of families but the very destinies of nations. With this trip, Margaret Sanger was to bring the force of a new idea, a new way of life to the Far East. "Since the coming of Commodore Perry," wrote Baroness Ishimoto,[1] "no American has created a greater sensation in the land of the Mikado than Margaret Sanger."

It was a hectic leave-taking, that last month. She made a dozen speeches between January 13 and 30 in a fast swing through the Midwest, organized a new birth control league in Reading, Pennsylvania, and attended a series of farewell luncheons and dinners in her honor. Carefully she noted on her speaking schedule—since money was an omnipresent problem—that each lecture had brought her a hundred and fifty dollars.

She rushed out to Peddie School in New Jersey to see Stuart and Grant. Stuart was a senior now, a handsome, stocky youth of eighteen who had followed in his uncle Bob's footsteps as captain of the football team and was preparing for Yale. He was well able to take care of himself. But Grant was only thirteen and new at Peddie. In the back of her mind was the thought of extending her trip through the Far East and up the Suez Canal to England, where she would attend the Fifth International Birth Control Conference in the spring. She dreaded being away from Grant all this time, a dread that reached back to Peggy's last illness. Why shouldn't Grant accompany her on the trip and reap a vast new education in their travels? "I had made up my mind beforehand," she admitted later, and despite the principal's objections to this break in school routine, Grant's shirts and shoes were bundled quickly into a suitcase and they set off for San Francisco.

Margaret Sanger undoubtedly had a secondary motive in having Grant accompany her. He would make a fitting chaperon. For the indefatigable Mr. Slee, who had followed closely on Margaret's heels for the last two years, now talked of carrying the pursuit to Japan. It had been a unique courtship. Possibly no two people had ever started out so far apart. But from the moment he had met her, this master of industrial organization and efficiency had decided, he admitted later to Dorothy Brush, "That's the woman for me, and I'm going to get her." All the past year, he had kept Margaret's office filled with flowers. He had telephoned her constantly, called at the

[1] Shidzue Ishimoto, *Facing Two Ways* (New York: Farrar, 1935).

office, at first skeptical of a movement—to his rugged masculinity, all feminists were "crackpots"—which devoured so much of the life of this fascinating woman.

One morning he wandered into the office at 104 Fifth Avenue and saw the mailbags, thousands of letters that came to Margaret every day from mothers all over the country. This was a sight that would delight any executive! But how inefficiently the mail was being handled, he grumbled. Right on the spot he reorganized the department—purshased a mechanical letter opener, a date stamper, set up a new system of filing, and turned in the old typewriters for a new supply of noiseless ones. That morning, the rugged entrepreneur of the Three-in-One Oil Company became a part of the birth control movement.

"She was the woman for you—because she was quicksilver." Dorothy Brush succinctly analyzed the courtship. "You never could quite catch her, and so she kept you fascinated always."

Slee had spent two years now pursuing her from lecture to lecture, following in her frantic footsteps from the office to the clinic, from New York to London. Now he saw the opportunity aboard ship to Japan of having two uninterrupted weeks with her. He gave her only a slight hint of his plan. Then at the last minute as he was seeing her off in San Francisco, he booked passage with her and Grant on the *Taiyo Maru*.

Always it seemed that giant obstacles reared in her path. She had requested a new passport from Washington for Grant and herself, and since time was short, instructed the State Department to send it directly to the consulate of the Imperial Japanese Government in San Francisco. But when she presented herself, the consul smiled politely and explained that his government had cabled that no visa could be given her. Why not? she demanded. Was she personally unacceptable? Or her lectures on birth control? The consul cabled his government and the answer came back: undesirable on both counts.

Yet her friends in the Kaizo group had already cabled her of the tremendous interest the announcement of her lectures had stirred. Let the Japanese Government try to stop her! Official censorship would only bring thousands more to hear her. Although her tickets had been canceled on the withdrawal of her visa, she discovered that the *Taiyo Maru* also stopped at Chinese ports; she immediately applied for and secured a Chinese visa. A day later she sailed, holding the same cabin that she had bought originally. "I felt the exhilarating flush that the prospect of a battle always starts in me," she wrote later.

Aboard ship were one hundred and fifty Japanese officials, the two chief delegates and their entourage of technical experts, who were returning from the Washington Disarmament Conference. Recognizing Margaret Sanger's name, many of them called on her with questions. Their interest in birth control was so great that a group asked her to address them in the dining room. After the speech, both Admiral Baron Kato, who headed the delegation and was later to be Prime Minister, and Masanao Hanihara, Vice-Minister of Foreign Affairs and later Ambassador to the United States, paid a personal call to express their admiration.

At Honolulu, where the ship docked for four hours, Margaret Sanger was rushed through a frantic afternoon of welcome and speechmaking. Garlanded with leis, she paid official calls on the Japanese, Chinese, Siamese, and other Far Eastern legations, was taken to a luncheon in her honor at the home of the Walter Dillinghams, and then hurried to a local hall, where she made an hour's speech to an overflow audience of Americans, Japanese, and natives in their bright Mother Hubbard dresses. From there a quick dash to the country club for tea, more garlanding with leis, and in the final few minutes, she officiated at the organization of a Hawaiian birth control league. Two Japanese reporters followed her through this afternoon and cabled enthusiastic accounts to Tokyo. As a result, Baroness Ishimoto wrote later, "The news and editorial columns of both Japanese and foreign language newspapers had been full of Mrs. Sanger ever since it had been announced several weeks before that she would arrive."[2]

The problem of her admission to Japan had now become the major topic of discussion among the passengers. Many of the delegation sent cablegrams to the Home Office and Foreign Office supporting her admission. Mr. Hanihara, strongly impressed by her views, cabled his government that birth control could not possibly impair public morals.

It had become a battle of cablegrams. Each morning the small, moon-faced cabin boy who came to Mrs. Sanger's cabin with early coffee brought the latest report from the wireless room. "Madam Sanger go in maybe. Yes, Japan Government let her go in," he would

[2]*Ibid.*

report excitedly. Ten minutes later he would be back, his face drawn. No, a new cable had just arrived. She would not be admitted.

"Thousand disciples welcome you," the Kaizo group cabled her. Messages came in from a dozen societies—the Medical Association of Kyoto, the Cultural Society of Kobe, the doctors of Nagoya, the Tokyo Y.M.C.A.—all asking her for lecture dates. The young liberals of Japan like Professor Isa Abe and Dr. Kato, head of the Department of Medical Affairs, who opposed the militarist block and its demands for a larger birth rate and Army, had stirred a tempest of debate in Japanese newspapers. Before she arrived, Margaret Sanger had become the most controversial figure in Japan.

Baroness Ishimoto wrote:

"The day she and Admiral Baron Kato, conference delegate from Washington, reached Yokohama on the same steamer, the baron's picture was diverted to out of the way corners of the Japanese papers while large photographs of Mrs. Sanger and her son Grant, who was with her, were featured as first class news. No group could come together, whether foreign or Japanese, in which she and her theories were not the subject of lively conversation."

When the *Taiyo Maru* entered the rain and fog of Tokyo harbor on March 10, the ship was immediately surrounded by a fleet of small craft—Police and Health Department launches, tenders for the mail, tenders for the newsmen and cameramen, seventy of whom, a record number, had come expressly to interview Mrs. Sanger.

The Japan *Times* described this scene the next day:

Was it Admiral Kato they sought? It was not. A dozen disgruntled shorthand men dropped out of the herd to take notes on the Envoy's address in the dining room, but the others flocked onward until they found the modest quarters wherein abode a modest little American woman and her handsome young son. Mrs. Sanger and the Cause of Birth Control was what the press of Japan was interested in—the Peace Conference was an old story.

For three hours, Margaret Sanger was interrogated in her cabin by government officials. Finally she was told that she might enter Japan if she agreed not to lecture publicly on war and population and provided that American Consul General Skidmore formally requested permission for her to land. She immediately sent Mr. Skidmore a cable and sat back to wait.

Then along the passageway came the tapping of wooden clogs. In Mrs. Sanger's cabin door stood a delegation of women from the New Women's Society of Japan—their pale white faces framed by perfectly coiffured black hair, their tiny, doll-like figures graciously bobbing and bowing like a picture from a fairy tale. Each of the twenty-five women represented one of the women's labor organizations. In halting English, their spokesman told Mrs. Sanger of the virtual slavery in which the industrial revolution of the past thirty years had plunged Japanese women and how dramatically the message of birth control had come to them. "When leaders say women need vote," the spokesman explained, "most women do not listen. When they say women need economic equality, most do not listen. But when women hear of birth control, then like the lightning, we understand."

Late in the evening, the ship docked at Yokohama. Still no word had come from the American consul general. "Not only did the representative of my government refuse to make a formal request for my admission," Margaret Sanger commented sharply, "but he did not even show me the courtesy of a reply to either of my messages." Baroness Ishimoto now boarded the ship with Mr. Yamamoto of the Kaizo group and Mr. Wilson of the British Embassy. It was Mr. Wilson, through a frantic hour of telephoning from the dock, who persuaded the British Government to vouch for Mrs. Sanger and secure her entry. "Mrs. Sanger was allowed to land in this country last night," wrote the Japan *Times* the following day, "after a series of negotiations that made the diplomacy of the Washington Conference look like child's play."

On the dock—and for the rest of her stay in Japan—crowds pressed around her. The efforts of the Japanese Government to stop her coming had only stirred public interest. She was taken to Baron Ishimoto's mansion, and for the next few days, clusters of people stood on the street waiting for her to appear. On March 12, the *Yomiuri Shimbun* reported: "The Police Department has sent several detectives and deputies to watch Baron Ishimoto's mansion, where Mrs. Sanger resides." On March 13: "Sometimes the police ride in a truck up and down in front of the house."

Margaret Sanger soon found that she had become the prime target of the new "Dangerous Thought Law," sponsored by the military and reactionary clique in Parliament, which sought to exclude from the country all ideas not conforming to ancient tradition. But letters from perfect strangers assured her that the younger generation had different views. "You will not judge us, who represent the majority of the Japanese people, by the obstinate attitude of the authorities," wrote one man on March 13. "Their thoughts are just one generation behind us."

On the second day, Mrs. Sanger went to the Chief of Police. She was received courteously, served tea though it was only ten in the morning, and learned that her book, *Woman and the New Race*, which had been translated into Japanese without her knowledge, had been read by almost everyone at Headquarters. But as to speaking in public—why, how could such "dangerous thoughts" be allowed when her book had already made converts in the Police Department?

She decided to go higher—right to the Minister of Home Affairs. But the Minister was out. She then went to the office of the Kaizo group, where the entire staff was called into a strategy conference. It was decided that she should go directly to the Imperial Diet. There, the same official who had greeted her at the Home Affairs office earlier informed her that the Minister had considered her case and decided to let her speak.

On March 14, Margaret Sanger addressed her first audience of eight hundred people at the Y.M.C.A. The hall was filled with prosperous-looking businessmen, students, shop girls, many foreigners, a sprinkling of Buddhist priests, and even two old women, babies on their backs, who paced the rear of the room, hushing the infants and trying to listen at the same time.

Her theme was the danger of exploding populations in Germany and the Far East. Germany, still at a starvation level as a result of the war, was already increasing its population at the rate of 700,000 a year. And Japan? Its greatest era of peace and prosperity had been from 1723 to 1846 when the population stayed at 26 million. Then came the Industrial Revolution. The population leaped to 33 million by 1872. Now it was close to 60 million and expanding at the rate of a million a year. How could all these mouths be fed? Over 2,600 Japanese had to live off each square mile of arable land, excluding volcanic, unproductive land, compared with only 466 people in England. If the population continued to grow, it could mean only starvation and catastrophe or a war of expansion. "Men and women of Japan," the Japan *Advertiser* reported her closing words, "I appeal to you . . . to make your women something more than breeding machines."

Invitations for lectures and receptions piled up on her. "Every evening, afternoon, dinner, lunch and morning taken until I leave Tokyo!" she wrote home. "I am now beginning to fill breakfast engagements."

The diligent correspondent of the *Yomiuri Shimbun* made a list of thirteen lectures, including:

> *March 16—Chamber of Commerce*
> *17—Peers Club*
> *18—Reception by liberals*
> *19—Real Woman's Society at Chutei*
> *23—Nagoya*
> *24—Kyoto Town Hall*
> *25—Society of Doctors at Kyoto*
> *26—Osaka*

At a dinner in her honor given by Baron and Baroness Ishimoto at the Imperial Hotel, to which came a hundred and fifty Japanese officials from the Home Office, the welfare departments, and the hospitals, Margaret Sanger for the first time discussed birth control. "My task it was," Baroness Ishimoto wrote later, "to stand at the entrance door and watch for police spies while Margaret Sanger was talking. . . ."

At such informal meetings as the Peers Club, the whole audience often sat on the floor on clean, fresh mats. "The room might be chilly," Mrs. Sanger wrote, "but a little charcoal burner was beside you and occasionally you warmed your hands over it. I liked the service and the food, which the maids silently brought all at once on a tray, covered over and steaming hot. After sake in diminutive porcelain cups, the group was ready to converse, and it was cozy and interesting. Often we did not get away until midnight because, although the discussion was carried on in English, each remark was translated for the benefit of those who did not understand."

Between lectures, Margaret Sanger studied the problems of Japanese women at first hand. Instead of the gaudy Japan of *Madame Butterfly* and the romanticism of Lafcadio Hearn, she saw that industrialism, which had come, not slowly as in Europe, but in the frantic space of a few decades, had left deep scars on the old feudal society.

It had brought no new freedom to women. Their low status, prescribed by ancient custom, was fitted to the ever increasing demands for cheap factory labor. Almost half the female population—13 million women and girls—were wage earners although only a handful had economic independence. Almost 75 per cent of the factory workers were women, many from the rural districts, practically "bought" by the mill owners under three-to-five-year contracts. When a mother wanted to scold her small daughters, she threatened, "I'll send you to the weavers."

In the silk-spinning mills of Nagoya, Mrs. Sanger saw over seven hundred girls, some no more than ten years old, twirling the slender threads from the cocoons and catching them on spindles. "They were pathetic, gentle, homeless little things," she wrote later, "imprisoned in rooms with all windows closed to keep them moist and hot." Their wages? Seven dollars a month, of which a fourth went for board!

In the cotton mills, the women worked twelve-hour shifts amid the deafening roar of machines. Dust and fine particles poured into their lungs. Many, she saw, were stunted, crippled things. And this misery always went hand in hand with the high birth rate. "I could not believe a country could contain so many babies," she said. "Fathers carried them in their arms; mothers carried them in a sort of shawl; children carried babies . . . boys with babies on their backs were playing baseball . . . even babies were carrying smaller babies!"

She explored every aspect of this feminine degradation, as if feeling it more deeply would give her added strength to fight it. Friends took her to the Yoshiwara or prostitute quarter of Tokyo, first to the cramped alleys of the "unlicensed" section, the endless rows of two-story houses where dark eyes peered through slits in the screen wall. "Working men were standing in the muddy roadways, chattering, scrutinizing the prices which were posted in front like restaurant menus . . ." she wrote. "Hundreds of lights behind paper windows seemed to flicker on and off constantly . . . The sordidness, the innumerable shining eyes made me quiver involuntarily."

Then she crossed the bridge to the licensed quarter and "seemed to enter another world. The houses were like large hotels . . . Through entrances as spacious as driveways men . . . strolled up . . . to view the photographs of the inmates, framed and not unlike those in the lobby of a Broadway theater. In some frames was only the announcement: '—just arrived, straight from ——. No time for picture.' "

Here was the very depth of woman's degradation that she had fought against so long. Here was the essence of man's uncontrolled instincts that stirred her to furious anger. "It made me feel helpless against the crowd of men swarming almost like insects," she said, "automatically reacting to the stimulus of instinct." For was this not the whole purpose of her fight—to control the blindness of human instinct, directing the life force toward the regeneration of the race, toward a planned and eugenic society?

Her strenuous schedule—ten lectures in the last week—now brought her down with pneumonia. Only in the last few days of her trip could she enjoy the simplified perfection of Japanese hospitality. One doctor in Kyoto had invited her and Grant to lunch. He called for them early, insisting on taking them to the art museum, not walking through miles of galleries, but just to view the select specimens of porcelains and one rare screen that he knew she would especially enjoy. After the luncheon, guests departed, new guests arrived, and with them a painter and his easel. Each guest made a single brush line of any shape or size on a large sheet of rice paper. Then the artist took his brush and with a few masterful strokes, converted this random mélange into a flower pattern, a lake, or a mountain scene. After an hour, the artist was replaced by a sculptor. Each guest was given a lesson in clay and his creation baked and glazed. Then there was ceremonial tea and a walk in the exquisite private garden, with a secluded nook or clump of trees for every mood. At dinner, there were new vases and flowers, new screens in the room. More guests arrived, and the conversation lasted until midnight, when Mrs. Sanger and Grant had to return to their hotel, since they were leaving for Kobe the next day.

The grace and abundance of Japanese hospitality was a wondrous thing. When she spoke at the Tokyo Medical Association, for instance, nothing had been said about remuneration. The next day, however, ten rickshas appeared with the officers of the society, laden with packages. She opened one lovely gift after another, a purse, a fan, a cloissoné jar. Then in the smallest package, tied in paper tape wishing her health, happiness, and long life, she found new bills in payment for her lecture.

She had now definitely decided to visit China as the guest of Dr. Hu Shih and go on from there around the world to the London Conference. Her few short weeks in Japan had laid the groundwork of the birth control movement. "I have never spoken with greater freedom, I have never had a more comprehending appreciative audience," she wrote later. "I have never felt such a complete rapprochement with my listeners . . . No matter how greatly my theory was opposed, there was none of the ranting bitterness I found so frequently in my own country—no priests denouncing me as an advocate of unbridled sex lust, no celibate clergy assailing me as the arch-apostle of immorality. Decency and consideration were shown to me instead of bigotry, abuse and hypocrisy."

Five hundred newspaper articles about her were proof of her impact on Japan. During the next month, out of 108 monthly magazines, 81 carried features on birth control. Under Professor Abe, a research group was formed to make a continuing study of the population problem. "No woman, foreign or native," Baroness Ishimoto wrote, "has ever been so welcomed by Japanese men as was Mrs. Sanger. . . . She appeared like a comet and left such a vivid and long-enduring impression on the Japanese mind that there is no possibility of reckoning the true value of her visit."

To her associates in New York at the Birth Control League Margaret Sanger wrote: "Japan has been put over, there is no doubt. Now for China!"

CHAPTER 17

Margaret Sanger and Grant sailed from Kobe through the Inland Sea, stopping at Fusan, Korea, and then crossing the Yellow Sea to China. Mr. Slee, who had been holding business conferences in Yokohama, had decided at the last minute—though the possibility of leaving Margaret had probably never entered his head—to accompany them. With Margaret separated all these months from her admirers back home, he had the opportunity at last to press his courtship. Slowly, imperceptibly at first, his dominating, executive efficiency had taken over all the details of the trip—the hotel and ticket arrangements, the handling of baggage, the planning of the route. Without yielding an inch of her personal freedom, for the first time she was actually enjoying the strong, masculine hand that was shaping her daily routine.

They made a striking pair, walking the deck together—Margaret Sanger, small, intense, the beauty of her wide-set gray eyes set off by the burning mass of auburn hair piled on top her head; Slee, tall and straight, an imposing figure with his white hair and ruddy cheeks, a face that clearly spoke tradition, authority, and decision. "An English squire right out of Sir Roger de Coverley," a friend described him. His old-world aura was emphasized by his bushy black eyebrows and the rimless glasses which he wore attached by a black band to a dapper waistcoat trimmed with piping. His eyes were dark and generally stern, for this was a man who had been brought up on the Bible, read the Bible to his children on Sundays, and said grace at every meal. The Bible, the Episcopal Church—and the Union League Club, too—were the foundations of his life. At aristocratic St. George's Church, where J. P. Morgan and other prominent families had worshiped, Slee had been the superintendent of the Sunday School for twenty-five years. "I nearly fainted when he told me that," Margaret said once.

They seemed to be worlds apart—could he ever understand her London exile or the Wantley circle? Yet in the two years he had pursued her, his growing interest in the movement had been genuine and touching. He was, in fact, the only man close to her in New York who stood firmly behind her work. This attention, the hours he had spent improving the efficiency of the office, the rock-like support he gave at every crisis, were naturally flattering.

All her misgivings would vanish in his smile—in the radiant personality that could not help cropping out from behind the gruff exterior; in his touches of chivalric tenderness, the flowers, the champagne he loved to order for her. He was a man of intense emotion who had been forced to bury his feelings for most of his adult years. His marriage had been bitterly unhappy—a beautiful and fragile wife had shut him out of her life and left him isolated and lonely. The three children had taken sides, isolating him even more. One son had left the Three-in-One Oil Company because he could not tolerate his father's rigidity. But this rigidity—the prayer meetings every morning, the years of fanatical devotion to his business and church—was only a refuge. At Margaret Sanger's touch, he unbent and flowered. Before they had left for Japan, she had casually mentioned how much she enjoyed dancing. Mr. Slee, who had never danced a step, promptly went to Arthur Murray's studio and enrolled for ten lessons.

He had changed her, too, this meticulous industrialist who with all his wealth still kept a pocketbook of his daily expenses, including each nickel carfare. He had, for instance, given her hectic, crowded schedule the discipline of time. In the whirlpool of those last weeks before leaving New York, she had often had trouble meeting him for luncheons or dinners at the appointed hour. "What kind of a watch do you use?" he had finally asked her. Oh, she had laughed, she never worried about watches, didn't even own one. She simply looked out her office window at the big clock on the building across the street. He had been visibly shocked at this. A woman in her position couldn't depend on someone else's clock. The next day, a package arrived for her at the office with a fine Patek Philippe watch, timed to the second and even giving the date. Now she was as devout a worshiper of split-second accuracy in her appointments as Mr. Slee. Sitting on deck at sunset as the ship plowed past the glowing

islands of the Inland Sea, Margaret thought how strange it was
indeed that when a year ago Juliet Rublee had commented on Mr.
Slee's ardor she had replied that marriage was the furthest thought
in her mind. Now with Mr. Slee's determined courtship, the subject
had become almost the focus of their conversation.

At Peking, they stopped at the elegant Grand Hotel, but her impression was "Dust, dust, dust! . . . Some of the streets were paved,
but the dust was suffocating . . . I bathed and bathed and bathed
in a desperate effort to get rid of the diabolical dust."

But the overwhelming fact of life in China, more overwheming
than the dust, was the people. Teeming hordes filled every street,
"millions of people with scarcely enough clothing to cover their
naked bodies . . . eking out a meager existence and [having] to
work twelve to fourteen hours a day to do even that," she wrote.
Here was the terrifying proof that poverty and mass breeding went
hand in hand.

In the ricksha boy, she saw the ultimate symbol of mass breeding.
"You could not set foot out of doors without being besieged by those
half-naked people, so weak, so underfed, so much less able than
the rest of us," she wrote. When they visited the Ming tombs at
Nankow, she was carried by three coolies in a sedan chair through
the arid, dusty countryside, ten miles to the tombs, ten miles back.
"These poor thin boys trudged all the way . . . I felt so sorry for
them I wanted to get out and walk . . . All the way they made
animal noises, 'Aah-huh, aah-huh,' nasal, interminable . . . It was
said that the average coolie lasted but four or five years—the remainder of his life he merely subsisted. I was submerged in a strange
despondency and questioned 'the oldest civilization in the world,'
which still, after so many thousand years, permitted this barbarism."

Always she had to reach out and touch this misery, understand
and assimilate it within her being. She grasped the enormity of this
tragedy as if her life had always been tuned to its hopes and sorrows.
At one of the cotton-spinning mills on the Yangtze outside Shanghai,
employing more than five thousand female workers, she saw hundreds of undernourished girls no more than eight years old. They
received five cents a day for ten or twelve hours' work. Mothers
brought their infants to the mill and put them to sleep in baskets
beside the machines though the air was choked with cotton dust.

In the streets of Shanghai, she was horrified by "innumerable
women with babies lying in the street begging." On one street

corner, a crowd was gathered around a woman leper. Mrs. Sanger thought the woman was dying. But she was only giving birth to a child—so meaningless an incident in this nation of rampant breeding that not one of the onlookers took the effort to call for assistance.

The cheapness of human life haunted her, made her physically sick. Girl babies in China, whose earning power was minuscule compared to the boys', were a drain on their parents. For centuries, Chinese women had limited their girl children by drowning or suffocating them. With the help of a newspaper reporter from the Shanghai *Star*, Mrs. Sanger studied the statistics. Each story of infanticide was like another death in her own heart.

The present alternative to infanticide was to sell the girl babies to the brothel-keepers—often at the age of three or four so that they could be kept at the brothels until they were old enough to begin working off the indentures. Shanghai alone was estimated to have a hundred thousand prostitutes. Mrs. Sanger visited one of the quarters with a local missionary and talked with a group of girls, none of them over twelve years old.

"They seemed like specimen cases in the devil's laboratory," she wrote. ". . . They belonged body and soul to the keeper and are never permitted to return to their native homes. Any attempt to run away, any insubordination is promptly met by the cruelest beating and torture—often the breaking of their leg bones so that it becomes impossible for them to stray . . . I went away sick in soul with doubts and pity."

Although she had scheduled no lectures for China, she could not remain silent. She had to speak out. Her own philosophy, with its mystic overtones that one constructive step, one hopeful word would bring some radiant, expanding force, bore a striking parallel to the work of Mahatma Gandhi. There was some limitless power to her touch, some universal ingredient that instantaneously reached the needs of those who heard her.

Dr. Hu Shih asked her to address the students of Peking National University. Only in his late twenties, this philosopher had been educated at Cornell and Columbia, spoke flawless English, and was considered the father of the Chinese Renaissance. He not only offered to be chairman of the meeting but to interpret for her, a signal honor.

Two thousand students and faculty crowded into the large hall of the university. Even standing room was filled—men had to perch

on the window sills. The very words birth control had transmitted
an electric current, as she had expected. For two hours, she spoke
and answered questions. Then she was escorted to a dinner in her
honor at the chancellor's home—a feast of bird's nest and quail soup,
fried garoupa, roast pheasant, and other luxuries that lasted until
one in the morning. A group of students, to whom she had given a
copy of *Family Limitation,* now asked permission to translate it
into Chinese and have it printed at their own expense. By the next
afternoon, five thousand copies were in circulation—the first flame
of birth control in China!

The message had spread to Shanghai, and the National Association of Education in China and the Association for Family Ref-
ormation asked her to speak. Before eight hundred members, she
described specific techniques of contraception. Later there was an
interview with representatives of fifteen newspapers.

She knew this was only the beginning, that China, with its impoverished millions, was "the best argument in the world for birth
control." The South China *Morning Post* concurred. In an editorial
after her speech, it stated: "From what we know of our customs, it
would be a hard fight, so hard that if it were won, the education of
the rest of the world would be a simple matter."

A hard fight—but there were auspicious signs. After she had left,
a letter from Chen Mai-cheng of Soochow told her:

*Ever since your departure birth control has become one of the
much discussed topics of the press and among the intellectuals of
this proverbially conservative land . . . [Your pamphlet] has been
translated into Chinese and published by myself. The first edition
enjoys a wide distribution in Shanghai, Peking, Nanking, Changsha,
and other cities, though with only a little publicity. The copies have
been practically exhausted. We are therefore considering the feasi-
bility of a second edition . . .*

She was due in London for the birth control conference. They
took passage on the S.S. *Plassy* for the long trip to Port Said, Egypt,
via Hong Kong, Singapore, and the Red Sea. She could sit on the
deck in the crisp breeze and try to forget China—"that land of
ghastly object lessons where pestilence, famine and war are the
loathsome substitutes for contraception in checking population
growth." But she was always part, in one way or another, of the
turbulence of the birth control movement. Before she had left New

York, Evangeline Adams, the astrologer, had insisted on sending her the "aspects" of her trip. Although Mrs. Sanger took these predictions only half seriously, she recalled that Mars would be in opposition at their arrival in Hong Kong. And there it was—a message from the Chief of Police to call at his office.

He was out when she called. Later the Chief missed her at her hotel. But at the dock at Singapore, British Intelligence summoned her to its office. They had heard that Mrs. Sanger was going to India and had been in contact with members of the Indian independence movement. She pointed out that if these members also happened to be supporters of birth control, it was pure coincidence. "I am only interested in one subject," she announced firmly. Besides, the whole question was academic since she did not have the time to make any speeches in India on this trip.

When they reached Cairo, Mars was still in opposition according to the "aspects" of the Adams chart—only this time the opposition took a sudden and frightening shape. Grant came down with dysentery. It was a serious case—his temperature shooting up suddenly to 104 degrees and remaining there despite the efforts of the attending Czechoslovakian doctor. It was a desperate moment for Mrs. Sanger—all the forebodings of Peggy's last illness rising up to haunt her as she stayed at his bedside day and night. She could laugh off the predictions of astrologers; yet there was always one part of her that heeded these distant voices. Just before their arrival at Shepheard's Hotel, the fortuneteller there had predicted an imminent death. Now the servants at the hotel assumed it would be Grant.

On the fourth day, with Grant's temperature still high, she waited until the doctor left for his office and then decided to act. Ordering a dishpanful of ice, she sponged Grant thoroughly in the frosty water. Two hours later his temperature was down to normal. Slee, who had grown tremendously fond of the boy, now took command. He insisted that he take Grant to Switzerland, where he could recoup his strength.

For months, Grant had been dragged from speech to speech, meeting to meeting. He had been whirled through the Far East and the Middle East and tasted all its exotic grandeur from the Great Wall of China to the Buddha's Temple of the Tooth at Kandy, crossed the Nile on a primitive raft to see the spot where Moses had been found in the rushes, and camel-backed across the Sahara to the Pyramids and the Sphinx. Although accustomed to the frantic pace of his mother's life, for a boy of thirteen, as he commented later, the trip "was like being dragged at the tail of a typhoon." The only thing he wanted now was to see Big Bill Tilden play at the Wimbledon matches in London and then return to the uncluttered security of camp and school.

Facing a crowded week at the Fifth International Neo-Malthusian and Birth Control Conference, Mrs. Sanger decided to send Grant back to the United States. Friends ran a summer camp for boys in the Poconos; they would take care of him for the rest of the summer. Grant was put on board the *Majestic;* Margaret Sanger returned to London to the patient and determined Mr. Slee.

He insisted that they be married immediately. But she wanted more time to think—time to assess this aristocrat of American industry against the poetic worlds of Ellis and De Selincourt. She spent a week end with Hugh and Janet at Wantley, and after she had gone, Hugh recaptured those moments in his shimmering letters. ". . . You utterly heavenly darling! . . . Sweet as the air of early morning . . . sweet as briar leaf, sweet as bell heather . . ." Again he wrote: "You shed beauty all around you wherever you go like the smell of a rose, only yours is lasting." She needed such moments. These trips to Wantley would always be a period of regeneration to which she would return again and again. Some part of her, the dreamer, the poet, would always belong to this place— but not the essential part, not the woman of action. That, she knew, was impossible.

She went to see Ellis at the old flat at Brixton. They sat quietly together by the small fire, for quiet had always been the language between them. He had grown even more gentle, more Olympian— his frosty blue eyes, burning yet peaceful; the flowing white beard; the craggy, slightly sunken cheeks. All these years since they had first met in 1915, they had written regularly each week. Each meant something to the other so lasting, so unshakable that neither could ever put it into words.

But Hugh had grasped it. "You darling woman, living his [Ellis's] work in the wonderful way you do——" Hugh had summed it up. "—Mother of his Cause—what finer child could possibly be born!"

"I sometimes think," Hugh wrote her, ". . . that you do not (because of a funny, darling streak of self-deprecation in you) quite realize how deeply he loves you: how much you mean to him . . .

You are in a very real sense (the realest) simply a part of his life."
And Hugh later described a day the three had spent together:

". . . *You sitting in the dining room is a picture stamped forever
on my memory with Havelock one large, shy beam of happiness
opposite; neither looking at the other; me brazenly staring at each
in turn. I, wholly, openly, unblushingly excited; and didn't care a
toss who minded. It was one of the happiest moments of my life and
will remain so.*

The link between them had grown stronger with the years. Yet
if a permanent relationship had been impossible in 1915 or 1916,
it was more impossible today. Ellis needed someone whose life
would be completely subordinated to his writing, his studies, his
daily needs around the house. Margaret's life would never be subordinated to anyone. It would be years before she could win the
birth control fight in America. Now she was carrying the movement
to the rest of the world. She could never separate herself from this
thing that was her very reason for being—even for the man she
called "the wisest man in all England."

What Ellis needed, he found in Françoise Cyon, the "French
woman" he had mentioned in letters to Margaret as early as 1918.
She had come to him first as a patient when the breakup of her
marriage to a Russian Army colonel had brought her to the verge
of a nervous breakdown. "You must not grudge my dear little French
woman the help and consolation she is able to extract from me," Ellis
had written Margaret. Later he described how Françoise "looks
radiantly happy when she comes to Brixton and says I am 'better
than a desert island,' a desert island being her idea of paradise."
Françoise had to struggle to make her living as a schoolteacher
and support her two sons, but she was able to bring Ellis the day-
by-day care and devotion that had been lacking in his life. "There
is no danger of the Irish woman you speak of," Ellis had written
Margaret in answer to her gentle chiding, "being dragged out of my
heart by any French woman." There was room for both, Margaret
knew, and it was better this way. Françoise was to become not only
his secretary but his constant companion.

If all these men, these poets and philosophers, even Ellis, the
giant of them all, could not bring her to the point of marriage, how
then could Slee, who seemed so many worlds apart?

But this very gulf actually drew them together. Marriage for her could mean no diminution of her personal freedom, no cessation in the exhaustive devotion that she gave the birth control movement. None of the others had offered these terms. None of them could give her real stability; none would make their own lives complementary to hers.

In this unique courtship that had lasted almost three years, Slee, the very essence of rugged individualism in his business, had gradually come to accept her on her own terms. It had been a battle of titans in its truest sense. She had always tested herself against the most demanding standards; life for her was a process of testing, whether in her work or her relations with men—her father, Sanger, Ellis—whose Olympian image was a challenge to her own strength.

Yet with all Slee's wealth, social status, and dominating position in his own business world, she had finally brought him to a complete acceptance of her own terms. She laid down a specific platform of personal independence, and he had agreed to it.

She would continue to lead her own life. She would be known as Margaret Sanger in the birth control movement and as Mrs. Slee only at social affairs. She would even keep a separate apartment from his. They would live in the same house but in two apartments, each having an individual key, taking nothing for granted—telephoning each other even for a dinner engagement. She had her own group of friends—intellectuals, writers, artists—who would probably not interest him. He had his business circle. They would entertain separately if necessary. He was a pillar of the Episcopal Church. She loved the opera, which he ignored. Each would make no attempt to interfere with the old pattern of the other's life.

He had an enormous Victorian mansion at Beacon on the Hudson —so sprawling that Margaret insisted she would be lost in its ghostly caverns. He agreed to sell it, and as a wedding present bought her a hundred acres around a willow-circled lake at Fishkill, where they were to build a new house she had designed herself. It was modeled, significantly enough, on the house at Wantley, as if in stone and mortar on the New York earth she wanted to enshrine some permanent vestige of the world of Ellis and De Selincourt.

Even financially, she would accept no compromise with her independence. He had the British attitude that the woman must be protected in marriage and offered to have a pre-nuptial marriage settlement made on her. Margaret flatly refused. She was proud of her ability to support herself, and Slee was openly impressed later when he accidentally opened a letter to her which enclosed a royalty check of twenty-five hundred dollars on one of her books.

Throughout so much of her life she had dealt with men of fire and intellect. Yet it was Slee's conservatism and integrity she admired most. He had built up an unimpeachable record in business. He was one of those men about whom you could say without triteness that his word was his bond. She knew that after he had accepted her terms he would never hedge. "I made it terribly hard for him," she once admitted. "I threw every obstacle in his path." Later there were times, it is true, when he almost rebelled.

Once, long after their marriage, when she had just ended months of grinding work in Washington in an effort to push through an amendment to the federal law on birth control, she was close to exhaustion. The bill had been defeated. All she could think of was to get away for a rest. She called up Slee at Willow Lake, the name of their new house, and suggested that he take her to Bermuda for a week. But he exploded angrily into the phone, "Here I sit alone in this big house, only servants as companions day after day. I could be sick; I could die in the night. You wouldn't know or care." He continued his outburst without giving her a chance to talk. Finally, without a word, she hung up the phone, called her secretary in New York to get her a cabin on the ship to Nassau departing late that afternoon, and sailed without even leaving him a message.

Slee immediately called back her Washington office, and learning she had gone to New York, concluded she was sailing for Bermuda. Repentant now, he booked passage on the Bermuda boat, found to his annoyance she was not aboard, and flew back to New York—only to find that her office still had no word from her. He then returned to Willow Lake to wait and think things out. "He knew he had been rude on the phone," she explained later, "but never in all his experience before with women had rudeness not paid! Here was a very different person to deal with. He put a bottle of French Cliquot champagne on ice, started a fire in the fireplace, took out his pipe, and ordered a good dinner. My week in Nassau had now ended. I, too, was jittery but rebellious. I realized how spoiled a man he was with a rough exterior but a great, gentle heart. He admired women who struck out on their own though in his heart he had not the faintest idea that any woman could make good without a man's guidance.

"Determined to take no nonsense, I finally caught the train two hours after his for Beacon. I took a taxi and told the driver to wait. I decided to pack up and leave if one word of complaint or one shout or blast greeted me at the door. I opened the door to see the handsomest man I ever saw in a velvet smoking jacket, smoking a pipe by the blazing fire, the police dog at his feet. He looked up, calling, 'Hello, darling, did you have a good time in Bermuda?' We rushed into each other's arms and laughed and partly cried. He dismissed the taxi with a typical aside: 'Damned extravagant when there are three cars on the place! Why should we quarrel when we care so much about each other?' he demanded. 'J. Noah,' I replied, 'you are English, oh so English, and I am pure Irish to the backbone for centuries. For three hundred years the English and Irish have fought, so we have just inherited the routine. But from now on, be careful. Never step on the toes of a redhead Irish woman!' "

What to many people seemed the most obvious reason for the marriage—Slee's wealth—was actually a negative factor in Margaret's eyes. It it certainly true that Slee gave generously to the birth control movement. Yet as one of their closest friends once pointed out, each time he gave a large contribution she treated him with momentary roughness, almost as if to prove that their relationship was totally separated from finances.

Far more important than money were the subsidiary appurtenances it could bring. Margaret had led a nomadic life for so many years, rushing from city to city, from meeting to meeting, that the security and dignity of a well-established home had become a strong need in her life. She was proud of Slee's position, of his commanding bearing and aura of authority that brought waiters in the most exclusive restaurants immediately rushing to his side. Further, the birth control movement had long since lost its radical character. It had gained international stature. It was attracting wide support now from leaders in the scientific, medical, and political worlds. The imposing home they would soon establish at Willow Lake would be a valuable setting to her work. That Christmas, Margaret had her picture taken in a distinguished gown and sent a print to De Selincourt. It was a striking pose, a pose that told the world, as Hugh wrote: "Yes, and I'll have you know I'm Queen of the Drawing Room too."

And what was the most important thing she gave Mr. Slee? He considered her the most beautiful, the most fascinating woman alive. He was wildly and unashamedly in love with her, and despite his earlier abhorrence of feminists, tremendously proud of the movement she led. Whenever they were introduced later at dinners or parties as Mr. and Mrs. Slee, he would always whisper to the person he had just met, "That woman is my wife. But she is also *the* Margaret Sanger."

But one factor stood out above the rest. At a party, a friend of hers, meeting Slee for the first time, once asked him quite bluntly after a few drinks what had brought Margaret and him together. "It's obviously an impertinent question, young man," Slee retorted, "but I'll tell you. Before I met Margaret, nothing important had ever happened to me. She was, and always will be, the greatest adventure of my life."

They were married in London before a Justice of the Peace, but Margaret insisted that no public announcement be made. She was still too concerned about the enormous diversity in their lives to be certain that the marriage would work. A few close friends, however, were notified, and De Selincourt immediately wrote her: "It's good to know that there's someone to look after you and cherish you all the time. Shall I like Mr. Slee?" he asked. Then he added from the deep wisdom of one who had already basked in her special radiance: "I don't see how I can help it (much as I want to hate him out of natural spite and envy) if he is much with you, for your beauty is so damnably infectious . . ."

CHAPTER 18

If Mr. Slee thought he could delay Margaret Sanger's return to the Birth Control League with an extended honeymoon, he soon found he was wrong. She insisted on sailing for New York in the fall. She had been away too long—on the quiet sea voyages, in the intensive periods of meditation where her plans and dreams were always hammered into blueprints for action, she had at last decided on one of the major steps of her life: the Clinical Research Bureau.

A leading factor in this decision were the letters that had been piling up in her office—almost two hundred thousand. Now they kept coming in at the rate of ten thousand a month. These were the letters from mothers all over the country, intimate, pleading voices, each of them touching the deepest places of her heart, fusing their need and urgency with her own flesh.

Each letter was a testament of pain and supplication. Here was a young mother of seven children, Mrs. A.R. of Vandergrift, Pennsylvania, who wrote on January 29, 1923:

. . . The doctor said when the last one was born that I should not have any more children, but when I asked him what I could do, he simply said nothing. I would rather die than have any more . . . Please, dear Mrs. Sanger, will you tell me what to do . . . ?

Here was Mrs. B.S. of Cleveland:

I have went to doctors and had illegal operations performed until I couldn't afford it any longer and then tried doing it myself until I'm afraid I'll have myself ruined . . . I am so nervous I just think I would lose my mind . . .

And a Michigan mother of twenty-nine:

I have had four living children and two are dead, one miscarriage and one stillborn and the other was dead when born . . . I lost

*my leg through childbirth . . . I have been married ten years and
I have had six children. Oh God, I wouldn't want any more.*

All these voices, echoing down through the years, emphasized
the necessity of the Clinical Research Bureau. Margaret Sanger had
always answered these letters personally until their volume had
reached such proportions that a special department of the league
with three secretaries had to be organized to handle them. At first,
she had sent each mother a copy of *Family Limitation*. Then as the
league had compiled a larger file of doctors friendly to birth control,
she had sent each mother the name of the nearest doctor—but "nearest" often meant a hundred miles—to whom she could turn for advice. But all this was a stopgap. The only fundamental answer to
this mass of human need and misery was a chain of birth control
clinics from coast to coast.

Mrs. Sanger had waited for this point in the historical evolution
of the movement. Eight years of struggle had gone into the preparation for this moment. People who considered her impulsive never
grasped the basic depth of her thinking. She had decided on the
clinical approach after careful analysis and meditation. She had
built toward it methodically. It had taken education and propaganda to emphasize the value of the clinics over the nonscientific
approach of Mary Ware Dennett and her Voluntary Parenthood
League which wanted contraceptive material available to everyone
as a gesture of free speech and information. By opening the Brownsville clinic, Mrs. Sanger had tested the law. In the Crane decision
of 1918, she had won some protection for the medical profession.
Now at last it would be possible to secure a medical director to run
the clinic.

She had long ago worked out the blueprint of what an ideal clinic
must be. "I saw the clinic not as an isolated social agency, but
functioning as an integral factor of public and racial health, forming
an integral part of all prenatal and postnatal agencies for maternal
and child welfare," she wrote. "I envisaged it as well organized as
the public school system. Indeed, from my point of view these sys-
tems of clinics were to be schools—centers, primarily in contraceptive technique, but schools as well for all problems of parenthood,
for men as well as for women . . ."

Since such a center would obviously come under immediate attack
from the enemies of birth control, she was convinced that it must
be kept separate from the American Birth Control League. Later

she would organize a board of advisors—such prominent doctors, scientists, and laymen as Dr. John Favill of Chicago, Dr. Adolph Myer, the Johns Hopkins psychiatrist, Dr. C. C. Little, President of the University of Michigan, Professors L. J. Cole and Raymond Pearl, and Mrs. Dexter Blagden and Mrs. Lewis Delafield. But for now she would have to take full responsibility for its financing and management. She would always have to take these major steps alone. "Never in all my life had I wanted money so desperately as I did during this period," she recalled.

After weeks of attempted money raising, she remembered the pledge that her English friends, Mr. and Mrs. Clinton Chance, had made two years back—that if she ever needed support for a major project she should call on them. She sent them a telegram and received an immediate telegram in return, pledging six thousand dollars to pay the doctor's salary.

It took additional months of search to find a medical director. To an enthusiastic young woman with the Georgia Public Health Service who volunteered, Mrs. Sanger wrote on October 17, 1922, giving a frank estimate of the risks involved:

. . . We would open the clinic on the authority of the Court of Appeals of the State of New York . . . this would be in the capacity of the physician's private practice, which means that if you would do clinical work, we would not advertise the opening of the clinic . . .

Now, I want to be perfectly frank with you and tell you exactly what I think; for I want you to come into this work with us in the same spirit that we are in it—and that is to give all you have and take the consequences for good or for bad. By that I mean there is a possibility of your going to jail, or at least of your standing trial, also, as you state yourself, of losing your New York state license . . .

On the other hand, for one doctor to stand up and assert her right under this legal opinion would give tremendous impetus and encouragement to thousands of other doctors throughout the country to do likewise.

Here was the crux of Margaret Sanger's whole philosophy of action—that progress could only come by a series of brave, often defiant steps, standing out as a symbol, a clarion call, and giving strength and direction to those who followed her.

This doctor agreed to take the post, and the center was opened

in January 1923 in two rooms in the same building as the Birth
Control League's offices at 104 Fifth Avenue. The choice of the
location was purposeful. Since the center would not publicize its
activities, its patients would consist primarily of women who came
to the league's office for advice and would then be directed immediately to the doctor.

On the door of the center was stenciled in black letters only two
words: "Clinical Research." The words summed up Margaret
Sanger's vision—that in its early stages the center would concentrate on the task of testing and evaluating the best methods of
contraception so that when other clinics followed, as she knew they
would, she would be ready to supply them with the most highly
developed scientific information. She saw it as "a laboratory . . .
dealing with human beings instead of white mice, with every consideration for environment, personality and background." It would
be an experimental bureau designed to demonstrate the practicabil-
ity of birth control clinics in all states and towns, to demonstrate
its influence as a social force and prove itself as a health center.

The file card on each patient was aimed at developing a complete medical and sociological study. Both the husband's and wife's
occupation, income, nationality, and religion were recorded. There
were questions on miscarriages, stillbirths, and abortions, whether
therapeutic, accidental, or self-induced. Mrs. Sanger was determined
to enlarge the whole area of sex knowledge in marriage. Thirty
years before such scientific researchers as Dr. Kinsey, the bureau's
questionnaires probed the patient's attitudes toward the marital relationship, coitus, and the relationship of menstrual periods to cycles
of desire.

In its first year, the bureau made rapid strides toward becoming
a study center for doctors, social-service workers, clergymen, and
Red Cross workers. The faculty of the Cornell's School of Home
Economics conducted special research there. One social worker of
the United Hebrew Charities of Chicago came for a day and stayed
for two weeks of observation. Of the first twenty-seven hundred
women who applied, only eighteen hundred were given contraceptive information since Mrs. Sanger insisted that the center stay carefully within the limits of the Crane decision. These cases formed the
basis of its first report—a report that was the focus of the Midwestern
States Birth Control Conference in Chicago on October 29, 1923.
The conference presented a list of distinguished speakers, including

Miss Jane Addams of Hull House, Judge Harry Olson of the Chicago Municipal Court, Rabbi Louis L. Mann, and Professors E. A. Ross, E. M. East, and C. C. Little. But it was the report that stirred the conference, for here at last was the first concrete evidence of the impact of birth control information, rigidly controlled and evaluated.

The Chicago Birth Control League under Dr. Rachelle Yarros and Mrs Benjamin Carpenter now decided to open its own clinic. It applied for a license. But the Health Commissioner of Chicago, Dr. Herman Bundesen, vigorously opposed the application, basing his arguments not on scientific grounds but on lengthy and impassioned quotations from the Bible. The league promptly went to the courts, and from Judge Harry Fisher secured a writ of mandamus that forced the city to grant the license. The judge's decision was a significant victory for medical progress. "Under our system of government," he stated pointedly, "courts cannot be called upon to officially interpret the Bible or to lend or withhold their processes to enforce Biblical injunctions."

The Chicago clinic, the second in the United States, was dramatic testament of Margaret Sanger's ability to infuse her dream with such devotion and radiant energy that it came to life in others with the same glowing intensity. She did not build her movement with paperwork. She built it with action and a spirit that produced action in whatever it touched.

In those first years "that remain in my memory as ones of smiles and tears, of heartaches and anxieties," she spent long hours each day at the New York center establishing the pattern of operation that would remain as an ideal through the years. Most women were frightened to step into this strange new world where science touched the most intimate moments of their married life. The waiting room was crowded—often as many as twenty mothers, each frequently bringing a brood of children. A dozen languages were spoken, but principally Spanish, Italian, and Yiddish. Mrs. Sanger soon employed a special interpreter to make these mothers feel at home. She gave explicit instructions to the nurse on duty. "We must welcome each mother as if we were placing a prayer rug before her. Think what these few minutes mean. During the time she spends at the center, the devotion, information, and service we give her can reconstruct her whole life."

Despite the opposition of the Catholic hierarchy, the center's records show that from its opening almost a third of the patients were Catholic. It took special courage, often an act of real desperation, for these women to come. In the early days, Mrs. Sanger herself took their case histories and instructed them sympathetically in the principles of birth control. One shy woman, who gave her age as twenty-eight, but whose reddened and exhausted face made her look forty, told how she had borne six children, one after another, until her health had reached the breaking point. The thought of another child had brought her almost to suicide. She had purposely fought with her husband to keep him away from her at night. The tension had become unbearable. Last night, she had walked back and forth along the river. "As a Catholic, I could not face the idea of suicide," she said. "I kept praying for God to give me the courage to jump. But I couldn't do it. This morning I read a small article in the newspaper about your clinic. It was like God's answer."

Mrs. Sanger asked one timid girl, obviously Irish, how long she had been married. "Long enough to have four kids," she said. She raised her blouse. "Look at me. Just past twenty-one and I've got scars all over my kidneys. Many nights, Jimmy would sleep on the floor and pray to God to keep him from temptation. The last pregnancy I was taken to the hospital for a Caesarean. It was so bad they were saying Masses for me. But I pulled through. Then the doctor said, 'You can't have any more. The next one will kill you.' I begged him to tell me what to do, but he said, 'I can't tell you.' Jimmy went to the priest and said he'd go away and leave his family before there was another child. He begged the priest to tell him where he could get the information. 'God should strike you dead,' the priest said. Jimmy said, 'But, Father, you prayed to God to keep my wife alive. The same God can't want to keep her alive and kill her with another child.' That night Jimmy asked a nurse he knew and she said to look up the Sanger clinic in the phone book. That's how I came here."

At the end of the clinic's second year of operation in 1924, Mrs. Sanger decided to enlarge its services by asking other physicians to give volunteer time and intensify the research into contraceptive techniques. She saw the necessity of replacing the present doctor in charge with a medical director of more experience and gynecological training. This was a drastic, perhaps a ruthless move. But if Mrs. Sanger was ruthless on occasions, she was motivated always by principle. With deep insight into the direction of the movement, she considered it essential to adhere rigidly to her long-range plan of action despite the sacrifice of a few individuals along the way. Subsequent events invariably proved her wisdom. In this case, the replacement of the first doctor by Dr. Hannah Stone brought the clinic an era of unparalleled progress and gave the movement one of its most distinguished leaders for the next eighteen years.

Dr. Stone, wife of the urologist, Dr. Abraham Stone, first met Mrs. Sanger in 1921 after the Town Hall conference and had served on the first advisory medical committee. An emergency meeting of these doctors was called. Where could they find a doctor with sufficient stature to run this enlarged program in the face of continued hostility from the medical profession? Dr. Stone quietly said she would take the risk. She would become medical director—and without salary.

She was then on the staff of the Lying-In Hospital. The director called her into his office and told her to abandon the clinic idea. "I must go ahead with it," she said. "My work in this hospital has convinced me of the medical importance of birth control." The director retorted bluntly, "No doctor at this hospital can be associated with birth control. Either you drop the clinic or give up your hospital position." She went home that night and wrote out her letter of resignation to the hospital.

The risk she took was soon borne out when her application for membership in the New York County Medical Society was tabled—and not accepted until years later, when birth control had achieved suitable respectability.

But Dr. Stone had the courage and faith to meet such challenges. She had "a madonna-like beauty which, coupled with her kindliness and graciousness, seemed a fitting complement to her position and inspired confidence in all who met her," Mrs. Sanger once said. "Her gaze was clear and straight, her hair was black, her mouth gentle and sweet." What fitted her so uniquely for this role, Mrs. Sanger said another time, was "her infinite patience, her attention to details, her understanding of human frailties, her sympathy and her gentleness."

With her husband, Abraham Stone, she was to make a balanced and expert team in the field of birth control and marriage counseling. Together they would set up marriage-counseling services at the Labor Temple and at Dr. John Haynes Holmes' Community Church and write *A Marriage Manual,* one of the most authoritative and widely read works in the field.

Not long after Dr. Stone became medical director, the number of patients increased so rapidly that Mrs. Sanger decided the center must have larger quarters. In an old brownstone house off Fifth Avenue at 46 West Fifteenth Street, she found an inexpensive basement suite. It was not the best neighborhood, the street constantly lined with trucks making deliveries to nearby lofts, factories, and warehouses. But the basement was converted into an efficient clinic with a large reception room and a smaller anteroom that became a playground for the children. For the first time, the secretary had a special room in which to take the patient's history. The doctors had individual consultation rooms, an examination room, and a treatment room.

The new center stayed open all day. As Dr. Stone brought in more doctors to assist her, two evening sessions were added—yet the waiting list was so long there was a two-week delay for appointments. The number of patients in 1925 totaled 1,655; by 1929, the number had jumped to 9,737. But these figures do not reflect the fact that each patient made an average of at least three visits. In addition, thousands of patients each year who did not qualify for birth control information under the Crane decision had to be turned away.

From Dr. Stone's 1925 report comes a concise picture of the average patient. Over 70 per cent of the families earned under fifty dollars a week, the average family income being thirty-six dollars. Thirty-eight per cent of the mothers were Protestant; 32 per cent Jewish; and 26 per cent Catholic. The urgent need for birth control information was demonstrated by the statistics on self-induced abortions. Out of 1,655 patients, these totaled 1,434, varying from one to as many as forty in one particular case.

Margaret Sanger had envisioned the clinic as the spearhead of the movement, slowly breaking down the hostility of the medical profession as it proved its scientific worth. This objective was well on the way toward being achieved by 1925. In that year alone, over ten thousand letters came to the clinic from doctors all over the country, requesting contraceptive information. The extent of this demand caused her to make a contraceptive session for doctors, directed by Dr. Stone, the focus of the Sixth International Birth Control Conference in New York in 1925. A thousand doctors tried to gain admission to this session—so huge a turnout that the hall rented for the occasion could not hold them and a second session had to be held.

What technique had Dr. Stone found most effective so far in her research? The answer was the diaphragm—the same technique brought back from Holland by Margaret Sanger in 1915—a vaginal device made in various sizes so that it had to be fitted specially to each patient after careful gynecological examination.

The diaphragm achieved its highest point of protection when it was combined with a chemical jelly. Mrs. Sanger had brought one jelly back from Germany. But because of import problems, the supply was small, and one of its ingredients, manufactured only in Germany, was too expensive to duplicate here. Dr. Stone and her husband, along with Dr. James F. Cooper, who had recently joined the clinic, were now working on other formulas, which would be "entirely harmless to the tissues and yet a reliable and efficient spermaticide."

From the 1925 conference, it was obvious that the rank and file of the medical profession was slowly giving its support to birth control—the prominent medical organizations lagging far behind. In general, they still considered Mrs. Sanger a propagandist; her name, they felt, had the taint of courtrooms and jails. If this criticism hurt her, she kept it carefully hidden and concentrated on the objective ahead. In her blueprint for the growth of clinics across the country, the support of the medical leadership was vital. The man whose support she needed most of all was Dr. Robert L. Dickinson.

Dr. Dickinson had been Senior Gynecologist at Brooklyn Hospital and Professor of Gynecology and Medicine at Long Island Medical College. Now, recognized as the dean of American gynecologists, he had retired to devote himself to the Committee on Maternal Health, a group of recognized authorities, backed by leading foundations, which laid particular emphasis on the problems of fertility and contraception. To get the backing of this committee would be like the final accolade.

At first, Dr. Dickinson believed the birth control clinic should not be an independent entity like the Clinical Research Bureau, but part of a major hospital. He had convinced seven New York hospitals to add a birth control information service. But by October 22, 1925, he was ready to admit that his approach was wrong. In a letter to Dr. C. C. Little, he stated frankly that "patients were shy of such

places and the doctors mostly timorous." In addition, he had been
deeply impressed by the 1925 report of the Clinical Research Bureau
at the Sixth International Conference.

During the next two years, long and complex negotiations were
carried on between Margaret Sanger and Dr. Dickinson to gain the
support of his Committee on Maternal Health for the center. Dr.
Dickinson insisted that the clinic must have more "representative,
responsible medical control." This, in effect, was a polite way of
saying that Mrs. Sanger's advisory board still did not include gynecologists and pediatricians of sufficient stature. But Dr. Little and
other nonmedical members of the board felt that they had taken
the early risks when few doctors would join them and they feared
that Dr. Dickinson might aim at gaining control of the center himself.

In 1927, Mrs. Sanger submitted a compromise plan which suggested that the center be completely separated from the American
Birth Control League, whose propaganda and educational activities
disturbed Dr. Dickinson. Even this plan was held in abeyance for
a year, until the center's 1928 report, prepared by Dr. Stone, completely won him over. A milestone in birth control history, the report
gave the center a new stature that had been Mrs. Sanger's goal all
these years. It was based on a three-year study of eleven hundred
cases—so thorough and controlled a study that Dr. Dickinson himself fought to have it printed in the March 21 issue of the *Medical
Journal and Record,* the first time that one of the leading medical
journals had touched the subject.

Dr. Stone's report was overwhelming proof of the efficiency of
scientific contraception. Of the two methods recommended by the
clinic, the diaphragm combined with some form of jelly, and the
jelly used alone, the diaphragm and jelly method had a record of
only 4 per cent failures, the jelly alone of 9 per cent failures.

In his laudatory preface to the report, Dr. Dickinson wrote: "I
believe this to be the first considerable and detailed study of the
efficacy of contraceptive measures combined with reliable follow-up
that has ever been made . . . This report constitutes a pioneer
contribution."

In 1929, the center was completely separated from the Birth Control League. In 1930, Dr. Dickinson gave it his final stamp of approval by joining its advisory board and threw the full weight of
his authority behind Mrs. Sanger.

It had been seven years since the center's founding, seven years in which Margaret Sanger, despite opposition, abuse, and apathy, pushed determinedly on. Few people knew the heartaches of those years; she rarely revealed her pain even to close friends. But in a few lines in his column in the New York *Telegram* on April 20, 1931, Heywood Broun caught the flame of that spirit which had turned a two-room center into a nationally recognized institution. "No living American has been assailed with more obscene abuse," he wrote. ". . . Hers was a forlorn hope and seemingly a doomed cause. She knew she was right and she just kept rolling along."

This spirit was not just confined to the New York center. It radiated and gave its strength to every member league. It turned hopes into reality in city after city. Chicago had been the second clinic. Then came the Maternal Health Center of New Jersey, which operated under Dr. Hannah Stone's direction. By 1928, there were clinics in Baltimore, Detroit, and Cleveland, and two new ones in Chicago. By 1929, Buffalo and Philadelphia added clinics; in California, Los Angeles had seven, Alameda County four, San Francisco three. By 1930, there were fifty-five birth control clinics in twenty-three cities in twelve states—an almost miraculous realization of the dream that had started with the Brownsville clinic and indictment and jail for Mrs. Sanger only a little more than a decade earlier.

CHAPTER 19

No one understood the two Margaret Sangers better than Hugh De Selincourt. "There is the stern Margaret devoted to a Cause who makes my knees shake to think of with awe and fear at her sheer tremendousness," he wrote her. "There is, however, the Margaret of jasmine tea and Rose Liqueur, the Margaret of exquisite dearness and loveliness. . . ."

In 1925, a decisive year in her life, the first Margaret was to achieve the final transformation of the birth control movement from its revolutionary heritage to a bold new scientific force that would soon shape the population of the world. The second Margaret would take title as the reigning queen of Willow Lake, her Hudson River estate.

Mr. Slee had given it to her as a wedding present—"a magnificent home which, it is said, will cost nearly a million dollars," reported the Poughkeepsie *Star* on February 18, 1924. This estimate was greatly exaggerated, as newspaper accounts about Mrs. Sanger were apt to be, but it was certainly true that Willow Lake was a show place of manorial proportions. The main house of local gray field stone sat almost at the edge of a large lake, rimmed by willow trees. It had three stories, with a slanting, gray-blue slate roof and exuded the unshakable solidity of sixteenth-century English manor life. The main floor was occupied by a handsome, beamed living room, a library, the dining room, breakfast room, and kitchen, with a sports room on the ground level. Four master bedrooms, two with fireplaces, an enclosed sleeping porch, and two servants' rooms were on the second floor. On a rise at a far corner of the lake was a six-room gardener's cottage, almost a replica of the main house, with additional servants' quarters.

It is not surprising that De Selincourt, in honor of J. Noah H. Slee, dubbed the house "Noah's Ark" and teased Margaret about her accession to manorial splendor by writing, "I shall come to see it in the autumn in a fur coat and a monocle and patent leather boots, driving my own automobile."

She and Slee kept a stable of horses and rode almost every morning before breakfast through the surrounding hills. No one, she always explained, could have ridden *after* one of her husband's typically British breakfasts of fruit, eggs, potatoes, and a wide variety of sausages and meats. Willow Lake, which also included a tennis court, was fashioned for entertaining. On week ends, in addition to her own guests, she held regular open house for Stuart and Grant and swarms of their friends, including the young ladies from nearby Vassar college.

Margaret Sanger's laughter filled the house on these week ends—one of her more poetic English friends, Harold Child, describing it as "the laughter of God," and another friend ascribing to it all the effervescence of bubbling champagne. An excellent cook, she made a particular specialty of mixing her salads for parties right at the table in the multicolored butterfly bowl she had brought back from China. Another tradition was the costume parties she had inherited from Easton Glebe. But she added an extra touch to H. G. Wells' revelry. For an evening in Indian costume, she prepared and cooked a complete and authentic Indian dinner—well flavored by her spice chest, to which friends continually contributed condiments from all over the world. The climax of these evenings—two occupations in which Margaret Sanger particularly excelled—was dancing on the grass and midnight swimming in the lake.

Although Slee's relations with his children had never been harmonious, she made a special effort to bring them and his grandchildren (for whom a special nurse was employed during the summer) to Willow Lake. "Her child relatives all adore her and think there is no one quite like 'Aunt Marg,'" Slee's daughter, Mrs. Elizabeth Willis, once wrote. "She is a regular fairy godmother who sympathizes with all their thoughts and feelings and makes their dreams come true."

Mrs. Sanger herself had planned and supervised the magnificent gardens which were Willow Lake's prize—the rock garden, the rose arbor, the delphinium garden, the iris path, and especially the large groves of lilac bushes a few hundred yards from the house which hid her private, elevated study, "Tree Tops." It was here she came to work—except for week ends, the house was completely absorbed in the work of the birth control movement. In this cottage among the lilacs, with its unobstructed view of the Hudson and the distant Catskill Mountains, she could cut herself off from the world, write articles and books, and give herself to that intense brooding which always preceded her major decisions.

Most days, even in the summer, Mrs. Sanger commuted the hour-and-a-half trip to New York. She was an exceptional organizer—writing out the day's menu and the orders for the staff early each morning before she caught the eight-thirty train, leaving Slee huffing and grumbling about "this damned nonsense" of keeping a beautiful house for your wife and then having her run off to the hot city to work with "a lot of crazy women."

Slee was convinced he could gradually wean her from her exhausting schedule in the movement. He was gruff and domineering—though many of Mrs. Sanger's friends rejoiced that he occasionally was able to take her off on vacation trips, usually on the plea that the trip was for *his* health. "Tell Mr. Slee I think he was sent from heaven," Mrs. Ackerman wrote her, "to keep you alive to see clinics all over the United States."

Actually it was Mrs. Sanger who slowly converted the indomitable Mr. Slee. It was a continuous and delightful tug of war, this marriage in which she set out to prove that a woman in love could still preserve her own independent life on her own terms. She never ceased to remind him that she had built a national movement and financed it before he had entered her life. Writing from San Francisco on one speaking tour, she pointedly described the "ten telegrams from places around here asking for dates and willing to *pay*. I could easily make another thousand dollars in two weeks and not work any harder than I have in the last three."

In New York, where they lived at 39 Fifth Avenue, one of those new luxury buildings springing up north of Washington Square, she maintained every clause of their compact of independence. They had separate apartments, with the kitchen and dining room in her suite. They telephoned each other for dinner or theater engagements or passed notes back and forth—a system, significantly enough, that had been adopted by that earlier woman rebel, Mary Wollstonecraft, who over a hundred years before when she was about to give birth to their first child, wrote hourly reports to her philosopher-husband, William Godwin, living a few blocks away.

Slee soon found himself involved deeper and deeper in the movement. In 1925, he contributed over fifteen thousand dollars to birth
control—in succeeding years, often far more. One project in which
she particularly wanted Slee's support was the retention of Dr. James
F. Cooper to lecture on birth control to medical groups throughout
the country. In a charming compact with her husband, formalized
by this letter, she persuaded him to pay Dr. Cooper's salary.

Feb. 2, 1925

To Noah H. Slee:
1925 is to be the big year for the break in birth control. If Dr.
Cooper's association with us is successful, I feel certain that the
medical profession will take up the work. When the medical pro-
fession does this in the USA, I shall feel that I have made my con-
tribution to the cause and shall feel that I can withdraw from
full-time activity. I shall still want to publish the Review *and take*
some interest in it and write articles and books on subjects allied
with BC.
Even should this not occur in one year, I shall be satisfied having
a Committee taking responsibility off my shoulder.
It is estimated that Dr. Cooper will cost about $10,000 salary and
expenses for 1 year. His work will be to lecture before Medical
Societies and Associations—getting their cooperation and influence
to give contraceptive information in clinics, private and public.
If I am able to accomplish this victory with Dr. Cooper's help, I
shall bless my adorable husband, JNH Slee, and retire with him
to the garden of love.

Sealed, signed and delivered,
Margaret Sanger

Mrs. Sanger not only did not "retire to the garden of love," but
that same year drew her seemingly iron-willed industrialist into the
very thick of the birth control fight by convincing him to become
treasurer of the Clinical Research Bureau.

2

The retention of Dr. Cooper was Margaret Sanger's first major
move in this "big year for the break in birth control." She was convinced that no other factor was more essential now than the support
of the medical profession. It was an objective that would take almost

a decade to accomplish—yet the plan she laid down now proved itself strategically faultless to the end.

Dr. Cooper, a distinguished-looking gynecologist who had been a medical missionary in Fuchow, China, and gave up a flourishing Boston practice to accept the post, had all the crusading zeal necessary to tackle the most apathetic doctors. In addition, he had the prestige which would make him welcome in any medical circle. The Birth Control League laid out the schedule of cities he would visit by writing ahead to those doctors who had already shown interest in the movement. But in many smaller towns he was a veritable pioneer, ringing doorbells from block to block to rally the support of local doctors.

In Nashville, Tennessee, he reported he was "footsore and weary" after interviewing twenty-six doctors and university medical professors in two days. "Birth control is needed here as much as anywhere, and the women want it, but oh, the indifference they meet." Often he stayed only a day in one town. "These one-night stands are certainly the life," he wrote from Marshall, Texas. "Marshall to Paris tomorrow. One hundred miles by bus. Real covered-wagon stuff." From San Antonio, he wrote Mrs. Sanger: "I glory in the pioneering work."

In most cities, however, he found large and appreciative audiences. Contraceptive information was still pitifully limited—even medical journals carried no articles yet. "A wonderful reception," Dr. Cooper reported from Atlanta. "Seven doctors called me up the next day and said my address was the talk of the town in medical circles." At Dallas, Texas, a public meeting was held right at City Hall. In Des Moines, Iowa, there was "a live group, anxious to work." From Greensboro, North Carolina, he reported: "The president of the Medical Society is the boldest man in town, and he sponsored the meeting. . . . I never saw such interests and requests to return. . . ." In that first year, Dr. Cooper covered twenty-four states; in 1926, he was to touch every state except Vermont.

The crucial question put to Dr. Cooper at meeting after meeting was: where could doctors obtain their contraceptive supplies? As a result of the clinic's studies, Dr. Cooper was recommending the diaphragm pessary combined with chemical jelly technique. But the supply of diaphragms was almost nonexistent. No company in the United States was manufacturing them. The U. S. Customs Law forbade their importation. The clinic could only obtain them through a few druggists who had the courage to smuggle them into the country—and from those staunch women of the Birth Control League who gladly became amateur smugglers on returning from their European travels.

The best diaphragms were made in Germany. Since they were available throughout Europe, many women supporters of birth control never returned from abroad without bringing a few dozen stuffed in their pockets, handbags, or muffs. One of the oldest and most revered names in the New York Social Register went through Customs with a large supply strapped around her waist. The league's office received frequent telephone calls, particularly at the end of the summer vacation period. "I just got back from England," a familiar voice would murmur. "Please send someone over for the jewels."

Although a German contraceptive company began to manufacture diaphragms in New York, Mrs. Sanger, with her unshakable faith that hundreds of clinics would soon be in operation, decided that a new company must be brought into the business. She asked Herbert Simonds, who was now an engineer in Boston, to survey the country's leading rubber manufacturers. But after months of interviewing one executive after another, he reported that no established house would touch so controversial a product.

The only alternative, she insisted, was for him to start the business himself. The challenge appealed to him. With a thousand-dollar investment, Simonds opened a small office and obtained a second partner who invested $432. Mr. Slee loaned them a few thousand dollars more.

Within a few years, they had built a prosperous company. Margaret Sanger had known they would. Yet she scrupulously refrained from entering the business herself, though it would have made her a millionaire. All through the movement she refused to touch any commercial venture, knowing how easily her enemies could use such a connection as a weapon against her. Still, when she was campaigning later for changes in federal legislation on birth control, these very smear tactics were tried. On one occasion, she retorted hotly, "Not long ago, I myself was offered nearly a quarter of a million dollars to speak on the radio for a chemical product." She turned down the offer flatly. At a party that same year, when she was desperately trying to raise funds for the federal campaign, a doctor came up to her and said, "I have a special admiration for you, Mrs. Sanger. I've always wanted to shake the hand of a woman who's made millions for others and is still passing out a tin cup for pennies for her own movement."

3

Ever since the Town Hall raid in 1921, the Catholic hierarchy had followed a new and more drastic policy in its opposition to birth control. It saw that Margaret Sanger and the Birth Control League were no longer irritating thorns; they were opponents of the first rank who must be crushed as quickly as possible. The new policy was to attack them at every opportunity—attacks that were usually launched through the Church's influence in the big-city political machines.

In Albany, New York, the attack came through Mayor William Hackett himself. The New York Birth Control League was holding its conference on February 20, 1923, at the Ten Eyck Hotel, with Mrs. Sanger scheduled to address the meeting that night when the Mayor at the last minute forced the hotel to cancel its booking—though the hall had been paid for. "Free speech might as well be a card in the hands of a conjurer," Heywood Broun described the incident acidly in his column. "Now you see it and now you don't."

As always, Margaret Sanger fought back with relish. Late that afternoon she telephoned one birth control supporter after another in Albany until she found a home large enough to hold the meeting. It went on that night as scheduled—an invitation even being sent to Mayor Hackett.

These attacks frequently used business as well as political pressure. When the 1923 convention of the Ohio State Birth Control League was scheduled for Cincinnati's Hotel Gibson, the local Knights of Columbus chapter warned the hotel that if it did not cancel the convention it would not only withdraw its own dinner but boycott all other events at the hotel. Despite these threats, the hotel, which had a number of Masons among its directors, stood by its commitment—though the Knights of Columbus eventually canceled its dinner.

Throughout 1925 and 1926, Mrs. Sanger conducted legislative campaigns to introduce birth control bills in New York, Connecticut, and New Jersey—campaigns where the Catholic opposition grew so bitter that in the New Jersey legislature, "Personal attacks were hurled across the Assembly chamber," the New York *Journal* reported.

In March 1925, Harvard's Liberal Club gave a luncheon in Mrs. Sanger's honor. Only fifty people had been invited but the table was eventually expanded to one hundred and fifty places, and hundreds more were turned away. Raging against her appearance in his bailiwick, Mayor Curley of Boston, reported the Boston *Telegram,* "declared war on birth control" and promised to remove the license of any hall that offered her its platform.

Mrs. Sanger could never be bullied—especially when her Irish blood was pitted against another Irishman. A few years later Boston's renowned Ford Hall Forum, hailing her as the "outstanding social warrior of the century," invited her to its annual dinner. Mrs. Sanger turned Curley's threats into a national joke by sitting in the speaker's chair with a large piece of tape across her mouth while someone else read her speech.

Although Jewish groups had been among the first supporters of birth control, there was still determined opposition from some of the orthodox congregations. When Rabbi Mischkind of New York's Tremont Temple invited Mrs. Sanger to speak, the board of trustees forbade her appearance. Rabbi Mischkind boldly stood his ground, resigned, and found another temple, where she was welcomed.

Through her own firmness in fighting back against every form of censorship, Margaret Sanger passed on to others some spark of her own strength. In Syracuse, when a meeting of the New York Birth Control League was scheduled for February 1924, the Catholic block in the City Council managed to have an ordinance passed making such meetings illegal. The league immediately began a house-to-house campaign to rouse the city. It took advertisements in local newspapers: "Free speech has been forbidden you! . . . Are you free Americans or are you subjects of Aldermanic rule?" This campaign encouraged Mayor Walrath to veto the ordinance. The Council's attempt to override the veto was beaten, and the meeting was held on schedule.

In Milwaukee also, Mayor Daniel Hoan stood firm against Catholic pressure when Mrs. Sanger was scheduled to speak. "The idea of stopping something because we do not agree is wrong," he told protesting Catholic groups. "If I forbid Mrs. Sanger a platform, I would have to do the same to you."

Always her policy in these tumultuous years was the simple instrument of action. When the attacks came, she fought back instantly without asking for sympathy or support. ". . . We have never wasted our time and energy whining about our constitutional rights to free speech," she wrote in the *American Mercury* of July 1924. "We have simply spoken out. We have asserted the truth as we have found it."

4

"I think of birth control," said one of Britain's outstanding biologists, Julian Huxley, "not only as something for the alleviation of distress in the present but as the means by which in the long run man can become trustee of the cosmic evolution."

Although it was for the alleviation of distress that Margaret Sanger had first spoken out as the protagonist of motherhood, "any social progress," she stated in her book, *Pivot of Civilization*, ". . . must purge itself of sentimentality and pass through the crucible of science." The year 1925 was to usher in the first stage of this process—a stage she would mark with her keen sense of drama by holding the Sixth International Neo-Malthusian and Birth Control Conference in New York.

Always before these conferences had been held in England or Europe. When she proposed bringing the conference to America, the executive committee of the Birth Control League was appalled. It would take far more money than they believed possible to raise— probably twenty-five thousand dollars. It would mean rounding up outstanding speakers and delegates in Europe and bringing them to New York. Mrs. Sanger brushed aside their objections. When the cause was right, money would follow. She herself would go abroad to line up the speakers. It was against all her principles to delay any major action because of problems of the moment. Accompanied by Juliet Rublee, she promptly sailed for England.

In London, John Maynard Keynes, one of the country's leading economists, entertained in her honor. Harold Cox introduced her at tea to such distinguished birth control advocates as Lady Wright, Lady Oxford, Lord Gerald Wellesley, and Mrs. Graham Murray. H. G. Wells, always tireless in her support, staged a dinner attended by what she called "the best minds in England behind the movement"—Lord Buckmaster, Sir Arbuthnot Lane, Sir Edwin Ray Lankester, Arnold Bennett, St. John Ervine, Walter Salter, and Bernard Shaw.

She had been particularly anxious to have Lord Buckmaster as a speaker—but the conference conflicted with the opening of Parliament. Instead, she secured Harold Cox, J. O. P. Bland, and Dr. C. V.

Drysdale for major addresses while Mrs. Pethick Lawrence, Sir Arbuthnot Lane, Sir George Knibbs, Arnold Bennett, Julian Huxley, Lytton Strachey, Keynes, Wells, and Ellis agreed to be conference vice-presidents. From Bernard Shaw came a witty and stimulating paper for one of the conference sessions. "Birth control," said Mr. Shaw, "should be advocated for its own sake on the basis that the difference between voluntary, irrational, uncontrolled activity is the difference between an amoeba and a man; and if we really believe that the more highly evolved creature is the better, we may as well act accordingly."

Once the groundwork of the conference had been laid, Margaret Sanger set out for "Sand Pit," near Storrington, Sussex, to which the De Selincourts had recently moved from Wantley.

It had been more than two years since she had seen De Selincourt, but he had written to her regularly every week. His love, reflected vividly in his letters, was never diminished by distance. Through Margaret, he seemed to touch the ideal of all womanhood. Through her his life came to full power—"quickening all my energy . . . making everything I care for more previous," he wrote her.

"You must know every atom I can show you," he told her in the midst of those years apart, "of the dearness, the spreading of your power and beauty . . . in the secret hearts of those who love you. . . ."

"I constantly . . . bless Havelock for ever having let me know such a woman existed," he wrote again, describing "that memory of you" as "some lovely perfume in one's heart, forever fresh."

As soon as Margaret reached England, he besieged her with invitations. "Sand Pit," he wrote, "waits for the benediction of Margaret's presence." It was all waiting for her—that "circle" where love was the start and end of life, those magic hours of music by the fireside, the walks on the moors, the talk, the poetry that lasted through the night.

Sand Pit was as hauntingly lovely as Wantley. The two-story house of local stone was four hundred years old—its magnificent oak beams and inglenook fireplaces all perfectly preserved. To the old sunken garden and pool, always the focal point of their life, the De Selincourts had added a whole series of new gardens on different levels, like a stairway of endless color against the tranquil backdrop of woodland silver birches.

They had tried so hard to keep the magic of those former days. But a shadow had touched them, violently and unexpectedly. In the two years that Margaret had been away, the circle had been broken and almost shattered by the very force which had created it. Its simple dedication to love had become agonizingly complex.

It was Ellis whose teachings had built the circle—the "King . . . divinely dear and human and worshipful," they called him. By the worst of ironies, it was Ellis who now recoiled from its practical consequences. De Selincourt's admiration—it was closer to worship—for Ellis had formed an obvious link between him and Françoise Cyon, Ellis' devoted friend. At first, this seemed natural. "I have come to love him," Françoise wrote in explanation to Ellis,[1] "better to unite you both who are friends."

But what had been a natural link between Françoise and De Selincourt turned suddenly to love—a triangle that was further complicated by Françoise's devotion to both men. ". . . I even failed to realize that I was embarking on having two lovers," she admitted.

Ellis was horrified. He refused to see either of them. "No letter, no suggestion of seeing him yet," De Selincourt mourned in a letter to Margaret on May 5, 1923. Françoise called those months "the bitterest ordeal of my life."

She besieged Ellis with frantic and passionate letters. He was the bedrock of her life. She had to have him back even if it meant giving up De Selincourt. But it took over a year. It was not until June 1925 that Ellis invited De Selincourt to visit him and Françoise at their summer cottage, not till August that De Selincourt could write that they had all "emerged from a sort of black hell out into the sunshine and light."

Margaret Sanger, of course, was not touched directly by this triangle. But she was well aware of the twists and turns of the currents of love which swirled through Sand Pit. No one had longed for her arrival more expectantly than De Selincourt. Yet unexpectedly it was Harold Child, gaunt, poetic, dark-eyed Harold, who gave a new and soaring wonder to this visit.

He pursued her all that week at Sand Pit. He followed her to London, filled her room with flowers, took her on long drives to Canterbury and the old English towns, and wrote her every day they were apart.

But their moments were numbered—she had to return to New York

[1] F. L. Delisle, *Friendship's Odyssey* (London: Heinemann, 1946) p. 366ff.

for the conference. It was always like this and would always be like this. They both recognized the fact, and perhaps this was what gave these moments the special intensity of an undiscovered land. In retrospect, it might seem a dazzling game. Few people, even her closest friends, could ever grasp it. Yet for Margaret, Wantley, and now Sand Pit, would always be an integral part of her life.

At home, to the rest of the world, she was the woman rebel, the crusader, the woman triumphant. Here she would always be the woman in love. She needed this in one way as much as she needed the tumult and struggle of the movement in another. It was a testing, a living out of her own faith in the power of love. "What man could help falling in love with you?" Janet De Selincourt wrote her. Now and later, Margaret hoped the question would have only one answer. If the spreading, the cumulative power of her love brought a fullness and completeness to those around her, she had lived her role.

5

Back in New York, refreshed by England and Sand Pit, Margaret Sanger threw herself into the final arrangements for the conference—fund raising, transportation and hotel accommodations for delegates, the schedule of meetings and round tables, the hundreds of last-minute details that had once overawed the league's executive committee. She was like a woman possessed, reaching the office at eight-thirty each morning and often staying almost to midnight. Even her closest associates, swept along in her furious energy, marveled that she could keep going month after month on four or five hours' sleep.

The Sixth International, opening in New York on March 25, 1925, had been conceived on a grand scale. Eight hundred delegates registered. Eighteen countries, including Austria, Czechoslovakia, China, India, Japan, Mexico, Norway, Rumania, and Russia, were represented. Professors came from twenty-four colleges and universities, delegates from seventy-nine religious and sociological organizations. "Representatives of the Episcopalian, Congregational, Unitarian, Baptist, and Jewish churches took their stand with physicians and scientists yesterday in endorsing birth control," reported the New York *Tribune* the day after the opening. Such influential clergymen as Rabbi Stephen Wise, Reverend Karl Reiland, and Dr. Charles Francis Potter led the religious vanguard whose gathering support was essential to the movement.

The conference had been planned to link birth control inextricably with the new science of population. Here was "the great experiment . . . the most important of all social efforts to bring order out of chaos," stated Mrs. Sanger in bringing this theme to the conference in her opening address. "For the first time in the history of the United States, men and women have come from other countries to these shores to consider the population problem."

Population and science—these were the goals that had brought the highest level of intellectual achievement to each conference session and round table. Professors Irving Fisher of Yale, James F. Field of the University of Chicago, and H. H. Laughlin and C. B. Davenport of the Cold Spring Harbor Station for Experimental Evolution led the discussion of eugenics. The sex and reproduction meeting was addressed by Professor William F. Ogburn and Dr. A. A. Brill. Population experts analyzed the danger spots of the world—Dr. Peter Tutyshkin speaking on "Does Russia Want Birth Control?", Dr. Johann Ferch on "Mother Clinics in Austria." The fundamental necessity of population control was summed up in J. O. P. Bland's speech. "The future destinies of our civilization," he warned, "must depend entirely upon whether the population problem is going to be solved either by birth control or mustard gas."

But it was the medical session on contraceptive techniques, open only to doctors and led by Dr. Cooper and Dr. Hannah Stone, that gave the birth control movement a new scientific stature and dignity in the eyes of the medical profession. News of this achievement was carried in eight hundred articles in papers throughout the country. Even more significant, as far as Mrs. Sanger was concerned, was the approval won for the first time from two of the profession's leading spokesmen. "I observed most of the thirteen sessions," stated Dr. Robert L. Dickinson, "and can bear witness to their dignity and reserve . . . to the weight of the papers . . . and lastly to the constructive character of the resolutions. . . ."

Dr. William Allen Pusey, ex-president of the American Medical Association, gave birth control the first support from this august body. "It is women who bear the penalties in injury, disease and death, and mental torture that are involved in unlimited childbearing. They have a right to know how they can intelligently—not crudely and dangerously—control their sexual lives."

On the last day of the conference, delegates from seven foreign nations met at Margaret Sanger's apartment to form the first international birth control organization. By unanimous vote, Mrs. Sanger was elected president. She insisted, however, that the position needed a scientist of international renown, and convinced Dr. C. C. Little, then head of the University of Michigan, to accept the nomination. Shortly afterward, they opened a London office—the Birth Control International Information Centre under the direction of Edith How-Martyn. The world movement had begun. "It took me nearly one year to recover from the strain, physical, nervous, and financial, of the Sixth International Conference," Mrs. Sanger wrote later. But long before she had recovered she was already pointing toward the next international goal—a second and even larger conference in 1927 which would bring the population problem to the very doorstep of the League of Nations in Geneva.

CHAPTER 20

In the last sweltering week of July 1926, Stuart Sanger and his uncle, Robert Higgins, made a hurried trip to Truro on Cape Cod where Michael Higgins had been living for the last ten years. Mr. Higgins, now eighty-four, had recently suffered a cerebral stroke which had left almost his whole body paralyzed and deprived him of the faculty of speech. The indomitable old man, however, refused to let such obstacles interfere with the process of communication. By the use of signals that he managed to blink with his eyelids, he insisted on showing the hospitality of an Irish philosopher to his son and grandson and carefully directed them to the recesses of a kitchen cupboard. There, despite the prohibitions of his doctor, he had stored away one last supply of the favorite tonic of his old age—a jug of local dandelion wine.

Margaret Sanger had given her father the Truro cottage. It was a comfortable memorial to his old age. The summer months on the beach were glorious, particularly when Stuart and Grant had come to spend their vacations with him. Then they had gone to college; he had become more and more isolated. For a while, Nan had lived with him—Nan and Mary were always the affectionate caretakers of the family. Then she too had left to take a job in Buffalo. Her replacement was Mrs. Powers, an impecunious but especially proper Bostonian who had become his housekeeper. The neighbors were convinced this partnership would blossom into marriage. But Mrs. Powers was too immersed in the past glories of her ancestors, five of whom had come over on the *Mayflower*. Almost daily, when she reminded him of her heroic past, he would make the same scoffing retort: "Who were they, anyway? A hungry crew. Nothing but un-desirables in their own country." It was a feeble effort at his old rebellion against the established order—but it must have disturbed Mrs. Powers enough to eliminate the possibility of marriage.

The town of Truro offered a poor stage to Michael Higgins. Once he had attracted the best brains of Corning to his workshop to hear his declamations on Henry George, Colonel Ingersoll, and socialism. But these taciturn Cape Codders were little interested in the radicalism of an old man. His only audience was the local grocer. Each morning, Higgins would plod into town to buy his provisions, the flamboyant lock of hair, now turned from red to white, still flopping grandly over his forehead. At the grocer's, he would deliver his daily oration, gather his provisions, and then head for home and the solitude of his books.

There was a haunting sadness to these last days—the once defiant voice that had no listeners, the stonecutter and sculptor who no longer touched his stone, the reformer, the politician without a platform. No one realized it better than Margaret Sanger. During the summers when the boys were at Truro, she tried to get up there for week ends when she could break away from the New York office. But these visits had grown fewer and fewer. Her father had given her the strength of his rebellion twenty-five years ago, and that was what she wanted to remember. Not the fading image, not the pale mirror of a past giant. Disillusion was always worst with people she had loved, whether it was Michael Higgins or William Sanger.

Higgins died peacefully that hot August, but even the end had its ironic sadness. He had wanted to be buried in the Corning cemetery next to the wife he adored. Margaret Sanger and the family escorted the body on the long journey across Massachusetts and down the Hudson River Valley. Joe Higgins was the last of them still living at Corning, and he insisted that his father lie in state for one night at his house. The ceremony might have been in the nature of an Irish wake, but Joe Higgins, a teetotaler, allowed no intoxicating beverages to pass his threshold. Whether it was this obstacle, or the forbidding aura of atheism and radicalism that still clung to Michael Higgins' name, not one of his old friends, not one resident of Corning, to which he had given so many hours of labor to bring free books to its libraries and better schools to its children, came to sit by the body that night.

At the nondenominational cemetery the next morning, Higgins was lowered into the grave beside his wife while hundreds of stone angels that he had carved looked on placidly from the Catholic cemetery not far away. He would have enjoyed this last small joke. Even in the presence of his own religious handiwork, he had stubbornly refused a religious funeral. No minister attended. No prayers were said. Higgins had remained an unswerving atheist to the end.

Except for Havelock Ellis, no man had exerted a stronger influence on Margaret Sanger than her father. In the first sixteen years of her life, he had passed on to her the dream she would pursue relentlessly —that out of the chaos of evolution, human beings had the strength to achieve their own perfectibility. For him, it was never more than a dream, but she would spend a lifetime turning the dream into reality. She was to achieve what he could never achieve—nor could Ethel, though she had once been as close to her father as Margaret, and they had both fought hard for his love. Margaret had won, of course, as she would always win what she set her heart on. She was proud of the fact and never underestimated its importance in her life. Many years later, when she was discussing a possible title for a biography, she laughingly suggested, *"Men I Have Loved."* A moment later she added, quite gravely, "Beginning, of course, with my father."

2

Thor Andersson, a Norwegian editor, once wrote Mrs. Sanger to ask that "you may permit me to call you the mother of the New World." It was a generous compliment from a European admirer— subsequent events would prove it was not exaggerated. She had been campaigning for the New World since her trip to Japan in 1922. Now, ten years before most politicians faced the issue, she saw the desperate necessity of bringing it to being before its enemies could launch the debacle that their policies must bring.

Significantly enough, although Margaret Sanger never entered the political arena like the suffragettes and other women crusaders, the fact that birth control held the key to the population problems of the world now plunged her into the very center of the whirlpool of international rivalry. As early as 1917 in the *Review,* she had analyzed the relationship between population expansion and war. What she saw now gave her even greater alarm.

At the Institute of Politics at Williamstown, Massachusetts, in 1925 she had heard a Fascist spokesman, Count Antonio Cippico, demand new land for an Italian surplus population that was growing at the rate of a half million children each year. Mussolini, envisioning new Roman legions throughout the Mediterranean, was exhorting Italian mothers to produce ever larger families. German nationalism was already stirring, the myth of a master race, which would grow from 66 to 90 million, already part of the Nazi blueprint. On the other side of the world, the danger was even more imminent. The Japanese military clique was demanding an immediate increase of 10 million in population to fuel the armies that would soon invade Manchuria.

It was a time for action, a time to stand up and cry the danger of these population policies to the world. For Margaret Sanger, it was never enough to analyze, to talk. A stand had to be made. This creative, spreading power of her will was the mainspring of all her work.

Although the scientists in charge of the international birth control organization had planned a conference in 1926, nothing had been done. Now Mrs. Sanger suggested to Dr. Little a daring and original plan—a conference of the foremost population authorities in the world to be held in Geneva in 1927, a conference of such scientific prestige that the League of Nations would have to accept the population problem as a key issue on its agenda.

A meeting of the planning committee was held at Willow Lake on June 9, 1926. Dr. Little came from Michigan, Clinton Chance from London. It was here that Mrs. Sanger in an act of significant self-effacement suggested that the conference should go far beyond birth control and concentrate on the widest range of population problems. Since the conference should attract scientists from every branch of sociology, demography, biology, and statistics, scientists who might demur at a connection with birth control, the very words birth control should not be mentioned. Margaret Sanger would organize the conference but her name would be kept in the background.

It was around a World Population Conference of this character that Mrs. Sanger put together an advisory council of international stature within a few months. Sir Bernard Mallet, formerly Registrar-General of Great Britain and president of the Royal Statistical Society, accepted the role of chairman. From England, the council had Professor A. M. Carr-Saunders, from Holland, Dr. H. W. Methorst, from France, Professor Leon Bernard. Only a few months before, Sir William Beveridge had scoffed at the idea of organizing so huge a conference in anything less than two years. "It certainly

takes you to make things move when you really get started," Professor Pearl wrote Mrs. Sanger admiringly.

The executive board of the Birth Control League, oddly enough,
did not share this enthusiasm. More and more during the past year,
the board had been dominated by a conservative bloc of club
women led by Mrs. F. Robertson-Jones. Mrs. Jones had been
brought into birth control from the League of Women Voters, and
had been trying to introduce the league's highly stratified and rigid
type of organization. The conservative block wanted a system of
executive board responsibility so that the decisions of any member,
even the president, would have to be debated and approved beforehand by the whole board. They put the Population Conference in
the category of impulse. It would not only take Mrs. Sanger abroad
for months but belonged, they felt, in a realm outside the league's
work.

The conservative bloc, moreover, was trying to introduce a new
financial policy. The league now had thirty local chapters throughout the country. They had advanced, it felt, beyond the pioneering
days when projects could be launched spontaneously without a
penny in the bank and only the faith and prayers of its members to
bring in the cash that was already spent. The league must operate
now on a well-planned budget—every dollar collected beforehand,
the bank balance always glowing with healthy reserves. Yet with all
these efforts to establish a sound financial policy, here was Mrs.
Sanger launching a world-wide conference that might cost the league
thousands of dollars.

Echoes of this dissatisfaction were not long in reaching Mrs
Sanger. She disagreed with the conservative bloc—but the demands
of the conference were so pressing she could not take the time now
to oppose it. It would be better to release the league of any financial or
organizational responsibility for the conference. In order to separate
the two completely, she would take a leave of absence from the
league and hand over control for now to the conservative bloc.
Mrs. Robertson-Jones, therefore, was elected acting president.

Mrs. Sanger knew that the Population Conference would keep
her in London and Geneva most of the following year. Mr. Slee
agreed to accompany her to Europe. There were few ties to hold him
in New York. He had recently sold the Three-in-One Oil Company
and retired a reasonably wealthy man. "I am glad he is with you,"
Edith How-Martyn wrote Mrs. Sanger, "as you will need all his

thoughtful administrations to keep you O.K. to the end of the conference and leave you smiling and happy when it is over."

Slee's participation in the movement had actually gone far past the point of thoughtful administrations. Month after month he had made up the deficit of the *Review* and financed Dr. Cooper's salary and expenses. He had not only poured large sums of money into the league, but as treasurer of the Clinical Research Bureau had brought the financial efficiency of big industry to its daily operations. A careful steward of every penny, he sent continual notes to members of the staff—one to Dr. Cooper, for instance, complaining of his excessive use of taxis and suggesting that "there are other methods of transportation."

Slee hated waste above all else. Once when he was vacationing in Hawaii, he sat and watched his friends riding the breakers on outrigger canoes. They finally convinced him to try the sport himself. He hired a canoe for an hour, but the first wave caught him broadside and filled the canoe with water, practically drowning him. He had never liked the water and liked it even less now—but he insisted on taking the canoe out again and again until he had used up his hour's rental.

This tightfisted exterior, however, was easily melted by numerous causes to which he gave generously—one of his favorites being members of the clergy who had lost their pulpits through misadventures with the feminine sex. To dozens of these each Thanksgiving and Christmas, he sent baskets of food and sizable checks. He kept a permanent rotary fund of twenty-five thousand dollars with which he financed the college or professional careers of boys and girls—an artist studying in Paris, a singer in Milan, a minister's daughter at an expensive eastern college. For years, he paid the school tuition of one of his wife's associates and for Hugh De Selincourt's daughter, Bridget, who wrote of him appreciatively: "He helps me believe in myself: the sort of way he trusts me and writes."

The most significant gift of all, however, would be made shortly after Slee and Margaret Sanger arrived in London. The occasion was Havelock Ellis's sixty-ninth birthday. The "King" was an old man now, a magnificent, white-bearded patriarch described in an issue of the *Review*—each February issue was devoted exclusively to his honor—as "silhouetted like a saint against the horizon of the dawning day. . . . the greatest benefactor of woman and of the human race." Yet for all the beauty he had given the world, he had received little in return. The royalties from his books had always been slim—the only considerable money coming from publication of *The Dance of Life* in the United States. He was still living in the dingy flat at Brixton; he was still burdened with the responsibility of supporting his two maiden sisters.

Ellis's birthday was the perfect moment for one final testament of love and appreciation. It was Margaret Sanger's plan to move Ellis out of Brixton to a house of his own in the country; to relieve Françoise of the drudgery of teaching so that she could devote full time to keeping house for him and acting as his secretary. It was essential, however, that the gift be arranged without injuring Ellis's pride. She decided to write De Selincourt, a graceful notion, not just for the excellence of his advice but because his involvement in the plan would help heal the breach between him and Ellis.

De Selincourt replied joyfully: "In all the wonderful happenings this year, this beats the lot: it's like a fairy tale, only more lovely: and for you to bring me in like you do, you miracle of dearness, by asking my advice, sort of, as though you needed it, you beloved darling, in doing a beautiful thing in a lovely, sensitive, INVINCIBLE way. . . . Who else but you—oh do it! do it! do it!"

De Selincourt advised that the approach be made through Françoise. Margaret wrote her, pointing out that Ellis desperately needed a secretary. Only Françoise could fulfill this responsibility. Would she give up teaching and take the equivalent salary, fifteen hundred dollars a year, to serve as his secretary? Would she convince Ellis to move out of Brixton if Margaret gave him a few thousand dollars to buy a house?

Françoise, in tears, brought the news to Ellis on his birthday—a scene that De Selincourt later described in a letter to Margaret: "Havelock . . . all beaming with happiness like a boy. 'How could one refuse what is so beautifully given!' He'd read *your* letter to her; he could appreciate its beauty . . . I wish you could have seen Françoise. She kept crying. I'm still too soft and moved and ridiculous about it all to give you any idea of the reverberations of delight of this dear creative action. . . ."

Ellis and Françoise selected a house at Herne Hill—he would always call it in the future "Fairy Tale House." De Selincourt went out to visit them and then wrote Margaret a description of how Françoise "sat down in each particular room and wept with joy: afraid almost to breathe lest she might wake up and find it a dream.

. . . You were so much, so beautifully, so rightly there all the time that I almost kissed the hovering presence that was you . . ."

"You have made Havelock ten years younger," De Selincourt summed up the gift in another letter. "I wish I could make you feel every ripple of delight that lovely action of yours is bringing and will continue to bring."

3

From the temporary London offices of the Population Conference, which Clinton Chance had provided along with a staff of secretaries and stenographers, Margaret Sanger plunged into the exhausting work of rounding up a list of delegates who would be the finest scientific minds in England and Europe. She had set her standards high—demographers, biologists, sociologists, and economists of the first rank—and she pursued this objective relentlessly. Often she would make a trip of hundreds of miles, in one case to Edinburgh, to secure one delegate, Dr. F. A. E. Crew, the biologist, whose experiments in making hens crow, had only recently filled the headlines. Slowly she added one distinguished name after another—Sir Humphrey Rolleston, John Maynard Keynes, and Julian Huxley from England, Sir George Knibbs from Australia, Lucien March and Andre Siegfried from France, Dr. Eugene Fischer from Germany, Dr. M. A. van Herwerden from Holland.

She made a special trip to Geneva to rent the conference rooms at the Salle Centrale for August 30—September 2, 1927. At the same time, she paid a call on the Siamese Minister, a devoted student of eugenics. She sent him a copy of one of her books, and he wrote her a letter of appreciation. Always preserving a keen sense of humor about her work, she added a penciled notation on the letter. "From a charming Siamese Prince, father of eighty children."

In Geneva, she opened permanent offices for the conference in a suite of four large rooms with a staff of seventeen secretaries and typists. Hotel accommodations had to be made for three hundred delegates. Interpreters and translators had to be hired who could handle scientific phraseology in a dozen languages, including Greek, Portugese, Japanese, and Chinese. The proceedings would have to be proofread, edited, and printed—all this would need highly skilled personnel, and Mrs. Sanger decided that she had better bring her trusted associate, Anne Kennedy, to Geneva to supervise them.

Mr. Slee, ever the faithful guardian of his wife's health, finally insisted that they should spend a month on the French Riviera. From there, she could still make occasional trips to the conference offices at Geneva and London.

He rented the Villa Bachlyk on Cap d'Ail between Nice and Monte Carlo. "From my room," Margaret Sanger wrote, "the sunrise was incredibly vivid—reds and yellows mixed with the glorious blue of the Mediterranean." The flowers, grown for the nearby perfume factories, covered the hillsides and made the air for miles around almost intoxicating with their fragrance. H. G. Wells was living at Grasse with Odette Keun. Margaret and Slee often drove up to see them and picnicked with them at the tiny mountaintop village of Eze, a favorite haunt of artists.

She wanted De Selincourt to share these moments of beauty and telegraphed him to come immediately. It was a vacation he never forgot. "Lord! What a heavenly time you gave me!" he wrote later. ". . . Our drive from Monte Carlo. Our little walks by the sea. The dinner at the Miramar. The poet in wreath and blue pajamas! The lunch at Cannes! The fierce cocktail party beforehand . . . the walk down from Eze and the lunch at Beaulieu! And the journey home! . . . Yeh Gods, how we laughed that night. Lord! I was proud to be sitting laughingly with the most beautiful women in that sumptuous room!"

The first stirrings of impending trouble now began to come from conference headquarters at Geneva. She hurried back. A week before the delegates were due to arrive, Dr. William H. Welch of Johns Hopkins, the dean of public health medicine in the United States, took her to lunch. He knew how many months she had labored to build this conference and warned her, "You may think your problems are over, but they aren't."

A day later, when the final list of delegates was compiled, the "machinations of these sinister forces," as she called them, first became evident. Months before she had sent invitations to the liberal scientists of countries like Italy whose population policies were already threatening the peace of Europe. She had expected the attendance of men of stature like Guglielmo Ferrero and Gaetano Salvemini. Instead, the Italian Government had forced Corrado Gini, the bombastic mouthpiece of Mussolini's Fascist theories, on the conference. Wanting only to prevent dissension, Sir Bernard Mallet had accepted Gini. He had made the same compromise in one Catholic country after another. From Spain, Belgium, France, and

Catholic Germany, he had accepted the most reactionary spokesmen. The storm finally broke on Friday before the scheduled opening of the conference on Tuesday, August 31. The proofs of the official conference program had just come to Mrs. Sanger's office for approval. Sir Bernard came in, inspected them over her shoulder, and then crossed out the names of Mrs. Sanger, Mrs. How-Martyn, and a dozen other associates who had worked almost a year on the exhausting details of the conference. Mrs. Sanger demanded an explanation. "The names of workers should not be included on a scientific program," he explained.

"But these people are different. They are as much experts in their own particular fields as the scientists."

It was soon apparent that Sir Bernard's explanation was only a pretext to hide a subtle move for domination of the conference by the Catholic countries. The delegates from Italy, Spain, Belgium, and Catholic Germany had demanded that no mention of birth control and Malthusianism should be made at any meeting or round table. Since Mrs. Sanger's name was synonymous with birth control, they insisted it be removed from the program. Again Sir Bernard had agreed.

This, of course, was a blatant corruption of Mrs. Sanger's original agreement with the planning committee. Their objective had been to make the population problem, not birth control, the focus of the conference. But to eliminate even Mrs. Sanger's name on the program approached the point of absurdity. As organizer of the conference and its principal fund-raiser for the traveling expenses of most delegates, her name had already been well publicized.

When news of this censorship reached the staff, the executive assistants, secretaries, and typists—all twenty-one of them—resigned in a body. In her letter of resignation, one executive assistant, Wilhelmina Breed, described Mrs. Sanger as "the heart and soul of this conference" and stated that "I cannot accept the injustice that no public recognition should be given for all your work."

But the issue, Mrs. Sanger insisted, was not recognition. Her name was not important. It was simply a tool through which the reactionary delegates were seeking to dominate the conference. In those agonizing hours while she pleaded with the staff to hold up their resignations, she determined that a stand, some sort of stand had to be made.

Julian Huxley and a group of younger English scientists argued her case before the advisory council. A compromise was finally proposed. She hated compromises—but almost two years of work and the hope of a dynamic population policy hung in the balance. For hours that Sunday, she pleaded with her staff to go along with her, and eventually won them over. Under the terms of the compromise, Mrs. Sanger's name would not appear on the program of the conference. Instead, she would be listed as a member of the general council in the final, printed proceedings.

One final attempt by the Catholic delegates to disrupt the conference was made on the day of the opening session at the Salle Centrale. Any delegate to the conference who had written a book had the right to display his work on the special book counter which had been set up in the lobby. A number of these books, quite naturally, were on the subject of birth control. As they entered the lobby that morning, a group of delegates from Italy, Spain, and South Germany marched up to the book counter and noisily demanded that these books be removed. When Mrs. Sanger appeared at the first sign of disturbance, they shook the books under her nose and repeated their demands with pompous gesticulations. She faced them coldly, saying, "This hall is for rent next week. Meanwhile, I will take no dictation from anyone as to what will be sold here." Mr. Slee arrived and planted his imposing six-foot-three figure at his wife's side. The books remained.

From that point on, the conference proceeded flawlessly to the highest levels of scientific analysis and debate. A brilliant succession of papers—the work of Lord Horder, Dean Inge, J. B. S. Haldane, Dr. C. P. Blacker, Lord Dawson of Penn, Dr. Edwin Bauer, Albert Thomas, Professor Henry Pratt Fairchild—made up an aggregate of scientific thinking that would be hard to surpass at any one meeting place. "An intellectual treat," the Manchester *Guardian* called these debates, "such as it is rarely given the ordinary mortal to enjoy."

Each morning at his breakfast table every delegate received a journal, printed in parallel columns of English and French, of the papers and debates of the previous day. It was the gift of the energetic Mr. Slee, who conceived, supervised, and paid for the journal himself.

At night, the delegates were brought together informally through a series of sumptuous dinners—one a steamer ride with dinner on board to the old château of Madame de Staël, another a supper and dance at Mrs. Stanley McCormick's Château de Prangins.

It was at the final dinner of the conference, the farewell dinner at the Hôtel des Bergues, when Mrs. Sanger's name was finally brought into the open by Dr. Karl Reiland, the rector of St. George's Church in New York, and honored by the whole assembly. Appropriately enough, it was Sir Bernard Mallet who made the tribute. At the mention of her name, Dr. Drysdale described the scene. "The whole company arose and thundered in her honor."

Mrs. Sanger, said Sir Bernard, "has devoted herself with absolute loyalty and wholeheartedness to further the interests of the conference that the great fundamental question of population should be discussed in a purely scientific spirit. . . . Mrs. Sanger may be proud to have contributed so greatly to this result by the real ability with which she has done her part no less than by her restraint and self-effacement."

Gray-haired pedagogues, titled peers of the world of science, professors, doctors, sociologists whose names were trade-marks in their professions—all rose to their feet to hail her, like any group of eager undergraduates, by singing, "For she's a jolly good fellow."

The tributes poured in during the next weeks. "The conference was a great success," wrote Professor Raymond Pearl, "and you are covered with glory because of what you did to make it so."

She had stood fast in her resolve to make the conference a symbol of scientific achievement, stood fast against the forces that would weaken or destroy its fundamental purpose of solving the coming crisis of population. It was neither a question of glory nor self-effacement. She neither wanted the one nor practiced the other. What she did always seemed to spring from a necessity so deep within her that it lost all personal quality and became instead the synthesis of what she liked to call the feminine spirit, radiant and triumphant.

The only question that mattered to her was bringing the central issue of the conference to the world—"whether a nation whose birth rate is too great for its resources has a right to seek to expand at the expense of less densely populated countries or not." These men of science, the finest minds available, had agreed that no birth rate is uncontrollable, that no nation had a right to use this as an excuse for expansion or war. Now let the world listen. Now let the League of Nations act before it was too late! Here was the fundamental principle of her life—to start the process of perfectibility, to let loose those ideas so true and necessary that they would stir people, per-

,haps only thousands at first, but eventually millions, to make the dream a reality.

Of all the newspapers who covered the conference—and there were hundreds—the Manchester *Guardian* probably best grasped this dream in an editorial which warned: "It is high time the world took stock of its position!"

Few statesmen heeded the warning, and Margaret Sanger wondered whether time had not already run out. In Rome, Mussolini had already proclaimed that "with a falling population, one does not create an empire but becomes a colony." The Population Conference had supplied the key to the population problems of the world. It was up to the League of Nations now.

CHAPTER 21

No sooner had she finished editing the proceedings of the World Population Conference than Margaret Sanger hurried off to Berlin for a lecture tour. Despite her close-packed schedule, she found time to help in the establishment of a birth control clinic in the working-class district of Neukölln. She was even preparing to leave for a lecture tour of India—the feverish energy accumulated during those months of work at Geneva carrying her to almost explosive heights before her health broke suddenly. She was put to bed; the doctors ordered a month of complete rest. Mr. Slee fussed over her patiently and then at her request went back to England "so as to leave me completely alone for a while . . ." she wrote De Selincourt. "I'm going to the mountaintop for the week to dream."

The mountaintop was at St. Moritz. She stayed in bed, reading and writing for a few days, then restlessly got up to skate and ski on the glistening slopes. But even this vacation was cut short. Disturbing letters began to come from New York. Anne Kennedy had returned, and her return had indirectly brought a culmination to the crisis which had been postponed by Mrs. Sanger's temporary leave of absence in the fall of 1926.

Mrs. Kennedy, by virtue of her long service as Margaret Sanger's chief lieutenant, had now become the target of the conservative bloc of the Birth Control League. She had gone to Geneva almost a year before to work on the Population Conference—a move which irked members of the conservative bloc since they had not been consulted beforehand. On her return, they had shown their displeasure by not re-electing her to the executive board, a position she had held for the last eight years.

It was now becoming obvious that the conservative bloc was determined to oust Mrs. Kennedy from the league. At the office, she was deprived of all executive function, refused the use of essential files, and harassed by continuous restrictions. Mrs. Rublee, also a board member, described the four women of the conservative bloc as "hard as nails and determined as iron." She wrote Mrs. Sanger on December 8, 1927, that "Anne's situation is so ghastly, so humiliating, so unbelievable that it is hard for me to write about it."

Mrs. Kennedy wrote Margaret Sanger: ". . . You are still president, and it is only on your authority I can pass in my resignation."

But the board acted on its own. At the December 12 meeting, without allowing Mrs. Kennedy a hearing, it drafted a letter terminating her employment by the league. The key sentence of the letter—"You have not shown yourself amenable to direction by the Board"—demonstrated the board's contention that Mrs. Kennedy gave her allegiance only and directly to Mrs. Sanger.

Mrs. Sanger was not consulted on the dismissal. From London, she had only been able to follow the case through reports from Mrs. Kennedy and Mrs. Rublee. She, therefore, wrote the board in blunt language: "I had every right to be informed of the pending action of the Board beforehand—to help if possible avoid the unpleasant and critical situation which has arisen."

Mrs. Sanger asked the board to delay final action until she returned to New York. Meanwhile, the disposition of the case was eliminated by fortuitous circumstance. Early in January, the executive secretary of Herbert Simonds' company left to set up a competing firm. Simonds offered the position to Mrs. Kennedy.

She had grown up with the movement. Ten years of her life had gone into it and few people outside of Mrs. Sanger were as closely linked to its development. She analyzed the situation with Mrs. Sanger. They both knew that the movement as a whole would benefit if the contraceptive industry could achieve the highest ethical standards in the eyes of the American Medical Association. With her unique knowledge of birth control, Mrs. Kennedy could play an essential part in helping Simonds' company meet these standards. They both agreed, therefore, that Mrs. Kennedy should accept the post.

But the conclusion of the Kennedy "case" was only a prelude to harrowing months of sadness and strife for Margaret Sanger herself. She had known two years back that the movement was changing. Now it was almost unrecognizable. This thing that had been built

literally out of her own flesh and blood had become a pale imitation
of principles and policies that were no longer hers. The fighting
spirit had gone out of it. In every department of the league, she
saw the process of petrification setting in.

She had built the movement on faith and action. Every forward
step, every new battle had been the result of decisiveness and daring against often impossible odds. No one counted the odds in those
days. She had always plunged ahead, transmitting to those around
her some spark, some touch of that intangible flame inside her that
swept others along with her toward objectives and pinnacles that
had seemed impossible to them before.

But she had outrun the others now. They had fallen back into the
conservative pattern of an organization that had tasted partial victory and was willing to settle for that. The executive board wanted
only safety. Instead of the expansion that lay ahead, they wanted
only to consolidate the gains of the past. Instead of faith and action,
they had substituted a new doctrine—the "doctrine of accountability."

She saw proof of it almost as soon as she returned to New York.
The league had taken a booth at the Parents Exhibition at Grand
Central Palace, an exhibition in which all civic and educational
agencies were participating. The booth had been paid for—but at
the last minute the Superintendent of New York Public Schools,
William O'Shea, threatened to withdraw unless the league was
banned from the exhibition. It was an old story—the bullying threat
of the Catholic hierarchy through political or civic channels. Mrs.
Sanger had stood up to these threats countless times before and
almost always defeated them. Now she immediately took steps to
hire a lawyer and obtain an injunction against any breach of contract by the exhibition.

But she was immediately informed that in her absence a resolution had been passed prohibiting action by one board member
without the agreement of the rest. She tried to reach the other
board members by telephone, but before she could gather a quorum
it was too late. The league's check for its booth was returned; the
exhibition had opened. "Our opportunity to force the issue had been
lost by our own delay and by the Board's timid indecision," Mrs.
Sanger concluded.

This "doctrine of accountability" was carried to the point of absurdity a few days later when she unhappily found that subscrip-

tion-renewal notices had not gone out to subscribers of the *Review,* and circulation as a result had fallen from thirteen thousand to twenty-five hundred. She accordingly told the bookkeeper to give fifteen or twenty dollars to the clerk to circularize the old subscribers. But this was impossible, she was told, under the board's new policy. Any expenditure over five dollars now had to have the approval of the full board!

She felt like a stranger in a land she never knew. The league had become a creature of routine and red tape. The conservative bloc, trained in the rigid school of the League of Women Voters, had brought the doctrinaire and highly stratified approach of that organization to birth control. But this was a revolutionary movement—a movement of constant change and struggle. Stratification, she knew, would slowly crush the strength from its body.

All this machinery of "accountability" had the obvious purpose of checking the daring, the impulsive quality of her own leadership. Some of her critics had called it a "one-woman movement." She would have been the last to deny that there was not some justice in the phrase. She had always acted quickly, dramatically, sometimes a trifle impetuously. She had had to make many decisions independently. But whatever she did, controversial or sensational as it may have seemed at the moment, always sprang from an instinctive and historically rooted grasp of long-range objectives. Invariably history had proved her right.

"These campaigns could never have been waged," she once pointed out, "had I been tied or hampered in my activities by individuals or boards or committees lacking the understanding, vision, or appreciation of these qualities. Experience had given me judgment which entitled me to a certain amount of freedom of action, and I could not well observe the dictates of people who did not know the subject as well as I did."

Behind this criticism of her being a "one-woman movement" lay an even more personal attack. The members of the conservative bloc were essentially women of social position. They felt that the time had come to make birth control palatable to the rich and socially elect. In their eyes, the movement had outgrown Margaret Sanger. She had sprung from the cauldron of political and social revolution that had swept the country at the turn of the century. Her approach, her motivation were still revolutionary. She had built the movement by challenging laws and institutions, by knocking down the established prejudices of society. Although her position had now placed her on intimate terms with such dignitaries as Lord Dawson of Penn and John D. Rockefeller, Jr., she maintained many of the rebel ideas of her youth.

What the movement needed now, the conservative bloc felt, was a new tone—a college graduate at its head. In place of indomitable rebels like Kitty Marion, the conservative bloc wanted to place the movement in the hands of women of leisure and position, young women of the Junior League, who would take on birth control as a social responsibility, as one of their expected duties along with settlement house and welfare work. The whole conception was repugnant to Mrs. Sanger. For her, the movement had always been like fire in the blood, consuming all her energy, interest, and often fifteen or sixteen hours of her day. Birth control "was not something that could wait on this or that mood," she stated. "Its interest came first in my waking consciousness, and was my last thought as I lost consciousness at night."

Even the conservative bloc's financial policy reflected this shift to quiet decorum. They instituted five- and ten-dollar memberships, giving them the advantage of a planned budget; but the major disadvantage was that once a member had sent in her yearly check she tended to disassociate herself from further work and responsibility. Mrs. Sanger had made even finances a part of the ever changing pattern of struggle and development. Each new objective she made a campaign in itself—dispatching telegrams or appeal letters to a few hundred of her most devoted followers, each bringing anywhere from a dollar to a thousand dollars for the immediate fight. "We were not like other organizations," she always explained. "We were a crusading group. We had to inspire, to expand, to bring people with us. We could not stand still on regular memberships."

The split between the conservative bloc and Mrs. Sanger's followers on the board of directors increased in severity all during 1928. Mrs. Sanger still controlled the board. But this was not a question of power politics. For Mrs. Sanger, leadership had to unite an organization in absolute purpose and devotion. It mattered little that her decisions could be enforced by vote when the bickering and dissatisfaction continued. "I can fight to the last ditch against the outside enemy," she wrote Mrs. Robert Huse, who had succeeded Mrs. Kennedy as executive secretary, "but to fight old friends, women that I have loved, respected and worked with, that I cannot do. . . . Such pettiness! Such small limited minds cannot lead the birth control movement . . ."

The split had finally reached the stage of personal attack. For Mrs. Sanger, who had built the movement from the depth of her love, from her mystical fusion with the aspirations of motherhood, the continuation of such internecine warfare was unthinkable. "I've been going through such unreasonable days—personal attacks by friends and foes," she wrote Hugh De Selincourt. "No longer the cause attacked but MS. Friends turn out of the air—nothing to account for it. . . . I'm left weak from the sadness of it."

The conservative bloc even sought to undermine her authority as editor in chief of the *Review*. A four-woman board of editors was named to run the magazine. Nominally, Margaret Sanger, given the title of chairman of the board, was in charge. But the ruse was too obvious to be tolerated. She handed in her resignation as editor, thus enabling, as she wrote, "the present management to assume the entire responsibilities for its policies."

Even at this point, she could have fought to eliminate the conservative bloc from the board. She had never avoided a fight. But a fight within the movement would soon explode into a public controversy. The league was too precious to her to have it chewed to pieces by her enemies in the press. There was only one other alternative, and through the agony of many nights, she came finally to this decision. She would leave the league. She would resign.

On June 8, 1929, Margaret Sanger submitted her letter of resignation, a letter without rancor or bitterness, which still pinpointed the basic issue—what she called "the danger of curtailing the initiative of individuals and deadening the creative interest which is essential to successful leadership." The conservative bloc had claimed that the movement had outgrown the "fanaticism" of its youth. "What some call fanaticism," Mrs. Sanger stated, "is never dangerous to the life of an organization as this one. Apathy and languid convictions are . . ."

But there was one thing she would not give up—the Clinical Research Bureau. Although affiliated with the league, the bureau had always operated under her personal control. It was, as nothing else, the crystallization of her dream. It was the final scientific expression of the need and want of motherhood that she had suffered, fought, and gone to prison for. "I did not regret the theoretical part of the movement going in to other hands," she stated, "but I would have been traitor to all that had been entrusted to me had I yielded the clinic to women who had shown themselves incapable of the understanding and sympathy required in its operation."

The five women who had worked side by side with her almost from the earliest days of the movement—Mrs. Rublee, Mrs. Ackerman, Mrs. Day, Mrs. Hepburn, and Mrs. Timme—handed in their resignations. Mr. Slee followed with his resignation as treasurer—but less politely. Caustically pointing out that in six years he had given the league over sixty-four thousand dollars, "for the benefit of the ideal Margaret Sanger had slaved for," he enclosed his check for three hundred dollars, "the last contribution I will make."

An era had come to an end—a sixteen-year era in which one woman, virtually alone at the start, had radically changed the social pattern of a nation. But an even more important era was about to begin. Margaret Sanger wasted no time brooding about the past. In her mind was already forming the outline of a new campaign that would take her on a fresh and daring course in the next decade. "Now that I am released from that deadening influence of petty whispering criticism," she wrote Mrs. Huse on February 28, 1929, "I am a new, vital being again, ready and free to forge ahead and fight as never before."

CHAPTER 22

Margaret Sanger had stood alone and embattled many times in her life, but all possible enemies seemed to have conspired against her that spring. The Birth Control League was split by dissension. Her son Stuart was ill, the old sinus condition that had plagued him for years suddenly becoming a serious mastoid case. Then as if they had been waiting for the opportune moment when one overwhelming blow could prostrate the whole movement, the Police Department and its political allies struck suddenly at the citadel and symbol of her work, the Clinical Research Bureau.

On March 23, 1929, a plainly dressed woman with a round, thickset face had come to the bureau and registered as Mrs. Tierney. To the nurse at the desk she stated that she was married, the mother of three children, the oldest being five. Her husband was a truck driver earning forty dollars a week and addicted to drinking. She was given an appointment for a medical examination on April 3. It was then that one of the staff physicians, Dr. Elizabeth Pissoort, found several pelvic disorders and recorded them on the chart. The patient's social and medical history indicated that she should not conceive too soon after the birth of her last child. Dr. Pissoort, therefore, prescribed a suitable contraceptive and instructed her in its use.

On Mrs. Tierney's return a week later, Dr. Hannah Stone checked the method prescribed and found that the patient had learned to use it correctly. The case was considered closed—only to be reopened with startling and violent suddenness when "Mrs. Tierney" returned on April 15, this time bringing with her a squad of seven policemen and using her real name, Policewoman Anna K. McNamara.

Margaret Sanger was about to take Stuart to the hospital for a mastoid operation when her telephone rang. It was her secretary, Anna Lifschiz, crying, "The police are here."

Mrs. Sanger rushed by taxi to the clinic. A police car stood ominously at the door. The Chief of the Policewoman's Bureau, Mrs. Mary Sullivan, had staged the raid. Dr. Hannah Stone, Dr. Elizabeth Pissoort, and three nurses were already under arrest. The door of the clinic was shut, the shade pulled down. "You can't come in," the policeman at the door announced brusquely.

"I'm the owner of this place," Mrs. Sanger snapped. "I intend to get in." The policeman turned to his superiors for orders, and they agreed to admit her.

The clinic was in chaos—detectives rushing back and forth "like chickens fluttering about a raided roost," she described the scene later. Fifteen women patients, most of them badly frightened, were sitting in the consultation booths. Policemen with pads and pencils were bellowing at them, trying to force them to give their names and addresses. Mrs. Sanger went quietly from woman to woman. "You won't be arrested," she assured them. "You don't have to give your name if you don't want to."

One detective had even tried to enter the room where a highly nervous patient with a bad thyroid condition was being examined. Dr. Stone had stopped him only by planting herself squarely in the door. Poised and dignified despite the policemen milling around her, Dr. Stone told Mrs. Sanger, "Only a few hours ago a visiting physician from the Middle West asked if we ever had trouble with the police any more. Oh no, we assured him. Those days are gone long ago."

Over the whole scene, Mrs. Sullivan presided like some high priestess at a long-awaited mystic rite. Margaret Sanger later described her face as "terrifying" and "flushed with anger." Standing in the center of the reception room, she waved her arms and shouted directions to the policemen. "She was giving orders to her minions in such rapid succession it seemed impossible to keep pace with them."

The patrolmen were removing everything they could lay their hands on—books from the shelves, diagrams and pictures from the walls, contraceptive materials from the cabinets. Then Mrs. Sanger saw Patrolwoman McNamara, working quickly from a list in her hand, removing the case histories of patients from the files. It was time to act, to stand fast against this rude violation of medical ethics.

These records contained the most intimate confessions of women who had come to the clinic. For the doctor, they were considered a sacred trust—not even the nurses having access to them. What a woman had revealed about her husband's venereal disease or insanity could easily be used for purposes of blackmail.

"You cannot touch those records," Mrs. Sanger told Mrs. Sullivan. The Head of the Policewoman's Bureau scornfully produced a search warrant signed by Chief Magistrate McAdoo. Nevertheless, Mrs. Sanger repeated that the removal of the records would result in "serious trouble."

"Trouble?" Mrs. Sullivan mocked. "What about you?"

"I can take care of myself."

"Well, this is my party," cried the policewoman, repeating the order to her aides to seize the records.

Mrs. Sanger immediately telephoned Dr. Robert L. Dickinson at the Academy of Medicine. Horrified by the seizure of the records, he called Morris L. Ernst, a lawyer who had already amassed a distinguished liberal record in civil-rights suits.

The patrol wagon had now arrived, and Mrs. Sullivan hustled the two doctors and three nurses out to the street. Mrs. Sanger called a taxi to take the arrested party to the Twentieth Street station, but the police insisted, although Dr. Hannah Stone suffered from a weak heart, that the journey be made by wagon.

At the station, Mrs. Sullivan ordered that the party be fingerprinted. The old anger arose in Margaret Sanger. Here it was twelve years after her own arrest at the Brownsville clinic when she had fought against the indignity of being fingerprinted with common criminals. That principle had to be protected even if it meant a new fight. Resist, she told the five women. Resist with every ounce of your strength even if the police try to force your fingers to the ink pad.

Fortunately Mr. Ernst arrived at this point and was able to convince the police to forgo fingerprinting. The women were booked for violation of Section 1142 of the Penal Code—the same statute under which Mrs. Sanger had been arrested at Brownsville but which had been so broadly interpreted in Judge Crane's decision that the clinic had operated under it unmolested since 1923. They were then taken to the Jefferson Market court. Magistrate Abraham Rosenbluth looked over the warrant and ordered each released in three hundred dollars' bond.

Those two days after the raid passed like a blinding nightmare for Mrs. Sanger. Stuart was operated on for mastoid the next day. She was due in Chicago for an important conference and lecture. The doctor insisted that she go, but "the going was the hardest thing (next to one) I ever did in my life," she wrote De Selincourt. She conferred quickly with Morris Ernst. They agreed that the greatest point of vulnerability in the Police Department's action was the seizure of the records. Mr. Slee's minister, Dr. Karl Reiland, was a personal friend of Chief Magistrate McAdoo. He arranged to have dinner with him that night and present the facts.

Mrs. Sanger rushed back from Chicago to find that the operation had been successful. "We think and pray and hope he is a little better and recovering," she wrote De Selincourt.

Meanwhile, Magistrate McAdoo, distressed at finding that the clinic search warrant had been signed automatically by him among the dozens placed on his desk, had immediately called the police and ordered the medical records locked in his safe. He was well aware of the storm that would break around the heads of those who had perpetrated the seizure. To the New York *Times* the next day he asserted that the raiding party "had gone beyond the authority of their search warrants."

The Police Department was already under fire for its ineptitude in a number of recent underworld killings, including the murder of gambler Arnold Rothstein. Now it was denounced by almost every New York paper. "If the police can seize doctors' and lawyers' general files without a specific warrant and paw over them in search of possible evidence," the *Herald Tribune* protested, "the privileged relation of doctor and client ceases to exist. The possibilities of abuse, including blackmail, are virtually unlimited."

The *Post* asserted that "Police Commissioner Grover Whalen has deeply shocked the civic conscience of New York in the raid made by his underlings." The Commissioner at this point, however, was not perturbed. He blandly told the press that he had no personal knowledge of the raid and that it was a "routine matter."

Despite Magistrate McAdoo's efforts, only about forty record cards and six books were returned by the police, leaving over a hundred and fifty cards unaccounted for. "What use the Police Department might have had for them," Margaret Sanger wrote, "or to whom they might have been of interest, no one can say—no one, that is, who *will*." But her investigation later revealed that several women patients "had received mysterious and anonymous telephone calls, telling them that if they continued to go to the clinic their cases would be exposed in the newspapers. They happened to be Roman Catholic mothers whose cards were taken and never returned."

The seizure of the records was decisive to the case, not just because the police had blundered legally, but because for the first time it roused the most prominent doctors and medical organizations in the city to the support of the birth control movement. Mrs. Sanger had waited many years for this moment. Morris Ernst told the *Times* that the seizure was "outrageous and threatening to the entire medical profession." Heywood Broun in his column of April 17 made an even blunter thrust at medical pride. "If the medical profession fails to resent the raid upon the Birth Control Clinical Research Bureau, the physicians of this city should all consult chiropractors in an effort to learn what ails their spines. The police descended on this dispensary as if it were a dive . . . Are the doctors of New York willing to have their files ransacked at the whim of any gardeniaceous popinjay [a reference to Whalen's omnipresent gardenia] who happens to be in the hole on a big murder case?"

The medical profession quickly demonstrated its determination to fight back. The august Academy of Medicine, where Dr. Dickinson had called a special meeting, attacked the raid as a grave menace to "the freedom of the medical profession within legal qualifications for care and treatment of their patients." The Academy's official resolution viewed "with grave concern any action on the part of the authorities which contravenes the inviolability of the confidential relations which always have and should obtain between physicians and their patients."

Equally important in its support of the clinic was the fact that the Academy's director, Dr. Linsly Williams, enlisted the help of five of the city's most prominent physicians to testify in court—in addition to Dr. Dickinson, two other renowned gynecologists, Dr. Frederick C. Holden and Dr. Max Mayer; the noted neurologist, Dr. Foster Kennedy; and Dr. Louis I. Harris, former Commissioner of Health of New York. Further, Dr. Williams sent a strong letter of protest to Commissioner Whalen for calling the raid a "routine matter." With the press, the medical profession, and a committee of such social luminaries as Mrs. William K. Vanderbilt, Mrs. Ogden

Mills Reid, Mrs. Cornelius Bliss, and Mrs. Henry S. Schley supporting the defendants, the Commissioner quickly changed his mind and
apologized for the remark.

Significantly enough, during the course of the proceedings and
the trial not one publication praised the police for their action. "To
me every step in the legal procedure following the raid," Margaret
Sanger wrote later, "was an amazing revelation of progress—the fruit
of long, steady plodding, the response of an awakened conscious
interest which up to then had been strangely silent."

The trial which opened on April 19 before Magistrate Rosenbluth
was crucial to the future of the clinic and to the movement itself.
A defeat at this stage could wipe out all the hard-won progress of
the last twelve years. Describing the courtroom, the New York *Sun*
noted that "the walls were lined with spectators and every available
foot of standing room was taken." Ernst's brilliant defense was based
on the 1918 Crane decision, which had ruled that a physician could
prescribe contraception if the health or condition of the patient warranted it. "If the doctor is acting in good faith, with the thought
that the birth control information will prevent disease, that is all
we have to prove," Ernst told reporters.

Under Ernst's cross-examination, Policewoman McNamara admitted that she had made three visits to the clinic at 46 West Fifteenth
Street with the definite purpose of deceiving the doctors. She pretended she was the mother of three children, aged five, three, and
one when actually she had two children in their teens. She had told
Dr. Pissoort that she wanted to avoid having more children and
requested a device to prevent conception. Dr. Pissort examined her
and found her to have rectocele, cystocele, retroversion, prolapsus
of the uterus, and erosions of the cervix—findings that were all confirmed by Dr. Hannah Stone.

Ernst then called on Dr. Harris and the other expert witnesses to
support these findings. On the basis of her history and physical report, they stated, Anna McNamara presented definite medical indi-
cations for contraceptive advice. This testimony under the Crane decision gave the clinic a seemingly unshakable defense.

But Ernst was determined to do more than hold the ground that
had been won in 1918. He wanted this decision to enlarge the whole
future scope of the clinic—to establish the clinic once and for all as
a vital factor in public health work, and to have the court include

the spacing of children as an integral part of the care of a mother's health.

Ernst called Dr. Harris to the stand. "The birth control clinic is a public health work," stated the doctor. As Commissioner of Health, he had made an intensive survey of the clinic and found it "quite in keeping with the spirit and purpose of the law and with the spirit and purpose of medicine, public health medicine."

When Dr. Harris pointed out that every woman coming for treatment is asked if she is married, and if not, is rejected by the doctors, Magistrate Rosenbluth demanded: "Does the clinic send out social workers to discover the truth of the patients' statements?"

"Did you ever know of a situation where a doctor dispatched a detective to find out whether his patient was married?" asked Mr. Ernst. A wave of laughter swept through the courtroom. Obviously annoyed, the magistrate ordered the courtroom cleared. As the spectators filed out, they shouted, booed, and sang, "Sweet land of liberty!" A delegation of women thereupon went to the office of Chief Magistrate McAdoo and protested the ruling. After the next recess, the public was again admitted to the trial.

To support his contention that the birth control law must be interpreted to include the spacing of children among those factors vital to a mother's health, Ernst again called on Dr. Harris. Were frequent pregnancies and births without proper spacing a serious danger? asked Mr. Ernst. Definitely, said Dr. Harris. "So far as the mother is concerned, it aggravates and may, in fact, precipitate invalidism; as far as the child is concerned, it increases the hazard to the next born child very decidedly."

For corroboration, Ernst called on Dr. Foster Kennedy. "I think all pathologists and gynecologists realize the advantage of women not having babies at too frequent intervals," Dr. Kennedy stated. ". . . The possibility of recuperation for the mother depends upon proper spacing."

Such testimony was irrefutable, and the actual result of the trial, as Mrs. Sanger noted, was "well known in advance." But even two days before Magistrate Rosenbluth's decision on May 14, Commissioner Whalen demoted Mrs. Sullivan as Chief of the Policewoman's Bureau and admitted that her fall was the result of the raid. She had not consulted him about it, he stated. A decision "so important," said the Commissioner, who not long before had called it "routine," should have been brought to him for approval.

Who then was the instigating power behind the raid the New York *Herald Tribune* demanded editorially:

First who ordered the raid and why? Police Commissioner Whalen is quoted as refusing to say who made the original complaint. Why? If outside bodies or individuals are directing the work of the police, the public has a right to know it . . . It [the clinic] has never concealed its existence or its methods. Yet it was raided without warning, and the police showed an evident animus against its staff. Why?

When reporters questioned Mrs. Sullivan, she stubbornly refused to reveal the reason for the raid. Asked if there was any connection with the Roman Catholic hierarchy, she stalked away angrily.

Mrs. Sanger, however, insisted on making her own investigation and later reported:

I employed the Burns Detective Agency to sift the affair. Approximately fifty per cent of our cases were being sent by social workers on the Lower East and West sides, a conglomerate of all peoples and classes, including Irish, Italians and other Catholics. So many had benefited and told their neighbors that others also were asking of their agencies how to get to our clinic. Catholic social workers at a monthly meeting with officials of the Church had sought guidance in replying to parishioners . . . Catholic policewomen had been summoned, Mary Sullivan had been chosen to wipe out the Clinical Research Bureau, and Mrs. McNamara selected for the decoy.

No official admission of these facts was ever made. But it is significant that the clinic raid was the last strong-armed attack on the birth control movement by the politico-religious hierarchy in New York. Magistrate Rosenbluth's decision in the case was too strong to leave any further loopholes for police interference. "The law is plain," stated the magistrate, "that if the doctor in good faith believes that the patient is a married woman, and that her health requires prevention of conception, it is no crime to so advise and instruct therein . . ."

The two doctors and three nurses were not only completely exonerated, but the Rosenbluth decision, "one of the finest we have ever won," Mrs. Sanger called it, gave an unshakable legal foundation to the immediate expansion of the movement. The unstinting support given by the medical profession and the Academy of Medicine made it dramatically clear that birth control was, Dr. Hannah Stone wrote, "an important public health measure and a valuable aid in the conservation of family health . . . and must be regarded as an important factor in modern preventive medicine." In the next eight years, the number of clinics throughout the United States and Canada would not only expand from 55 to 374, but birth control would become an integral part of the public health services in many states.

As she had done so many times before, Mrs. Sanger had turned defeat into victory, a victory that transmitted to the whole movement an impetus and strength ushering in the greatest decade of its growth. "Margaret Sanger is a great and gallant woman," Heywood Broun wrote in fitting testimony to the climax of the trial, "and her work for welfare will be remembered when Grover Whalen is no more than 'Don't you remember that little fellow who was Police Commissioner for a while?'"

The publicity alone resulting from the raid brought so many new patients to the clinic that the waiting list now extended for months. Mrs. Sanger saw the necessity both of enlarging its services and housing it in a building of its own, so that it was no longer dependent on an outside landlord. In 1930, therefore, a whole building at 17 West Sixteenth Street was purchased as the gift of Mr. Slee. A four-story, red brick mansion of gracious pre-Civil War architecture, furnished with tasteful parquet floors, chandeliers, and fireplaces in every room, it provided the ultimate in friendly hospitality that Mrs. Sanger wanted for its patients as well as ample room for enlarged clinical, research, and office facilities.

The raid even had its ironic denouement. A few months later Policewoman Anna McNamara, who had listened anxiously in court to the medical analysis of her ailments, all reported in the public press, came once again to the clinic. This time, however, she came not as a policewoman but humbly to ask Dr. Stone's aid in the diagnosis and treatment of her case.

CHAPTER 23

In those dark months of conflict within the Birth Control League, Margaret Sanger had been editing the letters which had come to her from the mothers of America—almost a million in the last decade—into a new book, *Motherhood in Bondage*. "These voices of maternity's underworld . . . a sort of Greek Chorus of mothers in Greek tragedy," she called them, made an incomparable sociological record. These were the voices of women who had cried out to her in their need . . .

I am asking you for the remedy to save me from this awful pain and sin of bringing children into the world without any way to care for them . . . How am I to work for so many little children myself with a crippled husband?

The four of us are huddled in a little room about eight feet square. At night there is no way of ventilating the place, and I think it's a crime. I think children deserve something better than that.

It's just one baby after another. I can't stand it much longer and work like I do, trying to keep a little to eat and wear. I pray you to help me.

All told, these million letters were probably the greatest outpouring of human need and yearning ever directed toward one person. They were the link between Margaret Sanger and motherhood, a mystical link through which she often seemed to exist solely as the voice of all these other voices.

The concept had long been growing in her mind—"My mind is always ten years ahead of my actions," she once said—that the link between her and these mothers could someday be fused in a final assault on one of the last major legal barriers to birth control. That barrier was Section 211 of the Federal Penal Code, the infamous Comstock law. It intimidated physicians, making them afraid to use the mails or common carriers to send or secure contraceptive information or supplies. It was an obstacle to the study of contraceptive methods in medical schools. It hampered research. It made public notice of clinical services illegal. For fifty-six years, it had been "silently shackling the lives of American women, perpetuating suffering and physical torture, and spreading the blight of biological tragedy because of its diabolical taboos," Mrs. Sanger stated.

As early as 1926, she had sent Mrs. Kennedy and Mrs. George Day to Washington to make a study of the possibility of amending this law. They had spent several months interviewing senators and congressmen as to how they would vote on an amendment. The results of these interviews had been published as a box score in the *Review*.

Now Mrs. Sanger was convinced that the time was propitious to draw up a new federal bill and campaign for its passage. She worked on the bill with a committee of medical experts. It would be a "Doctor's Bill." Its specific purpose would be to open up the mails and common carriers to information and contraceptive materials which were sent by doctors, hospitals, and druggists for the care of their patients. In brief, it was based on the most scientific principles—to give any doctor in the country the right to secure the birth control materials he needed in his practice so that he could give contraceptive help to patients who requested it.

To put the "Doctor's Bill" through Congress, Mrs. Sanger now organized the National Committee for Federal Legislation for Birth Control. It was a giant undertaking—the establishment in a few months of an organization far larger than she had built in the American Birth Control League over many years. Although it had branches and clinics in other states, the league had always essentially been a New York movement. The National Committee, however, was to cover the country. It was to reach into every city and town, to rouse the mothers of America in a concerted chorus of angry protests against this legal barrier to their freedom, the Comstock law, and in support of the "Doctor's Bill." Here was Mrs. Sanger's ultimate vision of motherhood in revolt. Through the National Committee, she would direct the yearning and needs of these million mothers— and eventually far more. The National Committee at its peak would gain the support of a thousand national organizations, speaking for 20 million women.

Margaret Sanger established Washington headquarters for the National Committee at the Hotel Carlton late in 1929. Then dividing the country into three major areas, she staged regional conferences, first of the New England states in Boston in October, then of the midwestern states in Chicago in November, and finally of the western states at Los Angeles in February 1930. Each region had its own chairman, each state its own chairman and vice-chairman, but the basic organization was centered on the workers in each congressional district. The support of so complex a system would require Mrs. Sanger to make 114 lectures to local groups and raise $41,315 in 1930 alone.

Most of her closest associates on the league's board—Mrs. Rublee, Mrs. Day, Mrs. Ackerman, and Mrs. Timme—had followed her to the National Committee. The Washington office was directed by Mrs. Hepburn. Mrs. Alexander C. Dick, who with her late husband, Charles Brush, had made the Ohio league a model for the country, was secretary. Mrs. Hazel Moore had left the Red Cross to become legislative secretary, concentrating on the votes of senators and congressmen in support of the bill. Mr. Slee, still treasurer of the clinic, now undertook the additional responsibility of financing the committee's field workers.

It was the women on the community level, however, who carried the fight to local organizations and their neighbors. One typical worker, Mrs. Fred Thompson of Tacoma, Washington, was to secure thirty-three resolutions for the bill from women's groups in her state and 2,450 individual endorsements.

Mrs. Sanger's basic strategy was to win the support of every key national organization behind the bill. A group like The General Federation of Women's Clubs often took years of relentless effort. Hazel Moore, for instance, was sent to Detroit to attend its national convention but was barred from distributing literature for the bill inside the convention hall. Undaunted, she stood on the street day after day handing out pamphlets to delegates as they entered. A southerner with a large quota of regional charm, she first concentrated on the North Carolina delegation and won them over in two weeks. During the next few months, she gained the support of a dozen others. At the following year's convention, she was able to win the first concession—a vote by the Federation to appoint a committee to study the "Doctor's Bill." Ceaseless campaigning among state committees in the interval finally produced victory the third year. The Federation voted 493–17 to endorse the bill.

From the start, Margaret Sanger saw that the religious bodies must be a major point of concentration. Each year, she attended dozens of religious conventions, often spending hundreds of dollars in travel expenses to get five minutes of speaking time before the delegates. Ministers who supported birth control, like Rabbi Sidney Goldstein and Dr. Charles Francis Potter, were assigned to contact their fellow ministers; step by step, they swung other congregations behind the bill. One of the first groups to support it by a resolution at its 1930 convention was the American Unitarian Association. In England, a major impetus came that same year when the Bishops of the Church of England sitting in conference at Lambeth Palace voted 193–67 in favor of birth control.

In 1931, the Special Commission on Marriage, Divorce and Remarriage of the Presbyterian Churches in the United States followed suit. Then came the Central Conference of American Rabbis and the Universalist General Convention.

In March 1931, the Federal Council of Churches of Christ in America, a parent body including 23 million Protestant members, brought the first overwhelming victory through its resolution that "the interests of morality and sound scientific knowledge and the protection of both parents and children require the repeal of both Federal and State laws which prohibit the communication of information about birth control by physicians and other qualified persons."

"This is a day of triumph for Mrs. Sanger," stated the New York *World-Telegram*. "It's just what I would have written myself," she jubilantly told the press. "It is a real testimony of progress."

For in its lengthy analysis of birth control, the Federal Council had come out in full support of the new morality for which Margaret Sanger had fought all these years—"based upon knowledge and freedom while the old was founded upon ignorance." The key sentence in the Federal Council's report proclaimed: "There is general agreement also that the sex union between husbands and wives, as an expression of mutual affection without relation to procreation, is right."

"A remarkable statement . . . remarkable because of the nature of the body from which it emanates, for the reverence as well as for the realism of its expression," editorialized the New York *Herald Tribune*. "A service to the morals of the nation as well as to its physical well-being," the *World-Telegram* called it.

Support of birth control by so respected and influential a body stirred the anger of Roman Catholic spokesmen. Father Charles Coughlin in his weekly broadcast called it "a surrender to the ideals of paganism." "Continue this practice," said Reverend Wendell Corcoran of Notre Dame University, "and the sons of the yellow man or the black one will someday fill the President's chair at Washington." Catholic doctors in Brooklyn and the Bronx met and organized for an open campaign against birth control supporters in their profession.

In the face of these attacks, the Milwaukee *Sentinel* warned: "The spirit of this guaranty [religious liberty] has been forgotten apparently by the very churches which throve under its protection. . . ."

In Washington, Mrs. Sanger, Mrs. Hepburn, and the rest of the staff worked month after month to line up congressional votes behind the bill. They trudged from office to office, sometimes shunted aside by secretaries, often rebuffed, insulted, or stalled, but eventually gaining their interviews. If a secretary continuously claimed that a congressman was out, Mrs. Sanger would post a special staff member outside his office to watch for his arrival or departure. Mrs. Moore, always tireless in pursuit, would often hide behind a pillar in the hallway and track her prey—usually a southern senator or congressman—as he rushed for the elevator. Once she had him cornered, she released a southern charm that was irresistible—knowingly shifting her accent from Virginian to North Carolinian as the occasion demanded.

During the height of the legislative campaign, as many as seventeen staff members were kept in Washington, and Mrs. Sanger worked them ruthlessly. One afternoon just before the "Doctor's Bill" was called in committee, she saw the necessity of getting out an urgent letter to key constituents of every legislator. The staff stayed all night—but twenty thousand letters got out.

"There were days—an awful lot of days," one staff member recalled, "when we didn't even have the time to wash our petticoats. We were all living at a hotel near the office—if we were lucky enough to get back there. I can't remember how many times I wanted to quit. Then Mrs. Sanger would come along and take us out for coffee. She'd talk quietly in that glowing way of hers and laugh once or twice and soon we were all laughing. In half an hour she could recharge us. We'd go back and work all night."

To introduce the first "Doctor's Bill" into the Senate, Mrs. Sanger had lined up one of the most venerable Republicans, Frederick Gillett of Massachusetts. Guiding the bill carefully through the maze of congressional procedure, he sent it to the Judiciary Committee whose chairman, Senator Norris, was friendly to it. Norris appointed a subcommittee for the hearings—Samuel G. Bratton of New Mexico, William E. Borah of Idaho, and Gillett. The hearings opened on February 13, 1931.

Two years of relentless effort had gone into this moment, two years of speeches, interviews, campaign tours to line up hundreds of national religious groups, and union, political, medical, and social organizations behind the bill. Mrs. Sanger stood up before the committee and quietly read off the impressive list. She was wearing a simple black dress with a turtle-neck collar that accentuated the glowing, luminous quality of her face. ("All those dresses from Paris, and you never wear them," Mr. Slee always complained. But she knew the dramatic value of simplicity.) A reporter from the Reading, Pennsylvania, *Eagle* later described the impact of seeing Mrs. Sanger in action for the first time. ". . . I still cannot believe this is THE Mrs. Sanger . . . She is slight, she is beautifully dressed . . . and although her history belies it, she doesn't look a day over thirty-four. How anyone could bear to commit her to jail for even an hour I can't imagine. Her face, sober or smiling, has a kind of wistful quality, and her lovely auburn hair turns up in a soft natural roll at the back of her neck."

In the hour and a half allotted to them, Mrs. Sanger called on authorities from every field—Dr. Charles Francis Potter on the moral phases of birth control, Dr. Sidney Goldstein on its religious aspects, Professor Roswell Johnson on eugenics, Professor Henry Pratt Fairchild on economics, Mrs. Douglas Moffat, speaking for the New York Junior League. The medical representative was the renowned Dr. John Whitridge Williams, chief obstetrician at Johns Hopkins. "A doctor who has this information [prevention of conception] and does not give it," he concluded, "cannot help feeling that he is taking a responsibility for the lives and welfare of large numbers of people."

It was the health of women and children that Margaret Sanger made the focal point of her testimony. Since the Comstock law was passed in 1873, more than a million and a half mothers had died from causes related to childbearing, the major cause being abortions. A study at the Clinical Research Bureau had shown that each woman had had an average of one abortion to every two and a half confinements. For the country as a whole, Dr. Fred J. Taussig had estimated an average of seven hundred thousand abortions a year—the great tragedy being that almost all could have been prevented by birth control.

"It is also roughly estimated that since the law was passed," she continued, "more than fifteen million children have passed out of life during their first year of infancy; many of them were children born in conditions of poverty and their mothers' ill-health. A great majority might have been living today had their mothers had a chance to recuperate from the ordeal of previous pregnancy instead of using up the vitality of the child before it was born."

The very crux of the "Doctor's Bill" was to abolish the necessity of abortions by making contraceptive information and materials available to the medical profession. "We believe that there is nothing to be gained by keeping such laws on the statute books," she concluded, "when they are known to be inimical to the personal health of mothers, to the family happiness, and to the general welfare and progress of the nation . . . Mr. Chairman, we want children to be conceived in love, born of parents' conscious desire, and born into the world with healthy and sound bodies and sound minds."

The next morning was allotted to those forces opposing the bill— the Society for the Suppression of Vice, now led by John Sumner, Comstock's successor; the Patriotic Society, the Purity League, the Clean Books League, and foremost among them, the Roman Catholic hierarchy. "These dogmatists, harking back to the Dark Ages," she wrote later, "summoned to their aid the same arguments that had been used to hinder every advance in our civilization—that it was against nature, against God, against the Bible, against the country's best interests, and against morality. Even though you proved your case by statistics and reason and every known device of the human mind, the opponents parroted the line of attack over and over again . . ."

As she listened to the tirades of the opposition, her anger grew. Here were these twisted minds, searching out every effort toward human advance, trampling hopes and ideals into the ground. She felt as though she had been plunged into some antediluvian age, into some fantastic kingdom out of *Gulliver's Travels.* Here was her old antagonist, she wrote, "not the Church of Christ but the Church of Rome, with its two thousand years or more of organization, of power, of secret intrigue and machinations, the Church that my father had combated when I was only a little girl, the Church that had obstructed every effort of human emancipation, every step towards the stars—the Church that had sent me to jail."

She had to speak out, to pin down these falsifications of the democratic process with all the strength that burned in her. "We are not imposing any legislation on the Catholics," she cried in rebuttal. ". . . They have a perfect right to use the method of self-control if they wish; but we do believe that we have just as much right under the Constitution to enjoy health, peace and the right to the pursuit of happiness as we see it . . .

"Regardless of religion, women come to us, desperate women, women trying to live decently, trying to avoid the conditions that unwanted pregnancy and too frequent pregnancy bring. These women come in equal proportions—about thirty-three per cent Protestant, thirty-two per cent Catholics, and thirty-one per cent Jewish women. They all come with the same cry: 'Give us a chance to space our children. It is not that we do not love children, because we do love them; but because we want to give them a better chance than we have had, and we know that another child born into this family only deprives the children that are already here of a decent living with the ideals that we have for them.' "

The two senators attending the meeting listened impassively. When the vote was taken, Bratton voted against the bill. Gillett was for it. Senator Borah, who had not even attended a minute of the hearings, killed the bill with his negative vote.

Almost two years of impassioned work seemed to have been lost that morning—yet before the day was over Margaret Sanger had given orders to get out a new mailing to field workers all over the country to start the fight for the reintroduction of the "Doctor's Bill" at the next session. "Life has taught me one supreme lesson," she wrote at that time. "This is that we must—if we are really to *live* at all . . . put our convictions into action. My remuneration has been that I have been privileged to act out my faith." Even in temporary defeat, the real victory was in action—perhaps slow, inching progress, but progress that she knew would bring eventual victory.

"When we look at the work she has done," John Dewey, the

eminent philosopher of Columbia University stated at that time, "I think we can begin to understand what that passage in the New Testament means about faith moving mountains."

2

The one retreat from the turbulence of Washington was always Willow Lake. It was Margaret Sanger's "jewel of peace," a friend described it. Inside its gates with the manicured lawns stretching to the lakeside, the path of blue irises that led to her "Tree Tops" study, she could instantly recapture the serenity and perspective that gave her leadership a quality of eternal wisdom. She ate her meals on the breakfast porch overlooking the lake. She worked at the small pavilion near by, her cocker spaniel, "Pepper," stirring restlessly at her feet. Her secretary and other staff members usually arrived at some point during the week end, bringing with them a thousand problems from the office. "As soon as we arrived," Florence Rose once said, "the weight seemed to drop from our shoulders. It was like a new gift each time—the serenity she gave us."

The pressure of the legislative campaign, which kept Mrs. Sanger in Washington or took her on speaking trips around the country, separated her more and more often from Mr. Slee. When she didn't turn up at Willow Lake for the week end, he would call her New York or Washington office and vent his anger into the telephone. "Poor dear," she once said. "There he sits home all alone. I always tell him what Ellis once said, that there ought to be a league for the husbands of famous wives."

Stuart and Grant too appeared less and less at Willow Lake. After graduation from Princeton, Grant had begun the intensive life of a medical student at Cornell Medical School in New York. Stuart lingered on a few more years on Wall Street; then he too turned to the study of medicine. The devoted and unpredictable Daisy, who had been Mrs. Sanger's maid for almost fifteen years, superintended the New York apartment, where Grant and two other students lived. Daisy, despite certain eccentricities that grated on Mr. Slee, would always be a fixture in Mrs. Sanger's life. Often she came up to Willow Lake to assist at a dinner party, and occasionally during the evening while the guests were seated around the fireplace, would drift into the living room and stretch out in a corner armchair, listening attentively to the conversation. "What are you doing here, Daisy?"

Mr. Slee would demand. "Gettin' an education. Just gettin' an education," she would answer.

Once when they were giving an Italian dinner at their New York apartment, Mrs. Sanger had laid in a gallon jug of Italian wine. Just before dinnertime, she asked Daisy to bring it out. "I don't know nothin' about any wine," Daisy murmured.

"Of course you do. I put it right on the bottom shelf of the main cupboard."

The bottle appeared a few minutes later—completely empty. "Daisy, what could have happened to that?" Mrs. Sanger demanded.

"Evaporation. Pure evaporation, madam," she explained.

Even with the demands of the legislative campaign during these years, Mrs. Sanger sailed for Europe in the summer of 1930 to organize the Seventh International Birth Control Conference at Zurich. It was "a period in my life," she wrote, "when I reached a height . . . from which I could discern the harvest of the seeds I had sown." In 1927, she had helped Dr. Martha Ruben-Wolf establish the first birth control clinic in Berlin. That one center had now expanded to eighteen. Reporting to the conference on the impact of her tour eight years before, Dr. Kan Majima, Japan's official delegate, described how "Margaret Sanger's visit laid the foundation for birth control work" and the opening of that country's first clinic.

Those were two seeds that had grown well. More had to be planted—particularly in the Far East. But there were special problems in those areas that didn't exist in the United States—the problem of the inexpensive and simple contraceptive that could be used by the great mass of the people in the out-of-the-way villages which might never see a doctor. That was why she had called this conference specifically to consider the scientific aspects of new birth control techniques. She had brought together 130 physicians and clinic directors from all over Europe and America to analyze new possibilities in the field of contraception.

New words were beginning to creep into the language of contraception—chemical contraception, hormonal control of fertility, spermatoxin. The words danced like dreams before her eyes. She had an intuitive vision into the future of biochemistry that always put her mind at least a decade ahead of the scientists themselves. Here was an enormous expanding movement that still depended on mechanical techniques that had been developed sixty years ago. She saw the imperative necessity of a search for new techniques, a search that was to absorb her for most of the rest of her life. There were rumors of a spermatoxin, an inoculation that would prevent pregnancy, being developed in Russia, but the most concrete explorations reported at the conference came from the young biologists and biochemists of Oxford, Cambridge, and Edinburgh universities. She was determined that the international movement must stand solidly behind their work. It would take time and money, lots of them. But she saw now the blueprint of the future. "One left the conference," she wrote, "convinced that here was the beginning of a new era in human progress. . . ."

3

Back in Washington, she launched a new campaign that would bring women all over the country immediately and directly into the fight for the "Doctor's Bill." Here were these thousands of letters from mothers that came to her office every month, pleading for birth control information. Why not have them write to their own congressmen? Why not bring this great mass of human need to the very legislators who were blocking passage of the "Doctor's Bill?"

To each mother who wrote her, she would now send a form letter, stating briefly: "I would gladly give you this information. But the law forbids it. Your Congressman now has the chance to change this law. Write him and tell him how many children you have living, how many that died, how many abortions you have had, and how much your husband earns. Tell him how desperately you need birth control information and want the 'Doctor's Bill' passed."

The results of these mailings were remarkable. On her visits to the offices of senators and congressmen, Mrs. Sanger would find dozens of these letters from constituents piled up on their desks. Once, walking through the tunnel which connects the House with the Senate, she stopped to ask a man for directions. He inquired what she was doing on the Hill and she described the "Doctor's Bill."

"Isn't that amazing?" he cried. "Just this morning I received a letter from a woman who's lived a few miles from me all her life." He pulled it from his pocket and read off the dismal list of abortions and children dead in infancy. "I've never read anything so awful— and at the end she says, 'Help me, help me by supporting Mrs. Sanger.'"

She walked with him back to his office, and he introduced himself as Senator Henry D. Hatfield of West Virginia. A few months later, Senator Hatfield became the sponsor of the "Doctor's Bill" at the next session.

As grass-roots support increased for the bill, so too did the almost frantic attacks of the opposition. At one hearing, Mrs. Thomas A. McGoldrick, representing the International Federation of Catholic Alumnae, asserted it was "the younger promiscuous generation, high school boys and girls" who financed birth control. "I heard one of the doctors of the Birth Control League say on a public platform a large percentage of the people who apply at the clinics are unmarried people. . . ."

Mrs. Sanger immediately challenged her to name the doctor. Mrs. McGoldrick remained conspicuously silent.

The lowest depths of vilification still remained to be reached by the radio priest, Father Charles E. Coughlin. In an outright attack on Mrs. Sanger's associates who had just spoken at the hearings for the "Doctor's Bill," he cried: "We know how these contraceptives are bootlegged in the corner drugstores surrounding our high schools. Why are they around the high schools? To teach them to fornicate and not get caught. All this bill means is 'How to fornicate and not get caught.'"

There was a shocked silence in the hearing room, then a quick murmur of angry voices. Some of the women who had come with Mrs. Sanger rose in their seats as if to move toward Father Coughlin. Mrs. Sanger held them back. Two men on the committee refused to sit there in silence and stamped from the room. "It was probably the greatest mistake in my life to hold those women back," Mrs. Sanger said later. "Here were these fine, decent women, standing for all that was best in motherhood, and they had practically been told to their faces that they were prostitutes. They were bursting with anger. I have never seen women so angry. If I had not held them back, they would have hurled inkwells at that man and struck him with chairs."

In 1934, the "Doctor's Bill" was introduced into the Senate by Senator Daniel O. Hastings of Delaware and into the House by Representative Walter Pierce of Oregon. Preceding it between October 1932 and October 1933 had come a lecture campaign of amazing intensity—826 lectures by thirty speakers from the National Committee. More senators and congressmen had been lined up behind the bill than at any previous session.

It was a moment of optimism—and some of Mrs. Sanger's supporters were even convinced that the bill could pass this year with the help of liberal Catholic support from an unexpected quarter. Dr. Joseph J. Mundell, they said, was ready to withdraw some of his major objections to the bill. Dr. Mundell was a key figure—Professor of Obstetrics at Georgetown University and adviser on medical legislation to the Catholic Welfare Council. Mrs. Sanger went to see him. Together they worked out a compromise. She agreed to change certain aspects of the bill; he agreed not to oppose others. "The compromise," she wrote later, "apparently suited everybody."

Then came his testimony at the hearings and an unexpected bombshell. He "deliberately betrayed us," Mrs. Sanger stated. Instead of supporting the revised "Doctor's Bill" as he had agreed, he testified blandly that no legislation on birth control was now even necessary. The reason—the release of new scientific studies which proved, he said, that the monthly fertile period in women could now be reckoned with almost mathematical precision, thus eliminating the necessity of using contraception. The studies referred to were *The Sterile Period in Family Life* by Very Reverend Valère J. Coucke and Dr. James J. Walsh and *The Rhythm of Sterility and Fertility in Women*, by D. Leo J. Latz.

The "rhythm method," as it was called, introduced a radical new aspect into the Catholic attitude toward birth control. Faced increasingly with the fact that a growing percentage of Catholics were making use of clinics throughout the country, the church hierarchy had come to the realization that some drastic step had to be taken to meet this trend. "Rhythm" seemed to offer a logical solution since, as Reverend Wilfred Parsons, editor of the Catholic periodical, *America,* explained: "It is not proper to refer to the theory as one of birth control when it concerns natural laws rather than the use of artificial means of contraception, which are condemned by the church authorities." This seemed to be drawing a fine distinction, for whether it depended on natural laws or not, "rhythm" still aimed at the same objective—the prevention of pregnancy. But the distinction was obviously enough for the Church. Dr. Latz's book carried the official imprimatur of the Church, as did another version, *Legitimate Birth Control,* which had the sponsorship of Bishop John Francis Noll of Fort Wayne.

The rhythm theory was based on studies of the reproductive cycle in women by Dr. M. Ogino of Japan and Dr. Herman Knaus of

Vienna. During this menstrual cycle, a woman matures one egg—
an egg that is ripe according to the general concensus of opinion
for at most a forty-eight-hour period. Since the male sperm cell also
lives no more than forty-eight hours, the theory assumes that conception is possible only around the time of ovulation. The problem
then is to find the exact day on which ovulation occurs. The eight
days of this period of ovulation are the fertile period. The rest of the
month are "safe"—a period when the woman is supposedly infertile.

Whether rhythm was the answer to the Catholic dilemma or not,
the more important issue was that no one had proved its accuracy—
nor has to this day. Mrs. Sanger, who stated that medical evidence
had shown it no more than 40 per cent accurate, immediately called
on the renowned Dr. Prentiss Willson, who testified bluntly about its
lack of medical standing. Dr. C. C. Little issued another statement
to the New York *Herald Tribune,* declaring that "There is no evidence from human or animal experimentation that it would be de-
pendable." Mrs. Sanger even challenged the Catholic hierarchy to
test the theory at the Clinical Research Bureau. "Our staff of fifteen
women physicians, nurses and experts will be placed at the disposal
of Catholic physicians if they will send their women to us," she
announced. No one took up the offer.

Mrs. Sanger was determined to use the Catholic advocacy of the
Latz book to her own advantage at the hearings. When it was time
for her to testify, she walked to the witness chair and very quietly
announced that she was going to read one of the finest statements
on birth control ever written. The statement was in answer to the
question whether married couples were obligated to bring into the
world all the children they could. "Far from being an obligation,"
she read from the book in her hand, "such a course may be utterly
indefensible. Broadly speaking, married couples have not the right
to bring into the world children whom they are unable to support,
for they would therefore inflict a grievous damage on society."

Where did this statement come from? From Dr. Latz's book on
rhythm, the very book that bore the Church's imprimatur, she told
the subcommittee. The point was obvious. Both Mrs. Sanger and Dr.
Latz were in virtual agreement on their objective.

For the first time since the National Committee had begun its campaign for the "Doctor's Bill," it was reported out to the full Senate
and placed on the unanimous consent calendar. Even to get this far
after all these years was like a miracle. Each day Mrs. Sanger and

her associates went to the senate gallery and waited. Then came the last day of the session, June 13. There were two hundred bills ahead of it. Every member of the committee who could squeeze into the visitors' gallery watched tensely as one bill after another was hurried through—some passed, some tabled, some sent back to committee. At last the "Doctor's Bill" came up and passed quickly, with no voice raised against it. It was the ultimate miracle.

There was still one more hurdle—a twenty-four-hour limit for any senator to ask for unanimous consent to recall the bill. They waited—but not long. Twenty minutes later, Senator Pat McCarran, a prominent Catholic, rushed from the cloakroom to the floor and asked for recall. Senator Hastings granted the request—practically a necessity since if he had objected Senator McCarran would have tried to block every bill he introduced thereafter.

The "Doctor's Bill" was referred back to committee and final death. It seemed like the end of a long road of heartaches and relentless labor—yet always Mrs. Sanger knew it was only the beginning.

If the legislative campaign had not yet convinced the Congress of the United States, it was slowly gaining the support of some of the most important bodies in the country. On April 21, 1931, the New York Academy of Medicine passed a formal resolution which demanded immediate changes in federal and state laws to exempt doctors from the prohibitions on birth control information. "The public is entitled to expert counsel and information by the medical profession," stated the resolution, "on the important and intimate matter of contraceptive advice." It was the first major medical group in the United States to come out in full support of Mrs. Sanger's National Committee. "Epoch-making is no exaggerated term [for it]," said the New York *World-Telegram*.

Then on November 12, 1931, the American Women's Association under the direction of Miss Ann Morgan became the first national women's group to honor Margaret Sanger officially with its medal of achievement. In its citation the association said:

. . . *She has fought a battle against almost every influence which in the past was considered necessary to the success of a cause. Against her stood the state, the church, the schools, the press and society. She has fought that battle singlehanded . . . a pioneer of pioneers.*

She has carried her cause without remuneration or personal reward other than poverty, condemnation and ostracism. . . . She has changed and is changing the entire social structure of our world. She has opened the doors of knowledge and thereby given light, freedom and happiness to thousands caught in the tragic meshes of ignorance. She is remaking the world.

The "Doctor's Bill" still remained unpassed, but a different kind of victory, perhaps even more significant, was being won. Commenting on the Women's Association award to Mrs. Sanger, the New York *Herald Tribune* stated: "Such is the common sense of what she has been saying, and so great the courage and conviction of her way of saying it, that people have at last begun to listen and believe." That was what Margaret Sanger wanted above all—the listening and the believing.

CHAPTER 24

"It is fate pushing you into the world work," Edith How-Martyn had written Margaret Sanger at the moment of her resignation from the Birth Control League. They were prophetic words. She was ready to reach out again beyond the boundaries of America. It had begun, of course, with the Japanese trip in 1922, then continued with the 1927 Population Conference and the 1930 Zurich Conference. Now she knew, with the deep, instinctive knowledge that always put her a decade ahead of her time, that the focus of birth control was shifting to the Far East. Once the objectives of the "Doctor's Bill" had been won, the dreams would lie to the East. That vast, immeasurable reservoir of human suffering was where the battle for population control, the new science of rational evolution against the chaos of the past, would meet its ultimate test.

She was drawn by the very enormity of the challenge. In India, two hundred thousand women each year died as a result of childbirth. The maternal death rate of 24.5 compared frighteningly with Great Britain's 4.5. Almost one and three quarter million infants died each year before their first birthday. Almost 97 per cent of the people did not eat more than one full meal a day, 95 per cent did not earn over five cents a day. Yet the birth rate was climbing at a frightening rate. Here was the ultimate agony of motherhood—a system where mass breeding engaged in frenzied competition with disease, starvation, and death. Here was a need so desperate that Margaret Sanger felt it inside her like a tangible, physical sickness.

But the international challenge was scientific as well as emotional. Since the first discussion of a biochemical contraceptive at the Zurich conference, she had been convinced that to bring birth control to these massive areas of illiterate populations would mean the development of new techniques—birth control so simple, so inexpensive and so safe that the remotest peasant in the smallest village could use it.

Russia had issued reports of a new spermatoxin, a sperm protein injection that could render a woman immune from conception for a period of weeks or even months. Here was the scientific dream that must be explored. Further, Russia was the great experiment, the first state where socialist theory was being hammered into reality, where the emancipation of women had been heralded, not just with political and economic equality, but a complete revolution in social values which, it was said, made birth control and abortion a service of the state.

Russia in 1934, India in 1935—these two trips with such diverse objectives and results would thrust Margaret Sanger irrevocably onto the world stage.

2

She made up a party of four for the Russian trip. Grant, about to enter his final year at Cornell Medical School, would observe the progress of medicine in the Soviet Union. Her secretary, Florence Rose, an efficient organizer in the office or field, and Mrs. Ethel Clyde, a veteran officer of the National Committee, were the other two members. Their small group made up just one unit of a much larger group, a guided tour known as the Second Russian Seminar. Mrs. Sanger had learned from friends of the problems of traveling in Russia except in an officially recognized tour with expert interpreters. She had scheduled many of her own side trips of investigation, but she would travel with the Seminar.

The Russians were a mass of contradictions, she found. "One moment I was irritated enough to tear them limb from limb, the next prostrate before their sincerity and zeal."

Russia's proudest boast—she heard it wherever she went—was that its children had been made its most treasured possession. Even her guide, Tanya, hardly over thirty, would always say, "Our hope is the young people." At Leningrad, Mrs. Sanger visited the Institute for the Protection of Motherhood and Childhood. It stretched for over a mile, one gleaming new building after another—hospitals, model clinics, nurseries, milk centers, and educational laboratories. The vast center was as impressive as its name.

The emancipation of women—at least of the new generation—had been accomplished with blinding speed. The trained and essential worker had been freed from the kitchen and nursery. Mrs. Sanger visited dozens of factories and offices in each city where mothers held jobs with equal stature and pay of men. Their children were scrupulously cared for and fed at adjoining nurseries and child centers.

The Revolution had brought sweeping new concepts of marriage and sex. Most significant of these was the legalization of abortions. Any Russian woman on application to her doctor could be admitted to an abortion center for a nominal fee. The operation was legal and respected. The woman suffered from no prejudice. She would return to her job in a few weeks with no loss in pay.

Mrs. Sanger went through one Moscow clinic, interviewing at least fifty patients. They had received the best medical attention. Their health was good. Soon they would return home to rest for a week or two. Some of these women had had five abortions in the last two years; one woman, seven abortions. How wasteful, how cruel, Mrs. Sanger protested! All this medical skill concentrated on an operation that involved danger, pain, and constant draining of the woman's health. Why this complex system of abortion clinics? Why not birth control?

Mrs. Sanger asked each woman if she would have preferred birth control to the dangers of abortion. "We hear of it, but we have nothing," each replied.

The frustrating paradox was that many Russian health authorities claimed that birth control information was available at women's clinics. But where? In Moscow and Leningrad, Mrs. Sanger visited fifteen hospitals with no results. At Stalingrad's vast new hospital, she asked the superintendent, a gynecologist who spoke fluent English, whether he gave contraceptive advice.

"I do not, but we have a department of consultation."

"May I see it?"

The superintendent took her down the hall, and they entered the department, where posters on the wall seemed to give ample evidence that birth control was being taught by the government. But the consultation room itself was locked. The superintendent called a woman assistant. "When I send patients over here, who takes care of them?"

"I do sometimes," the assistant said. She let them into the consultation room. Mrs. Sanger saw the same display cases she had seen everywhere, the diaphragms and other contraceptive techniques, moldy and cracked, probably untouched for years.

"When patients are sent over," she asked, "what equipment do you use?"

"We have nothing," the assistant said. "We've asked and asked Moscow, but we get nothing."

The superintendent was embarrassed. "How long has it been since supplies have come?"

"Two years."

"Well, what about the patients I send over here?"

"We just tell them to go home and wait. We have nothing for them."

It was tragic, Mrs. Sanger realized. This amazing set of contradictions. This apparent blueprint for birth control, when the government actually ignored its own objectives despite the fact that the Soviet Union had increased its population by 20 million people since the downfall of the Czars.

She was determined to wring from the highest Soviet official an official statement on population policy. In Moscow, she met Sherwood Eddy, the author and authority on Asia, and Louis Fischer, then living in Moscow and writing for the *Nation*. They invited her to a joint interview with Dr. Kaminsky, the Secretary of the Commissariat of Public Health. Ushered into an enormous room with high windows and a banquet table laden with afternoon tea, they questioned the doctor briefly and then Mrs. Sanger broke in: "Has Russia a population policy, Dr. Kaminsky? Has she formulated any program for the rate of increase of her people?"

The interpreter did not even pass the question to his chief but leaped to his feet, crying, "Malthusianism! We will not have Malthusianism here! We can have all the children we want, and Russia can do with twice the population she now has."

She waited for the outburst to subside. "I asked Dr. Kaminsky a simple question," she said. "I said nothing about Malthusianism. Russia has five- and ten-year plans for agriculture and manufacture and everything she makes. But what plan has she for the most important issue today—the rate of population growth?"

This time Louis Fischer whispered the translation to Dr. Kaminsky, and the doctor replied, "If I understand correctly, you are asking if there is a policy from the biological or economic point of view."

"I know you have a fine technique of abortions," she said. "Four hundred thousand abortions a year certainly indicate that women are trying to control the number of their children. But abortions in my opinion are a cruel method because no matter how well they are done, they are an exhausting strain on the woman. Do the legality of abortions and their widespread use indicate any population policy of the government?"

Dr. Kaminsky's answer was short and curt. "There is no policy as to the question of biological restriction. For six years, we have had a great shortage, not only of skilled workers but of labor in general. Now the only question is the increase of population."

There it was—the demands of the Soviet Union's rapidly expanding economy had taken priority over previous plans for birth control. There was one more factor. The Soviet Government, already fearing the threat of Hitler's Germany, had begun the build-up of its armed forces, a build-up that necessitated the highest possible birth rate. The demands of history seemed to have conspired against the fulfillment of a once-promising birth control program.

Margaret Sanger's search for the new biological contraceptive, the spermatoxin, made her frustration complete. In Leningrad, she found old Professor Tushnov, who had helped develop the spermatoxin. He welcomed her politely. Yes, he had conducted experiments with the injection on many women, the majority of whom had been rendered immune from pregnancy for periods of three to five months. But now the government's policy had halted the experiments. All laboratory technicians were being removed from pure research and transferred to more immediate scientific projects. The government had even banned the publication of all information on the spermatoxin under penalty of arrest and allowed no dispatch on it to foreign newspapers that had not already been printed in the Soviet Union.

She won one concession from Professor Tushnov—permission to take a copy of the spermatoxin formula back to the United States and test it there. She left Russia, taking an Italian liner from Odessa and meeting Mr. Slee at Naples. As soon as she got back to New York, she secured a grant from a major public health foundation to test the serum. The grant was made to the University of Pennsylvania, where for two years the spermatoxin was used on animals. The results were unconvincing, the experiments mismanaged, Mrs. Sanger concluded. One day she would renew her search for an efficient spermatoxin. The dream was to pursue her for the next fifteen years—the dream of a chemical contraceptive that would bring birth control to the most remote corners of the world.

3

India was different. India waited expectantly for Margaret Sanger. Not only its nationalist leaders like Jawaharlal Nehru, but many educators and philosophers saw the crucial necessity of birth control. She had met Rabindranath Tagore in New York in 1931. "In a hunger-stricken country like India," he had stated, "it is a cruel crime thoughtlessly to bring more children into existence than can properly be taken care of, causing endless suffering to them and imposing a degrading condition upon the whole family." The editor of the *Journal of Marriage Hygiene*, Dr. A. P. Pillay, had long supported Mrs. Sanger in his magazine. Recently he had started distributing birth control information from centers in Calcutta, Madras, and Bombay.

But it was the All-India Women's Conference, speaking for 12 million Indian women but voicing the aspirations of millions more, whose invitation brought Mrs. Sanger to India. Last year's conference had passed a resolution approving birth control in theory. Now its leaders wanted Mrs. Sanger at the December conference to help put across a more practical resolution and launch a working birth control program. They also wanted her to make a speaking tour of India. Her presence would be a flame here.

Mrs. Sanger's trip would be sponsored by the Birth Control International Information Centre, that vigorous organization with headquarters in England which had grown out of the 1927 Population Conference. Its executive secretary, Mrs. Edith How-Martyn, immediately left London for India to make the advance arrangements. Mrs. Sanger sailed from New York for England on the *Normandie* on October 23, 1935, accompanied by Anna Jane Phillips, a young newspaper woman who would act as her secretary.

In London, Harry Guy, chairman of the council of the Information Centre, gave her a testimonial dinner of regal proportions at historic Barbers' Hall. The high-ceilinged paneled hall, once the dissecting room for the Guild of Barbers four hundred years before, glistened with heavy silver plate on its long dining tables. The plate had been given the Barbers by Queen Anne for state occasions. The large Royal Grace Cup was the gift of Henry VIII.

At the center of the head table in his high-backed chair above the rest of the diners sat Mr. Guy. On his right was the guest of honor, Margaret Sanger. Next to her was the eminent physician whose steadfast advocacy of birth control had brought public acceptance so quickly in England, Lord Horder, physician to the Prince of Wales. The guest list was equally impressive—the Countess of Limerick, Lord and Lady Wellesley, Lord and Lady Walker, Lady Denham, Lady Minter, Sir Harold and Lady Mackintosh, Mrs. Harold Laski, H. G. Wells, and Arthur Rank, among others.

Following ancient ritual, the toastmaster proclaimed: "Pray, silence for the King!" The Royal Grace Cup, filled with red wine, began to make the rounds, followed by the silver finger bowl, a gift to the Barbers from Queen Anne. Then came the toast to the President of the United States, and finally a toast to Mrs. Sanger, proposed by Lord Horder in recognition of "her long and courageous battle for a principle which every intelligent person now accepts as the basis of a new and finer civilization."

"Margaret Sanger," said Harry Guy in his testimonial speech, "is one of the few people in the world upon whose forehead, as in the fairy stories of our childhood, a silver star shines brightly."

She sailed on November 9 on the *Viceroy of India* and landed at Bombay under a steaming Indian sun. They had felt the touch of her coming. Fifty of the city's leading physicians and eugenicists waited on the dock for her. They welcomed her with garlands of flowers hung around her neck. Photographers and newsmen crowded around. By the time she reached the Taj Mahal Hotel, she looked, as she noted later, "more like a bridesmaid than a propagandist."

That night she was honored at a reception by the officers of the Bombay Medical Union and the dean of the medical faculty of Bombay University. The next afternoon, she addressed a public meeting at Cowasji Jehangir Hall, the largest in Bombay—looking down at a white sea of caps worn by the followers of Gandhi, the hall packed.

There was an enthusiastic press; every Bombay paper covered the event. She was invited to speak on the radio. Lord and Lady Braybourne entertained her at Government House. The Bombay Corporation asked her to address a meeting convened in her honor. The Mayor himself introduced her. What she had to say about municipalities and birth control aroused such interest that shortly afterward the Corporation set up a special committee to establish contraceptive services at municipal hospitals. A few months later a free clinic was opened in the cotton-mill area of the city, with the Mayor leading the ceremonies.

But the real objective in India, she knew, was to reach the untold millions of workers and peasants, cut off from the main stream of life by illiteracy, ignorance, and superstition. Many days she spent just walking through the tenements of Bombay—the chawls, those huts of corrugated iron, three walls, and sometimes pieces of rag or paper hung in front in a feeble attempt at privacy, no windows, no lights or lamps. Here two or three families often lived in one small room, adults and children alike on the edge of starvation. She would often stop and ask the mothers through her interpreter how many children they had and how many more they wanted. Invariably there was the same cry, "No more. Please, no more."

"If at any time I should feel tired and wonder whether this campaign in India is worthwhile," she wrote to friends back home, "I should only have to walk five minutes through the side streets . . . and look at the teeming masses of poverty-stricken, starved men, women and children to be spurred on to an even more grim determination. . . ."

Many doctors and officials, though inclined toward birth control, told her frankly that she could never break through the wall of ignorance to reach these women. But Mrs. Sanger was convinced that once they had glimpsed the radiant, spreading power of birth control they would understand. One of the most cynical of these doctors had taken her to a welfare center in a poor district of Baroda. At least twenty-five women were in line. "These women," the doctor said, "have been brought up to the duty of having children. They are so shy they would not listen to anything on birth control."

Mrs. Sanger said, "There's a woman with a sickly baby. How old is she?"

"Twenty," the doctor replied.

"How many children has she?"

"Three."

"Did she have any more?"

"Two died."

Speaking through her interpreter, Mrs. Sanger asked the woman, "Would you prefer to wait until this baby is strong and well before you have any more?"

Before the woman could answer, everyone on line had converged around Mrs. Sanger, their hands together in supplication, asking almost in a chorus, "Can that be done? If this foreign lady has something like that, that is what we want."

Afterward the doctor admitted to Mrs. Sanger, "if I hadn't heard it myself, I wouldn't have believed it."

4

Dr. John Haynes Holmes had written Mahatma Gandhi, requesting an interview for Mrs. Sanger. Gandhi had answered by courier letter to the ship at Bombay. "Do, by all means, come whenever you can, and you shall stay with me, if you would not mind what must appear to you to be our extreme simplicity; we have no masters and no servants here."

It was to be a meeting of giants. The Mahatma's spiritual leadership of the Indian masses had launched a revolution in every phase of the political, economic, and social life of his country. No man sought power less, yet none held more in India today. From his primitive ashrama in Wardha, some mystic web of influence reached out to thousands of remote villages. She understood this power. She saw the infinite possibilities of the meeting. "So numerous were Gandhi's adherents, so deep his influence," she wrote, "that I was sure his endorsement of birth control would be of tremendous value if I could convince him how necessary it was for Indian women."

Her trip to Wardha, and the rest of her tour, required a servant, or bearer, to secure railroad compartments, make the beds, purchase food at stations, and carry the blankets, sheets, soap, and towels that by necessity were part of the private equipment of every railroad traveler. From Cook's travel agency, therefore, she secured Joseph. Dressed always in a black alpaca coat and colorful turban, speaking not only Hindustani but Bengali, Tamil, and English, he immediately became her devoted adviser. He slept outside her door at night, brought her tea in the morning, and accompanied her, despite her protests, on even the shortest trips across the street. His respect for her reached new heights when he heard they were to visit Gandhi.

They arrived at Wardha by train, Mrs. Sanger, Anna Jane Phillips, and Joseph. It was a tiny village in central India with no post office and no stores, mainly inhabited by "untouchables." Gandhi had sent a tonga for them, a covered, two-wheeled cart drawn by a cream-colored bullock. There were no seats. Sitting flat on the bottom of the cart, they were pulled leisurely along the dusty road to the ashrama.

Describing this first meeting with Gandhi, Mrs. Sanger wrote: "He rose to greet me, smiling from ear to ear . . . Perhaps even more exaggerated than his pictures was Gandhi's appearance: his ears stuck out more prominently; his shaved head was more shaved; his toothless mouth grinned more broadly, leaving a great void between his lips. But around him and a part of him was a luminous aura. He has an unusual light that shines in his face; that shines through the flesh; that circles around his head and neck like a mist with white sails of a ship coming through. It lasted only a few seconds but it is there."

It was Gandhi's day of silence. Mrs. Sanger, therefore, went out to inspect the industries connected with the ashrama—the oil press, cotton-growing, paper-making, the irrigation system of simple turn wheels. "Gandhi," she noted, "is experimenting with foods, trying to find out the most economical for the village people and the most nourishing. The great majority are living a life of starvation. When you ask a villager how things are going, he points to his stomach and says, 'Sahib, stomach too long empty.' "

In the evening, they had supper on the veranda of Gandhi's house. Everyone sat on the floor, shoes removed, food placed on trays by attendants—bitter green purée, raw onions cut up in cream, hot vegetable soup, hot milk, dry flapjacks, a fresh orange, and vegetables and rice. No one ate until prayers were said, a chanting prayer to a lullaby-like tune. After supper, Gandhi wrote Mrs. Sanger a note, inviting her to walk with him in the morning at 6:30 A.M. and to have their first talk at 7:30.

She was up at six the next morning, and they walked to the village, Gandhi maintaining a sprightly pace, dressed in his customary white robes and sandals, and carrying a staff. Two other women guests accompanied them. "They deemed sacred every moment they spent with him," Mrs. Sanger noted. "Men, women and children waited for him as he passed, several prostrating themselves as to a holy person."

At seven-thirty promptly—Gandhi had a passion for promptness— they had their first talk, sitting on the roof in the early sun. At three that afternoon, they talked again, Gandhi sitting in the burning sunshine with a white cloth over his head. Their conversation was frank —yet almost every sentence showed the complete divergence in their viewpoints.

While Gandhi agreed with Mrs. Sanger that "no nation can be free until its women have control over the power that is peculiarly theirs," he could not accept birth control but only the most rigid and saintlike continence as a solution. Women, Gandhi insisted, must "learn

to say 'No' to their husbands when they approach them carnally."
He saw the necessity of family limitation but demanded: "Why
should people not be taught that it is immoral to have more than
three or four children and that after they have had that number they
should live separately?"

Mrs. Sanger continued to protest that this "advice is not practical.
. . . It leads to divorce. . . . The average marriage contract assumes that the marriage relationship will be harmonious." But no
amount of debate could bridge the gap between them. Mrs. Sanger
insisted on a differentiation between "sex love and sex lust." "Sex
love," she stated, "is a relationship that makes for oneness . . . and
contributes to a finer understanding and a greater spiritual harmony."

Gandhi's thinking, however, was so dominated by his concept of
lust that he could not admit the existence or possibility of a higher
relationship. Even Mrs. Sanger's seemingly irrefutable testimony
from leading neurologists and psychiatrists as to the danger of enforced continence in marriage could not sway Gandhi. "When you
make up your mind to follow a code of ethics," he insisted, "you
must determine to sacrifice health and ease. There are things more
important than health; things more precious than life and well-
being."

"Mrs. Sanger did not bring away St. Gandhi's complete endorsement of her work," *Time* magazine reported with understated
cynicism. It was not only that he could not support birth control; he
could never really grasp it. Here were two world figures whose
humanitarian and spiritual aspirations had brought them millions of
followers. Yet their approach to one of the most fundamental problems of life was a universe apart.

Mrs. Sanger stood for an evolutionary science that carried the
psycho-sexual pragmatism of Freud and Ellis into the practical
arena of marriage. She aimed toward the spiritual heights of sex love,
"a new thing . . . as we evolve in our higher consciousness," that
"stepladder towards God" she wanted the new motherhood to build.
This would be the final triumph of the "feminine spirit." This was
her mission.

And Gandhi? He was rooted to the inexorable discipline of nega-
tion which admitted no psycho-sexual link between the body and
the mind, but relentlessly pushed the body into greater and greater
insignificance while the mind advanced toward its ultimate unity
with the eternal. "After reading his autobiography," Mrs. Sanger

wrote, "I thought I saw the cause of his inhibitions. He himself had had the feeling which he termed lust, and now he hated it. It formed an emotional pivot in his brain around which centered everything having to do with sex." Later she added: ". . . I am convinced that his personal experience at the time of his father's death was so shocking and self-blamed that he can never accept sex as anything good, clean or wholesome."

5

She set out now on the tour that would carry her ten thousand miles to eighteen key cities. She would address sixty-four meetings, hold dozens of additional conferences with city officials, medical societies, and social workers.

In Calcutta, she spoke at Albert Hall. "Every inch . . . was occupied, and the audience comprised a distinguished number of ladies and gentlemen of the city," reported the Calcutta *Advance.*

At Benares on December 14, she lectured to the local branch of the Indian Medical Association. Here she showed two important films, produced for her before she left the United States. One, *The Biology of Human Reproduction,* the work of Dr. Robert Chambers of New York University, included the finest microscopic photography yet achieved. The other, made by Dr. Abraham Stone, was a detailed description of contraceptive techniques, a training film for doctors and nurses. Both pictures were acclaimed at Benares—and at every succeeding medical meeting—and were a constant stimulus to the support of the medical profession.

At Allahabad, Mrs. Sanger was the guest of Madame Ranjit Sitaram Pandit, Nehru's sister. Her home was the intellectual center of this seething university city. The student audience jammed the hall. When Mrs. Sanger announced at the end of the meeting that free birth control literature would be distributed, a phalanx of students rushed toward the platform. She had to throw the literature hurriedly into the crowd to avoid being swept off her feet.

At Agra on December 18, she addressed the women medical students and then went sight-seeing at the Taj Mahal. It seemed, she noted later, "to breathe the essence of beauty . . . a perfect simplicity. I stayed until the sun sank, and in the afterglow, the marble shone in a mystic effulgence like something in another dimension reflected in the still, translucent pool."

She was the state guest of the Maharajah Gaekwar of Baroda during Christmas. A progressive ruler of 2.5 million subjects, he was already instituting a program of compulsory education and the abolition of caste restrictions. Her train arrived at three in the morning, but she was met by the Maharajah's secretary in regal dress and housed with full state honors—Mrs. Sanger assigned seventeen servants, Anna Jane Phillips a mere five.

The next morning she was escorted to the palace to meet the Gaekwar. The Maharani, he told her, was only recently out of purdah and already actively engaged in promoting health centers. "You must get her interested in what you're doing," he said.

Mrs. Sanger showed the two documentary films to the Gaekwar and his wife and gave a round of lectures at the State General Hospital and before other medical groups. Her host and hostess were deeply impressed. When Mrs. Sanger was about to leave, the Gaekwar told her they had selected a gift—perhaps a jewel, Mrs. Sanger hoped fervently. Instead, two servants led out a baby elephant. Slightly shaken, she thanked the Gaekwar but assured him she couldn't get it back to the United States. Don't worry, he insisted. He would arrange for it to be shipped at his expense on her boat. Later, when illness forced her to return by plane, she notified the Gaekwar with relief that it would now be impossible to take the elephant. It was all right, he said. The elephant would be waiting. No matter how long before her return, they would keep it for her.

At the end of December, Margaret Sanger reached Travancore for the All-India Women's Conference. In this semi-independent southern state, she was the guest of the Maharani of Travancore. The Maharani was the titular head of the Conference. But the majority bloc of delegates were actually led by Mrs. Rustomji Feridoonji, a Parsi from Hyderabad.

In her own state, Mrs. Feridoonji already directed an organization which sent doctors, nurses, and midwives directly to the poorest inhabitants of the remotest villages. Now she was determined that the Conference should set in operation a similar plan for birth control. With her, Margaret Sanger worked out a detailed blueprint for the distribution of contraceptive literature and materials as well as gyneplaques for demonstration purposes. Here also was an unequaled opportunity to test a new development in inexpensive contraception—a foam powder made of rice flour, developed by a

New York chemist, which would give the poorest family contraceptive protection for a year for twenty cents.

The resolution supporting this plan was to come before the Conference the next morning at nine. But at seven the Maharani, obviously distraught, called Mrs. Sanger to her palace. Her position as president of the Conference, she explained, was complex and delicate. The social secretary of the Royal House was a Catholic. She and other Catholic delegates had threatened to walk out if the resolution was passed. Couldn't Mrs. Sanger, she pleaded, speak on a subject other than birth control?

Mrs. Sanger was appalled. Here were the same tactics that she had been forced to battle all these years in the United States. Politely she explained to the Maharani that she had been invited to the Conference specifically to support the resolution. The needs of millions of Indian women were more crucial than the opposition of a handful of Catholic missionaries. The Maharani accepted the decision gracefully. Despite the conflict, she would preside in the chair this morning to keep "the debate full and free."

It turned out, however, to be a violent meeting. "All the red tape and influence of the Royal House and the ingenuity of a small and active group," Mrs. Sanger wrote her friends back home, "were put into play to defeat the resolution." Significantly enough, not one Indian woman opposed it. The whole opposition consisted of Eurasians who were Catholic converts.

Their arguments were the same worn stereotypes that Mrs. Sanger had been answering for twenty-five years—almost a psychological obsession with the lust and passions of men—"the same old arguments . . . as though a phonograph record had been passed around the world," she noted. Hour after hour, these phrases were hurled in the faces of the Indian delegates until they were exhausted answering them. Finally one Indian woman, a mother herself, stood up and quietly pointed out that this talk of lust all seemed to come from a group of spinsters who had become experts on the passions of men. The Conference broke into laughter. The opposition wilted, and a vote was called which supported the resolution 84–25. The Conference had achieved its goal and adjourned that afternoon although the Catholic bloc walked out.

She was off again the next day, maintaining the same tireless pace she had set from her arrival in India. At Madras, she addressed the All-Indian Obstetrical and Gynecological Congress, the first of its kind in India. On January 13, 1936, she addressed the Neo-Malthusian League of Madras; on January 14, the Malabar District Medical Association—then in rapid order the University Union at Bangalore, the National Education Society of Mysore, and nursing and medical associations at Hyderabad.

All through India the medical profession—as in perhaps no other country—was alive to the necessity of birth control. "Doctors come from all over the south of India," she wrote home from Trivandrum, ". . . asking me to come to their towns and cities to help get things started. I gave demonstrations in my room, in the dressing room, in the car, and in the anteroom of the Conference." Manjeri Sundaram, a young doctor from Calicut, rode all the way on the train with her to Madras in order to have the time to persuade her to speak in his city.

With each group, Mrs. Sanger left gyneplaques and contraceptive materials. In key areas, she arranged for test projects of the new foaming rice powder. Altogether forty-five medical societies made plans to establish birth control programs. Fifty birth control information centers were set up at public hospitals and clinics.

Always she made birth control not just an instrument of science, but a flame of hope for women who had never known the meaning of hope. When she took the train from Trivandrum, a poorly dressed young Indian woman kept glancing at her shyly. At last, the woman came over. She had traveled fifteen hundred miles to see Mrs. Sanger—her first trip from home. At the Conference, she had been afraid to interrupt Mrs. Sanger's crowded schedule of meetings and visitors. So she had followed her to the station and used her last money to buy a first-class ticket in the same car.

The woman was only twenty-seven—yet she had already had seven children, three of them dead. She had been desperate after the illness of the last child. She could never live through another pregnancy, she said quietly; she had to know how to prevent it. There in the railroad compartment, Mrs. Sanger gave a private lecture on contraception and supplied the woman with literature and materials. "I will never forget the gratitude and happiness in her face," Mrs. Sanger wrote later, "when, saying goodbye, she folded the palms of her hands before her face and bowed her head in the simple and dignified salute that in India takes the place of a handshake."

Even statistics—the fifty birth control centers—did not tell the full story of Mrs. Sanger's impact on the country. Even the news-paper coverage—"Never at any time have I seen more space . . . devoted to a discussion of birth control than during the past two months," she noted.

It was a new spirit that swept India. "These women appreciated, as no women have in the Western world, with the exception of the Scandinavians," Mrs. Sanger reported later, "that fighting for and obtaining the vote was insignificant as compared with fighting for and obtaining knowledge about their own bodies and freedom to shape their own destinies. . . . These newly aroused women have realized that they cannot fight for their country while they are en-slaved by maternity."

To a reporter of the *World-Telegram* on her return to New York she stated: "We were able to accomplish more in the few months that we were in India than we have been able to do in the twenty-two years of our work in the United States."

6

She was making it a world movement in its most literal sense. From India, she circled through the Far East. Rangoon, Burma, Feb-ruary 4 . . . meeting of doctors and public officials. Malaya, Feb-ruary 10 . . . meeting at the Penang branch of the British Medical Society, address to the nurses of the General Hospital and Maternity Hospital, demonstration at one of the largest maternal welfare centers, radio speech. Hong Kong, February 18 . . . luncheon and tea in her honor, public address at the Hong Kong Hotel, lecture, Chinese supper and conferences with Dr. Arthur Woo, past presi-dent of the Chinese Medical Association—all in twenty-four hours.

In the midst of this frantic schedule, she was taken ill. The pain was agonizing, but she gave herself codeine and went on with the lecture. Afterward, a woman doctor on the reception committee took her upstairs for an examination. It was a gall bladder attack. Dr. Woo, her host, rushed her to Memorial Hospital, where she stayed for two dismal weeks of fog, rain, and cold. An operation was post-poned until her return to the United States, but she had to give up the rest of her lectures and conferences in China and the Philippines.

She was still in a seriously weakened condition when she arrived at Tokyo. The militarists were in power. Birth control, lumped under the heading of "dangerous thought," was being suppressed. Dr. Majima, who had started a clinic after her trip in 1922, had been imprisoned on a birth control charge and spent four months in jail. Still Mrs. Sanger insisted on holding a press conference and conferred at length with Baroness Shidzue Ishimoto and other birth control leaders. A photograph of her and the Baroness, reproduced in poster form as the "photo news" of the week, was displayed in hundreds of Tokyo shop windows with the caption: "The Margaret Sangers of America and Japan."

She had hardly reached Honolulu and registered at the hotel when Dr. Muriel Cass of the welcoming committee was on the telephone. Despite her illness, Mrs. Sanger had agreed to a lecture series in Hawaii. Dr. Cass arrived at the room, bringing another doctor. "All we want you to do," she told the doctor, "is to give Mrs. Sanger something to keep her going. She's got eight lectures to deliver."

With quiet efficiency, Dr. Cass had Mrs. Sanger completely isolated—her meals brought to her rooms, no visitors, no telephone calls allowed. Everything was done to conserve her strength for the meetings. Dr. Cass took her to each lecture by car, rushed her back to the hotel, and put her to bed. "I felt like a poor old war horse," Mrs. Sanger wrote, "being fed the last measure of oats."

Mr. Slee had come to meet her at San Francisco. It had been six months since he had seen her. He was distressed by her lengthy trip, worried about her health. "He had been traveling with one of his old cronies from the Union League Club," she recalled. "It was a well-matched pair. He was a widower, and J.N. practically a widower."

But Mr. Slee had not lost his obsession for efficiency. She had brought back so many gifts and packages that he purchased a huge trunk in which they could be shipped home. He supervised the packing, making use of every inch of space. That bulky tiger rug for Grant, for instance. That could be wrapped around the large box of Darjeeling tea she had bought to give as gifts. When they got back to Willow Lake, she quickly sent some of these prized packages of tea to her friends. No letters of thanks were received, no mention of these gifts. Finally she opened one of the remaining boxes of tea—it was reeking with camphor from the tiger rug. Mr. Slee's efficiency had gone too far this time. The magnificent Darjeeling was nothing but mothball tea, hideous, worthless, unfumigatable mothball tea that had to be thrown away.

CHAPTER 25

It seemed hard to believe that 1935 marked the twenty-first anniversary of the birth control movement—twenty-one years since Margaret Sanger had first cried out against biological sex slavery in the *Woman Rebel*. She had accomplished in that short time so sweeping a revolution in the social patterns of the nation that, as one writer in *Survey* magazine put it, "to the discerning young college girl of today, Margaret Sanger's heroic battle on the question in 1916 seems as far back as the Civil War. . . ."

The officers of the National Commitee decided to mark the occasion with a dinner, a "Coming of Age Dinner." It would not be a celebration—not with the campaign for the "Doctor's Bill" approaching a feverish climax. Rather it would be a symbolic closing of ranks behind the final drive for federal legislation. The guest list would be drawn from the nation's outstanding women. The speakers would be Harriet Stanton Blatch, the veteran feminist, Amelia Earhart, Dorothy Thompson, and Pearl Buck, who had just returned from China after receiving the Pulitzer prize—women who had made their mark in every field. To carry the symbolism of feminine emancipation to its conclusion, the dinner was scheduled for the birthday of that greatest emancipator, Abraham Lincoln.

Mrs. Sanger herself was out in Arizona while the arrangements for the dinner were being made. She had taken Stuart to Tucson to recuperate. After five years of sinus and mastoid operations, complicated by the fracturing of a bone over one eye when he was hit by a squash racket, he faced yet another operation. His mother protested. Instead of surgery, she insisted Stuart try the warm, dry climate of Arizona.

They took a pink adobe house out where the desert meets the foothills. The days were sunny and translucent, the nights crisp.

Stuart improved almost immediately. She loved it there in the Catalina foothills and "felt such a part of the whole." She would get up early before the actual dawn when "you beheld the gold and purple and then the entire sky break into color. In the evening the sunsets were reflected on the mountains in pink-lavender shades; sometimes the glow sprayed from the bottom upwards, like the footlights of a theater, until the tips were aflame." When she left, she looked back regretfully at "the indescribable Catalinas, on which lights and clouds played in never-ending change of pattern."

She arrived back in Washington to find the dinner committee jubilant. The dinner was sold out; twelve hundred reservations had been made. Further, a significant precedent had been set. The Columbia Broadcasting System had agreed to carry the speeches on its national network—the first nation-wide radio coverage for birth control. Then, just six days before the dinner, the "Doctor's Bill," which had been introduced this year into the House by Representative Walter M. Pierce of Oregon, was killed in committee by a vote of 15–8. The National Committee's headquarters was plunged in gloom. Many women wanted to postpone the dinner; some to cancel it completely.

Mrs. Sanger opposed both alternatives. The dinner would go on as scheduled. Instead of bemoaning a temporary setback, the dinner would serve as a send-off for a new and bigger legislative campaign. That night, she told twelve hundred cheering guests that fifty field workers would be sent immediately to every section of the country to gather a million signatures in support of a new "Doctor's Bill." She asked for a $100,000-war chest. The new campaign would start tomorrow. "That," said an Associated Press dispatch, was Mrs. Sanger's "declaration of war" against the tabling last week of the Pierce bill.

It was this indomitable will, this unflinching belief in the ultimate triumph of the feminine spirit that Pearl Buck eulogized in her testimonial speech to Mrs. Sanger.

She started the fire of a great freedom, and it will not burn down and no one can put it out because no one has ever been able to put down that sort of fire.

. . . No cause ever fought has been fought against more stupid, blind social prejudice, not even the cause of the people against the divine right of kings, nor the cause of equal suffrage, nor any of the battles of freedom.

. . . The most important thing that Margaret Sanger has done has been to bring into the light of science and common knowledge a matter which involves every human being vitally. . . .

. . . I give my admiration to Margaret Sanger today, therefore, not only because she has been a pioneer in a great scientific and humane movement . . . but because she has dared to attack fearlessly a false attitude of mind . . . a serious refusal to recognize life as it is. . . . It is sure that her name will go down in history. . . .

2

A few weeks later Mrs. Sanger was up in Boston to address the Massachusetts Federation of Women's Clubs. The Boston *Traveler's* front page banner headline announced: POLICE CENSORSHIP FOR MRS. SANGER. The meeting was transferred to the home of Mrs. Charles Peabody in Cambridge. The Cambridge police chief assigned a policewoman to the meeting "to see that all utterances and statements . . . are strictly in keeping with the law." Mrs. Sanger refused to be intimidated. The next day the *Traveler* announced that the police had backed down, had never sent its censor to the meeting after all.

Such intimidation had to be fought at every step, Mrs. Sanger told the leaders of the birth control movement in Massachusetts. They had been operating several clinics in the state despite the shadowy netherland of Massachusetts law, under which the question of their legality had never been decided. The attitude of the leaders was to let well enough alone, to operate the clinics quietly under police sufferance. Mrs. Sanger insisted that the law must be attacked and tested in the courts. This was her philosophy—to constantly enlarge the scope of the movement's freedom by hammering away at legal blocks. This was what she sought in the federal field through the "Doctor's Bill," a clear-cut definition of the rights of the medical profession instead of constant fear of government interference.

To introduce a new bill into Congress, Mrs. Sanger now got the support of Senator Royal S. Copeland, former Health Commissioner of New York, and the colorful congressman from Oklahoma, Percy L. Gassaway.

Congressman Gassaway spoke out for the bill at a luncheon in his honor. The father of fourteen children, he told how "seven of my children died and I lost my first wife in childbirth. So I am convinced that if birth control information had been available, as it will be if my bill is passed, our children would have been stronger and my wife would have survived. . . . If we were as reckless to the interests of our cows, sows, and mares, it wouldn't be long before they became a scrub bunch of stock. . . . The slow progress of birth control legislation is due only to political cowardice. The mothers of this land are entitled to information that will give them the right of self-preservation."

March 9, 1935 . . . the country was writhing in the worst agony of the depression. "Birth rates among families on relief are becoming the concern of governmental agencies as relief rolls reach the twenty million mark," the New York *Times* reported. ". . . Babies are arriving at the fastest rate in the classes 'least capable of the responsibility,' says one report. . . ."

Margaret Sanger had already proclaimed the urgent necessity of birth control through relief and public health auspices. The year before she had held an American Conference on Birth Control and National Recovery in Washington. The government had shied away. Relief, its principal weapon, was only a temporary palliative, she insisted. In Texas, for instance, with 140,000 persons in need of relief, there were only 80,000 W.P.A. jobs and no facilities to take care of the others. In Columbia, South Carolina, the monthly food average for persons on relief was $7.96, with some assistance from surplus food commodities. In Arkansas, the maximum relief was $12 per month per family; many parents deserted their children so that they might be placed in institutions.

Margaret Sanger spoke in Providence, Rhode Island, on April 9 and again demanded birth control assistance for the unemployed. "A nation with 22 million on the relief rolls and a population which has increased 5 million since the depression will pass on to the coming generations a greater debt than the millions spent to feed the needy if relief officials continue to ignore birth control."

From the mail that poured into her office day after day, she had a firsthand picture of the ravages of unemployment. "In the Manhattan headquarters of the American Birth Control League and in Mrs. Margaret Sanger's Washington lobby office," *Time* magazine reported on April 8, "are huge stacks of requests for birth control help—from relief workers and administrators, from city managers, probation officers, public health workers, and officials of CCC camps."

This need, this urgency she transmitted to her staff at the National

Committee. "You would stop up at her apartment for a quick break-fast," one of them recalled, "and leave with an armful of work that would last a month." She swept her associates along with her own strength. During the Russian trip, Florence Rose was ill in bed in Moscow. Mrs. Sanger was in Copenhagen. She telegraphed her sec-retary, asking her to meet her the next day in Copenhagen for a conference. "I could hardly move," Miss Rose said, "but somehow I dragged myself out of bed. The things we would do for M.S.!"

Mrs. Sanger combined an unwavering toughness with radiant gentleness. She could interrupt a whole conference schedule because of a lost dog. Once when Florence Rose, accompanied by her Scotty, was driving Mrs. Sanger to an important speech, the dog somehow escaped from the car as they stopped for gas. They had gone many miles before discovering the loss, but Mrs. Sanger in-sisted on turning back. Miss Rose refused and drove on to the meet-ing hall. Mrs. Sanger, however, would not begin her speech until her secretary had returned to the gas station, found the Scotty safe, and then telephoned the news to the meeting hall.

By the end of 1935, the campaign for the "Doctor's Bill" had reached an unparalleled peak of intensity. Field workers were com-pleting the collection of a million signatures in three hundred cities in thirty-five states. The number of national organizations, which endorsed the bill, had risen to 949—the latest additions being the American Neurological Association, the National Federation of Temple Sisterhoods, and the Pasadena Council of Social Agencies.

The trend of national support, the increasingly vocal force of public opinion which Mrs. Sanger had labored for seven long years to crystallize behind the bill, showed a definitely optimistic upswing. A *Fortune* magazine survey revealed that 63 per cent of the Ameri-can people now favored birth control, 23 per cent opposed it. At the beginning of 1936, the National Committee's latest tally esti-mated that 37 senators favored the "Doctor's Bill," 18 opposed it, 22 were noncommittal; 107 representatives were favorable, 46 op-posed, and 91 noncommittal.

3

Margaret Sanger never fought on one flank alone. All these years while she had thrown her main strength into the legislative cam-paign, she had been quietly conducting a secondary battle in the courts. "In the United States we almost never repeal outmoded legislation in the field of morals," her lawyer, Morris L. Ernst, stated,[1] "We either allow it to fall into disuse by ignoring it . . . or we bring persuasive cases to the courts and get the obsolete laws modified by judicial interpretation."

Mrs. Sanger had grasped these principles early. From the time of her first indictment for the *Woman Rebel*, she had seen that the courts were more sensitive instruments of social progress in birth control than the legislatures. Judges, on the whole, were alive to the pressures of social change and public opinion. In 1916, she had mobilized the public and the press behind her so strongly that the government had finally dropped its indictment in the courts. With the Brownsville clinic, she had deliberately tested the law and won from Judge Crane's 1918 decision an extraordinarily favorable construction of the New York statutes. She had forced the 1921 Town Hall raid into court, thus making an open display of the bumbling of her adversaries. As a result of the 1929 clinic raid, Morris Ernst had won another dramatic advance for the movement. Almost every advance in birth control, in fact, had stemmed directly or indirectly from a victory in the courts.

This, then, was the motivation behind that most critical of all cases —the United States versus One Package. It had its origins back in the 1930 Zurich Conference when Mrs. Sanger had seen a new Japanese pessary demonstrated and requested that samples be sent to New York. The package, however, was seized by the New York Collector of the Customs under the terms of Section 305 of the Revenue Act—actually part of the Comstock law which had been divided up and distributed through the Federal Code. Here was a unique chance to test the law as it pertained to the free flow of information to the medical profession. Mrs. Sanger had another package sent from Japan by a Japanese doctor. This time, however, January 9, 1933, it was mailed to Dr. Hannah Stone. Again it was seized by Customs. Dr. Stone, with Mr. Ernst as her lawyer, now carried her claim to the courts.

The One Package case did not come to trial until December 10, 1935. Another significant case meanwhile was being fought through the courts, involving a book, *Contraception,* by Mrs. Stopes, which had been confiscated by Customs. It was a serious medical treatise, dealing with birth control in scientific terms. Ruling in Federal District Court that the law could not exclude an authoritative book

[1]Ernst and Gwendolyn Pickett, *Birth Control in the Courts* (1942), p. 15.

that did not fall into the classification of immorality or obscenity, Judge Woolsey ordered it returned to its addressee.

This decision ruled once and for all, said Morris Ernst, that in the importation of birth control publications "legitimate use was to be the determining factor. No bar was to be raised against research, and legislation directed to other ends would not be permitted to hamper the modern practice of medicine."[2]

The One Package case was brought to trial before Judge Grover Moscowitz in the U. S. District Court just a few months, significantly enough, before Senator Copeland and Representative Gassaway introduced the "Doctor's Bill" into Congress. The government had staked its whole argument, not on whether the pessaries would be used for legal or illegal purposes, but on its claim that Section 305 barred from importation all articles for "the prevention of conception."

Mr. Ernst contended this was an unreasonable construction of the statute. He introduced an impressive battery of medical authorities— Dr. Frederick C. Holden, Dr. Foster Kennedy, and Dr. Louis I. Harris among others, who described the many conditions under which contraception should safeguard the life and health of mothers and children.

Judge Moscowitz was obviously impressed by this testimony. Dismissing the suit and ordering that the package be delivered to Dr. Stone, his decision on January 6, 1936, was an unqualified triumph for birth control.

The government immediately appealed to the Circuit Court of Appeals. Speaking for the Court in its decision of November 30, 1936, Judge Augustus N. Hand upheld the lower tribunal. He pointed out that Section 305 and similar statutes all had their common origin in the Comstock law. "Its design, in our opinion, was not to prevent the importation, sale, or carriage by mail of things which might intelligently be employed by conscientious and competent physicians for the purpose of saving life or promoting the well-being of their patients. . . ."

Mrs. Sanger's supporters were already hailing it as "the greatest victory in birth control history." Morris Ernst called it "a legal triumph" and "in a very real sense, too . . . a medical triumph." She insisted, however, in waiting to see whether the government would carry the decision to its ultimate stage, the Supreme Court.

[2]*Ibid.*, p. 29.

The "Doctor's Bill" had just been killed once more in committee. She had seen too many seeming victories melt away in her hands.

Up to the last minute, she toured the country—even this final crystallization of public opinion could bear on the government's decision to appeal or not. On November 14, she spoke in Rochester before the City Club, on November 16 in Buffalo, where one reporter described her as standing "upon a brilliantly lit stage in a demure black gown, as gentle and feminine a feminist as ever breathed." Mrs. Sanger, he continued, "hurled facts in the face of a remarkable audience that was at least one half male."

She went on to Colgate University and Brattleboro, Vermont; jumped to Chicago for a tour of the Midwest; then to Dallas and El Paso, where she helped organize a new clinic. She lectured at Chandler, Arizona, where Mr. Slee awaited her, took a short vacation there, and finally wound up the tour with speeches at Chester, Wilkes Barre, Easton, and Bethlehem, Pennsylvania.

She was still traveling when the decision came. On January 29, 1937, Attorney General Homer Cummings announced that the verdict of the Court of Appeals would not be carried to the Supreme Court. The government would accept its ruling as the law.

She hurried home for a conference with Morris Ernst, Charles Scribner, and other legal advisers of the birth control movement. Their analysis of the court decision was summed up in Mr. Scribner's terse statement: "You have accomplished a great deal more by this decision than by amending the law."

What specific new freedoms had the birth control movement won? The decision not only gave physicians the right to import contraceptive materials, which was the *raison d'être* of the case. It went much further. It opened up the mails—not just from overseas but the domestic mails—for the transportation of contraceptive materials and literature to and from doctors and other qualified persons. The decision, as Dr. Hannah Stone wrote in the *Nation,* "once and for all establishes contraception as a recognized part of medical practice and removes the last legal barriers to the dissemination of contraceptive knowledge."

It was a time for jubilation. After eight years of grinding, relentless effort, the National Committee, celebrating amid tears and laughter, closed its Washington office on March 1. Margaret Sanger announced proudly in the *Birth Control News:* "The decision . . . may be acclaimed as the close of one epoch and the dawn of another. It brings to an end the sixty-three-year reign of muddle and tyranny inaugurated by the so-called Comstock legislation enacted in 1873 and clarifies once and for all future time the position and rights of the American physician in the legitimate use of scientific contraceptives . . ."

4

Now all honors were heaped on Margaret Sanger almost simultaneously. On January 24, 1937, at the same Town Hall where, ironically enough, she had been forbidden to speak sixteen years before, the Town Hall Club awarded her its annual medal. "The cause conquers because youth is for you," Pearl Buck told Mrs. Sanger in her testimonial speech. On the face of the medal were the words: "For contributing to the enlargement and enrichment of life."

On June 10 came the final triumph. All through the years, though the country's leading medical groups had insulted or ignored her, Mrs. Sanger had stuck to her fundamental doctrine—that contraception must be taught and administered by the doctor. At last, "smashing a twenty-five-year taboo," as one newspaper described it, the American Medical Association in its Atlantic City Convention gave birth control its recognition and support. The A.M.A. resolution stated that doctors should now be informed of their legal rights in the use of contraceptives. It established a committee to analyze new methods of contraception. It initiated studies to promote public education in fertility and sterility.

Margaret Sanger was at Willow Lake that June morning when she saw the headlines in her morning paper. "Here was the culmination of unremitting labor since my return from Europe in 1915," she wrote, "the gratification of seeing a dream come true. . . . In my excitement I actually fell downstairs."

At last, almost two years after her gall bladder attack at Hong Kong, she had the time to enter the hospital for a long-delayed operation. She had always ignored the ailments of her body. In the early days of the movement when she was suffering from tubercular glands, she had gone out night after night for speaking engagements despite a 103 degree temperature. A few years back she had been stricken with arthritis in Switzerland, forced to hobble around on crutches. The doctors feared she would be crippled for life. She refused to accept their decision. She saw another physician in England

and started a new treatment. In three months, she was walking normally.

"The human limitations which apply to most of us," Dorothy Brush, an old friend, once wrote, "just never apply to her at all. . . . She treats her body like a Victorian child—it must be seen but not heard; if it aches, it must ache in silence."

At New York's Harkness Pavilion now, she had the gallstones removed. The operation was successful. Friends, trying to hide their concern, waited to see her, including H. G. Wells, who had just arrived in America. "You are one of the loveliest and best people that I have ever met . . ." he wrote her affectionately.

After a week, she stirred restlessly in the confines of her hospital room. Everyone seemed to be sitting back, riding joyously on the huge wave which had carried the movement to its recent triumphs. At Colgate University, Professor Himes, sizing up Mrs. Sanger's impact on these last two decades, stated: "No reformer in human history—and I weigh my words well—no reformer has lived to see the things she stood for so completely brought about."

Words like that, flattering or not, made her uneasy. The Court of Appeals decision was simply a tool for further accomplishment. Without immediate action to give it breath and life, it was only a static page. She summoned her secretary and dictated a memorandum, a memorandum that went out immediately to all her supporters, field workers, and clinics.

"Make known to hospitals, relief agencies, and philanthropic and public health officials that the decision . . . frees their hands. . . . Call on public health officials and ask that birth control instruction be included in their services. Establish clinics. There are today approximately 320 birth control centers in America. I look forward to seeing not twice that number but ten times that number at the close of 1937."

CHAPTER 26

The One Package decision now made it possible to launch a daring plan she had been developing in her mind. It was the poorest women, the lowest strata of society, particularly in the rural areas of the South and Southwest, that had never been reached by the clinics. The one agency which penetrated the remotest areas was the public health services of these states. Previously, the federal law had been an obstacle to the free flow of contraceptive information to public health doctors. That obstacle had been removed. What she envisioned now was birth control as a state responsibility. Why shouldn't mothers go to public health state clinics for contraceptive protection as freely as they sought typhoid immunization or maternal health care?

Here was a new challenge that immediately outweighed the urgings of her medical advisers that she take a long rest. "Mrs. Sanger seems to thrive on struggle," one doctor said. "I don't think she'd have an appetite for her next meal without it." She would not disband the National Committee now. Its network of field workers and almost four hundred voluntary county and congressional district committees would be kept intact and transformed into a new organization—the Education Department of her Clinical Research Bureau.

The southern drive was favored immediately by three factors. The more advanced states were already concerned about the rising birth rates of their poor white and Negro families. Roman Catholic influence was negligible here—there would be a minimum of religious opposition. Finally, three of Mrs. Sanger's associates and friends were willing to give strong financial support—Mrs. Albert Lasker, Dr. Clarence Gamble, and particularly for work among Negro groups, Miss Doris Duke.

Mrs. Sanger had first met Dr. George N. Cooper, director of preventive medicine for the North Carolina Board of Health, on one of her speaking tours. A former country doctor who had tended thousands of poor mothers in their one-room shacks, he had long been distressed at the high infant mortality rate of his state. He immediately grasped the potentialities of Mrs. Sanger's plan. "We'll make birth control an integral part of public health medicine," he said. In 1937, he began to establish birth control services in the state clinics. Within a year, he had so enlarged the program that no family in the state was further than fifty miles from a public health clinic.

The next year South Carolina, followed by Alabama, adopted the program. Eventually Florida, Georgia, Mississippi, and Virginia all brought birth control service into their public health clinics. Seven states—an impressive triumph, it would seem. But Mrs. Sanger soon realized that a fundamental weakness limited the whole conception of public health birth control. The techniques used all these years by the big-city clinics, particularly the diaphragm and jelly, were too complex, too expensive ever to gain widespread acceptance among the poor and uneducated mothers of rural areas. In many parts of the United States, just as in the vast, overpopulated nations of the Far East, the universal acceptance of birth control would depend on the discovery of a new technique—inexpensive, simple, reliable, and psychologically acceptable. This new birth control "pill" or injection, whose attainment would pursue her relentlessly for the next fifteen years, would be the future pivot of the movement.

There was a new urgency in these years that came from farther west. 1939 . . . the dust-driven, impoverished caravan of migrant fruit workers, pushed from their lands in Oklahoma and the Southwest by drought, plague, and depression, had descended on the rich fruit valleys of California. Their boxlike homes, often windowless shacks without water or sanitary facilities, dotted the great fruit ranches. Epidemics were common; medical care almost nonexistent. The Federal Security Agency was rushing to complete new camps for them. Nurses were sent to care for the mothers and children. The high birth rate only complicated the already serious medical problem. Girls married as young as fourteen and often had ten children before they were thirty.

One young nurse, Miss Mildred Delp, who had been sent by the F.S.A. to these "Okie" camps, saw that the overwhelming need of these mothers was for birth control information. They not only

knew nothing of contraception; they were almost completely ignorant
of the anatomy of their own bodies. One perceptive grandmother,
discussing her daughter Sara, said, "I've had thirteen myself; got
fifty-three grandchildren. If Sara is goin' to work from kin-see to
cain't-see every day, she ought to stop havin' kids a spell."

With no experience in teaching contraceptive techniques, Mildred
Delp wrote to Margaret Sanger in New York, pleading for information and supplies. Mrs. Sanger came herself. She brought an efficient
plan for extending the birth control program to the migrant camps,
with a large supply of contraceptive materials and teaching techniques including a set of gyneplaques, the soft rubber reconstruction
of the female genital organs which had proved so successful in
India.

Soon notices began to appear on the bulletin board of migrant
camps:

> OLD TIME DANCE TONIGHT
>
> TYPHOID VACCINATION THURSDAY
>
> BIRTH CONTROL CLINIC FRIDAY AT 4

All meetings were voluntary, but the mothers were soon organizing
them on their own initiative. At one peach ranch, the teacher at the
ranch school announced the birth control meetings by pinning slips
to the dresses of the girls. Miss Delp was only a shade over five
feet; often she had to climb on a table to be heard. At each meeting, she described the fundamentals of birth control, then interviewed individual mothers to discuss their cases and teach the
technique in private.

Less than a year afterward, Mrs. Sanger's west coast field worker
visited Miss Delp at one of the migrant camps and wrote back to
New York: ". . . The thing that gave you a real thrill was to watch
the expressions on the faces of her old migrant friends at the camp
as they greeted her." By 1940, the Federal Security Agency had
extended the birth control service to twenty-five of its camps in
California and Arizona.

2

It was inevitable that Mrs. Sanger's new Education Department
would conflict with the status quo so treasured by the old Birth
Control League. The National Committee had confined itself strictly
to federal legislation; the Education Department leaped enthusi-

astically into a whole series of new projects. It not only developed birth control services in the South and the migrant camps of the West, but worked with any state or local group that wanted to found a new clinic, test new methods of contraception, or challenge the antiquated birth control laws of the state—projects that the league often considered part of its own domain. The Education Department was less concerned about tact than the immediate necessity of setting a flame to the countryside.

In California, for instance, Mrs. Sanger's representative, Gladys de Lancy Smith, was busily organizing the migrant worker birth control units and other recent clinics into an efficient state-wide group. But the league already had its own state organization headed by Dr. Harold Trimble. Appalled at the competitive aspect of their campaigns, Dr. Trimble called on Miss Smith and protested, "But Miss Smith, you cannot build an organization around a personality."

"It is because I have come into the field in the name of Margaret Sanger," she retorted, "that there has been aroused stimulus and aroused interest in birth control . . ."

The name of Margaret Sanger—somehow the old guard in the league's executive office could never grasp the fire it stirred! Even now, as in 1929, the executive director of the league complained that "we may in time convince Mrs. Sanger that the movement has progressed beyond the stage of 'rugged individualism.'" But it was this very "individualism" that brought a glitter and excitement to whatever she touched. A woman in San Marino, California, who had worked for her for years before finally meeting her wrote: "It so often happens that when an ideal is known in the flesh, the illusion of greatness is dispelled . . . Such has not been the case with you, for you shine always with a steady light—there have been no shadows. . . . Accept my gratitude and reverence."

The Sanger name had such magic that when the league sent out literature or requests for financial assistance it was flooded with letters asking why Mrs. Sanger was not among its officers. An expert from one of the major professional fund-raising organizations, Kenneth Rose of the John Price Jones Company, was called in to tackle the problem. After a detailed survey, he complained it would be almost impossible to run a national fund-raising campaign without Mrs. Sanger's name.

The rapid development of clinics had made the existence of two separate organizations even more complex. There were almost six hundred clinics now—171 in public health services, 92 in hospitals, the rest affiliated either with the league or the Clinical Research Bureau—occasionally with both. It was obvious, Mr. Rose reported, that amalgamation of the two organizations was an immediate necessity.

It took long, detailed negotiations between the joint committees to achieve this final amalgamation in 1939. Mrs. Sanger did not oppose the move. She had felt for the last three years that the pioneering days of birth control in the United States were almost over. Even the name of the new organization reflected this change— called first the Birth Control Federation of America, it became in 1942 the Planned Parenthood Federation of America. Even the address to which the combined organization moved—the statesman-like solidity of 501 Madison Avenue—signaled the ringing down of the curtain once and for all on the volcanic and pioneering past. *The Journal of Contraception* which had been published by the bureau all these years under the devoted editorship of Dr. Abraham Stone became *Human Fertility.* A new era had arrived—an era when the planning of the total family, incorporating such related aspects as marriage counseling, psychological guidance, and infertility research, had replaced the impassioned crusade for what Mrs. Sanger called "an enslaved motherhood."

In the new organization, Margaret Sanger was elected honorary chairman. A prominent physician, Dr. Richard N. Pierson, was made president. All functions of both organizations—clinics, state leagues, country committees, and field workers—were immediately unified, all that is, except the Clinical Research Bureau. The building in which it was housed had been given to Mrs. Sanger by her husband. The bureau and its services, the thousands of women who passed through its doors, were a part of her blood stream and her being. Its operation, she insisted, must remain her personal responsibility.

She was ready to turn completely now from the national movement to the Far East, to what the Lasker Award Committee later called— with no exaggeration—her "plans for a planet."

3

China was still the unknown challenge. Her trip there in 1921 had been brief. She had long wanted to return. Now she was invited personally by the China Medical Association at the request of

Madame Chiang Kai-shek. She sailed with Mrs. Dorothy Brush; Florence Rose had gone ahead to prepare the way. But the trip was haunted by bad luck. First she slipped on deck and broke her arm. The ship's doctor set it badly. In Tokyo, it had to be broken and set again. She had been booked for a few speeches in Japan and her friends begged her to postpone them. But with the cast on her arm still wet, she set out by train for the first stop on her schedule. The pain was intense. It grew worse each hour, and finally she had to turn around and return to Tokyo, leaving Mrs. Brush to give her speeches. Then she received a wire from Florence Rose in Shanghai. The city had just been bombed, Miss Rose almost hit by a bomb that exploded in front of the restaurant where she was eating.

It was impossible to go on to China. Japan's military dictatorship was ruthlessly preparing for a major war. Japan's birth control clinics were shut down, women like Baroness Ishimoto placed under close surveillance, and later jailed. Mrs. Sanger, unhappily accepting the fact that her plans for the Far East would have to be postponed, returned home.

She and Mr. Slee went out to Tucson and bought a comfortable, rambling house in the Catalina foothills. She had grown to love this city, the mountains that surrounded it, the vast silences of the desert, the never ending play of shadows and color outside her windows. The Birth Control Federation in New York routed all important memorandums to her; she was, as always, consulted on key decisions. Yet for the first time in thirty years she was separated from the day-by-day turbulence of the movement.

It was Havelock Ellis's eightieth birthday on February 2, 1939. She wanted to make it a memorable landmark. In addition, many friends wanted to join her in a gift. He had been writing less and less in the last few years, and she knew that it was money he needed above all else. She sailed for England and went to see him at the new house that she and Slee had given him—"the home of homes," Françoise called it, ". . . for it was the most intimate . . ."

She had collected almost three thousand dollars, but it had to be presented without offending Ellis. She found him in the revolving sun hut in the garden where he loved to work. He looked old; he had not been well that winter. His skin was almost translucent—the radiance seemed to be shining through.

"Havelock," she said, "all your friends in America begged me to bring their gifts to you. Mrs. Rublee wanted to give you some peach trees for the garden, but of course they would have been too cumbersome so I had to bring the money for them instead." Another friend wanted to buy him a library of new books. But who could select for Ellis? A third friend wanted to buy a complete set of the greatest symphonies but was afraid to duplicate Ellis's own collection. A fourth wanted to buy a painting, but dared not impose his taste on Ellis. She ran down the whole list and then said, "Havelock, I could not bring what they wanted. Instead I have brought you their best wishes in this envelope," and she put the money quickly in his pocket.

He smiled up at her gently and said, "Margaret, you are the most wonderful of women and the most practical of women."

She must have seen the farewell in that smile. It was only a few weeks later that Françoise wrote her that he was running a slight temperature. He could not retain food, not even an egg in milk or a boiled egg. He lived mostly in bed that spring, growing steadily weaker. He tolerated the doctors who were sent in, but after all he was a doctor himself. He knew his symptoms; he was ready. On the evening of July 8, he had a slight heart attack. The doctor came and left. Ellis felt better, and at eleven, Françoise came to chat with him and smooth his pillow. A few minutes later she looked in; he had already died, quietly, imperceptibly.

"Havelock Ellis dead!" Bernard de Voto exclaimed in *Harper's*. "It was as though Mt. Everest had died."

For Margaret Sanger, the strongest thread that had run through her life—twenty-five years since that cold December evening in 1914—had been broken. His invincible voice had illuminated the mind of the world, had ushered in a new era of sex knowledge. What had De Selincourt told her? ". . . You are a woman on his level, the embodiment of his ideas . . . living his work in the wonderful way that you do—Mother of his Cause . . ." But it had been more than that, more than any of them would ever understand. The ultimate of beauty through the art of love—that is what she had wanted and Ellis above all the others had helped her find. "The peaceful and consoling and inspiring elements of love," he had called them. Even an ocean apart from him, separated often for years, it had been like another world within a world—"a hitherto undreamed of world," she had once said. But she could not mourn; she could only honor what she had possessed.

It was a time now when loneliness came often. On July 10, 1941,

Dr. Hannah Stone died of a heart attack. She was only forty-seven. Her heart had been weak as far back as the 1929 clinic raid, but she had kept the knowledge to herself all this time. "Countless women silently call her blessed," Dr. Ira Wile said.

The scope of Dr. Stone's achievement had a visual monument in the file of a hundred thousand medical histories at the clinic. It was a staggering scientific feat. More than anything else, it had raised the birth control movement to the dignity and stature which had at last won the support of the American Medical Association. But a case history was more than a folder. It was a woman in need whom Dr. Stone had touched with "the divine grace that is Hannah," Dr. Wile called it. Except for Mrs. Sanger, no one had given herself so unsparingly—all those years as medical director, as a volunteer without salary.

She had become the outstanding authority on contraceptive techniques in the country. With her husband, she had pioneered in marriage counseling. She had coauthored with him the authoritative book in the field, *A Marriage Manual*. She had helped organize and develop many of the country's finest clinics.

When the body was brought to the funeral chapel, Margaret Sanger sent out telegrams to friends and associates everywhere to join her beside the bier. It was a rare gesture—those men and women who loved her, keeping her company during that long night, sitting beside the body in a final vigil. Later there was a memorial meeting at the Community Church at which Mrs. Sanger, Will Durant, and Dr. John Haynes Holmes paid their last tribute. "In her face, her mien, her manner, her voice, her whole presence," Dr. Holmes said, "there was a sweetness and light, a dignity and grace, a generous compassion which combined into the very essence of what we mean by 'character' in its truest and purest sense."

It was not many months later—just before Christmas 1941—when Mr. Slee was stricken. He had been finishing a drink on the terrace when David, the butler, found him lying on the floor. Mr. Slee insisted that he had slipped and would let no one help him to the dining room. But after dinner when he left the table he fell again. They put him to bed though he continued to protest this "damned nonsense." The next morning he was taken to the hospital. He still had trouble walking, but no injury had been revealed by the tests.

He seemed to recover, and in the spring, they returned to Willow Lake. Then it happened again. This time it was a stroke that left him partly paralyzed. He wanted to be back in Tucson, to bask in the warm sun. They took another house, closer to the center of town on Elm Street, more convenient to the constant medical attention he needed. Mrs. Sanger gave up all outside work now. He wanted her with him constantly. He had a buzzer device built with a long cord so that no matter where he moved in his wheel chair he could sound the buzzer and reach her ear instantly. He chuckled slyly over this mechanical wonder, as if in these final months he had at last discovered the secret of having his wife all to himself.

His closest friend in Tucson was the Reverend George Ferguson. Slee called him "St. George"; the minister called Slee the "Dragon." "I remember going over to see him one day after Dr. Stuart Sanger had complained that he was doing nothing for himself, that he had to take some exercise to flex his muscles," Dr. Ferguson recalled. "I had some tennis balls in my pocket, and I said, 'Dragon, once when I was sick and had to exercise my hands, I would squeeze these balls. It's a good exercise; please try it.' He looked at me carefully and said, 'St. George, who do you think you're fooling? I know I'm going to die, and I want to.' Then his eyes lit up and he smiled and said, 'Besides, why should I take exercise when I've got Margy and all these women to look after me? I've had to wait a long time for this.' "

Every afternoon the nurse went off for a few hours at four o'clock. Mrs. Sanger would sit and talk or read to him. Once she said, "J.N., here you've been a pillar of the church all your life, a supervisor of the Sunday School. Yet not once have you asked me to read the Bible to you." He answered slowly; it was often an effort to talk now. "Whatever my life has been will have to stand on its own. I know I can't do anything to make it up in these last few weeks."

One afternoon he asked suddenly, "Margy, was I ever married to anyone before you?"

"I burst out laughing," she recalled, "and said, 'Are you joking? Of course you were married.' 'Who was it? I can't remember,' he asked. I told him who it was and how young and beautiful she was. 'Did I have any children?' he asked. At that I laughed again and said, 'You surely know that.' And I named all three of them. 'Where are they?' he asked, and I told him. Then he said: 'Well, Margy, all that may have been true but I do not remember any of it. Only since I first saw you do I remember anything. I can see it all clearly—the way you wore your glorious long hair piled on top of your head, the way you held your head on one side, always listening, always a good listener. I can remember every detail of our first lunch together, every place we went, everything we did. It seems that only since I knew you have I begun to live.'"

He died on June 21. ". . . He was more than ready to go and did not want to live," Mrs. Sanger wrote Anna Jane Phillips, "so I am glad for him that he slipped so peacefully away at the end, and I could not wish him back." The body was cremated, as he had directed. A service was held at Tucson's Grace Episcopal Church.

Stuart and Grant, who were in the Army and Navy now, were able to fly back for the funeral. "I'll never forget you," a friend wrote Mrs. Sanger, "as you sat in church with Stuart in khaki at your left and Grant in his white navy uniform at your right, and you so small and defenseless in the middle."

The ashes were taken to Fishkill for a memorial service in the cemetery that Mr. Slee had loved. Dorothy Brush wrote the eulogy:

. . . What a stir you will make up there! How you will send the lackeys flying. First thing, you'll have them all putting 3-in-1 oil on the heavenly gates. You liked to frighten people with your gruff ways, but you were always all bark and no bite . . .

. . . You doubtless sent St. Peter a telegram, saying you'd be at the gate at such and such a time and to be sure to have it open for you. You reserved the best suite on the most comfortable heavenly cloud with cross ventilation, and told the management to be sure your harp and crown were home from the cleaner's in plenty of time. And when you did arrive, if everything wasn't as you thought it ought to be, you would be sure to shout in an outraged tone, 'Where's Margaret?' Then you'd remember, dear Noah, and heaven wouldn't be heaven after all . . .

The ashes were placed in the plot at the Fishkill cemetery that Mr. Slee had purchased many years before. Even that gesture—the stone, waiting and in place, while he was still in the prime of life—was typical of his everlasting planning and efficiency. Mrs. Sanger recalled, smiling, how once long ago they had been talking to a stranger on the train to New York, and Mr. Slee had introduced himself, and the stranger had asked if he was related to the Slee in the Fishkill cemetery. "Related, hell!" her husband had grunted, obviously enjoying the shock on the stranger's face. "That's me!"

Mr. Slee had been eighty-two, a little older than Ellis, a little younger than Michael Higgins. They lived long and well, these men who made up her life. She had not realized till then how deep the loneliness would cut, how much strength she had really drawn from him during all those years. "He was one of the last of the rugged individualists," she told Dr. Ferguson. "But it was all outside toughness. Underneath he was a child."

4

Her philosophy would be tested in many hard hours now. The war had increased her loneliness, had taken both sons far away. Grant was in Seattle, waiting to join his ship in the Pacific; Stuart in Florida, expecting orders for the European theater. When the Germans invaded Poland and France, she had opposed World War II as bitterly as she had cried out against the first war in the editorial columns of the *Woman Rebel*. Her hatred of war was passionate, intense. She ignored its roots in the economic and political framework of history. She saw it only as the evil eruption of exploding populations. It was the total abnegation of the feminine spirit.

To an old associate in the movement, Mrs. Henriette Posner, she once wrote: "Henriette, we send the genius of the youth, the life blood of the race, to fight old men's battles, and leave behind the maimed and the feeble-minded to propagate the race." Only after Pearl Harbor did she abandon her pacifist position.

She had tried long before to get President Roosevelt to enunciate a population policy for the United States. In 1936, she had visited him with a delegation of women at Hyde Park. "How can any country avoid war without a population policy?" she had demanded. The President had waved at her with his cigarette in its debonair holder and said, "Don't worry, neighbor. I'll get the answer for you." But he never did. She was convinced that the Roman Catholic grip on big-city Democratic politics had blocked any move by Mr. Roosevelt for an American population policy. Later she had been incensed when the Children's Bureau in Washington had threatened to cut off funds for North Carolina when that state decided to make birth control a part of its public health service. Her misgivings about the Roosevelt policy were increasing. "Some outstanding people, who have no prejudices whatsoever against the Roman Catholic hierarchy," she wrote to H. G. Wells, "are beginning to have grave feelings as to their power and influence over F.D.R. as well as their influence in our State Department."

She continued to hammer at the question of population and

Roman Catholic influence in her letters to Wells. "The thing that fills my heart with sadness," she wrote on September 19, 1942, "is that great minds like yours and others that are writing up peace plans either do not recognize the importance of the population problem, or are appeasing the R.C.'s by not mentioning the subject."

It was fortunate that in these years of war and loneliness she could lose herself in her family. Stuart and Grant had both married, one to a nurse, the other a doctor. Stuart had the first child, a daughter. Mrs. Sanger was touched when the child was named Margaret. Her own Peggy still remained a deep hurt in her consciousness. No matter where he was—even on ship in the Pacific—Grant always managed to send a telegram or message to his mother on Peggy's birthday.

Later the Stuart Sangers had a second daughter, Nancy. Little Margaret, however, always remained proud of her priority, and when she learned to write, signed her letters to Mrs. Sanger, "Love from your first grandchild." Grant and Edwina had their first son, Michael, in New York before he left for the Pacific. Eventually they would have a total of five boys and a girl.

There was plenty of time now to get acquainted with her grandchildren. Mrs. Sanger went with Barbara and the child to Palm Beach, where Stuart was stationed before going overseas. Later she went to Coronado, California, where Edwina lived after Grant shipped out. Her sons were compiling fine war records. She waited anxiously for each letter. Grant's ship had seen heavy action, Stuart was in the Battle of the Bulge. Invalided back to England, he insisted on postponing his discharge so that he could tend the battle casualties who overflowed the hospitals.

She sent regular food packages to H. G. Wells. Although a bomb had fallen almost opposite his house at Hanover Terrace, he refused to budge. He was alone. He was sick—kidneys, diabetes, heart trouble, catarrh. She begged him to come and stay with her at Tucson. "One winter out here," she wrote on May 5, 1944, "and we guarantee ten good, vigorous years of your life. If you don't believe me, write to the Chamber of Commerce . . ."

But H.G. clung to his house and kept a stream of wry telegrams flowing to Margaret and other friends: "Come over quick. Won't last long." And again: "Last big chance. Really dying."

At last, there was peace! Mrs. Sanger in a fervent cry, which could have been the cry of all mothers, wrote Juliet Rublee: "Good news.

Stuart is out of the Army! I am on my knees in gratitude to God that this has happened."

As soon as she could get a passport, she sailed for England. She found Wells still at Hanover Terrace, hanging doggedly to life. He dozed in the sun parlor, tried to read his paper, played the phonograph. Occasionally his nurse would take him down to the garden, where he would sit, wrapped in flannels, wearing dark glasses and a battered Panama on his head. He had survived the war, he chortled. He beamed happily, describing this personal victory over the demons of the air and all their bombs. She sat quietly, listening to the fervor of this indomitable giant calling on his last reserves. She had reached him in time, that was all that mattered. On August 13, 1946, he was dead.

They were all gone now, these deepest roots of her life. Ellis at Brixton and Wivelsfield; Slee and Willow Lake; Wells and Easton Glebe; even the Sand Pit circle, even Child and De Selincourt. She stood alone. What had De Selincourt written her not long before his death? "You are . . . the free woman, gentle, lovely and victorious; the creator of new life. " It would be that now, the hardest of all tests. Not an end, she promised, but one more beginning—the best of all.

CHAPTER 27

They were usually wrong about her, even her closest friends. Watching those years at Tucson while she lost herself in a whirlpool of parties and dinners, someone described that period with Emily Dickinson's line, "How dreary marbles after playing crown." Of course, she deserved the rest, they said. She was past sixty now. Why shouldn't she be the city's No. 1 socialite, have industrialists, statesmen, and ex-ambassadors at her dinner table? Why shouldn't she enjoy the homage due a great woman crusader in retirement?

What they did not know, even some of her closest friends, was that this was only a period of transition. Retirement, age—none of the ordinary limitations could hold her. She was ready to break free once more, to build now the greatest dream of all. What was age? Debarking from a ship at Sweden in 1946, a slightly officious passport clerk rattled off the routine questions. When he asked her age, she gave him some figure—what did it really matter?

"But that isn't the age recorded on your passport, madam," he protested.

She looked at him quizzically, tilting her head in that old familiar pose. "It isn't?" Astonishment in her voice. "But then it never is, is it?"

She was timeless, like a force in nature, her spirit detached from the limitations of her body. When Dorothy Brush had visited Tucson a short time before, they had gone out to meetings and dinners nine nights in a row. On the tenth evening, Mrs. Brush went to bed and announced that nothing could budge her from the house. "What's the matter?" Mrs. Sanger asked, concerned. "Are you sick?"

"Of course, I'm not sick. Just exhausted."

Such a possibility had never entered Mrs. Sanger's mind. "Are you sure you're not sick?" she demanded. She was not satisfied until she had brought Dr. Stuart Sanger over to examine Mrs. Brush and make certain that anyone foolish enough to pass up a good dinner party was not running a temperature.

2

The debris of war had given frightening intensity to the need for population control. At the World Population Conference at Geneva in 1927, few had listened to Mrs. Sanger. But they understood now. Germany's maniacal adventure in *lebensraum*, Japan's conquest of the Far East in its hunger for new lands and markets for its overcrowded islands were the ultimate, terrifying proof of the relationship of population and war. Now that it was time for remaking the world in a better image the necessity of birth control, particularly in the Far East, was clear.

Japan's population problem was desperate. Almost sixty million people had been crowded into those islands during Mrs. Sanger's 1922 trip. Now the population was almost 80 million. The birth rate had increased from 29.4 per thousand in 1940 to 34.3 in 1947. At the same time, the health program of the Allied armies was cutting the death rate from 32 per thousand in 1945 to 14.6 in 1947. Again the familiar specter—more people being born, more people living longer, 3,131 people being fed on one square mile of arable land compared with 259 in the United States.

India's population had increased by 50 million—more than the whole population of England, Scotland, and Wales between 1931 and 1940. Five million more mouths had to be fed every year now. Where was the food to come from? As it was, 60 per cent of the country was living on two cents per person per day. To make the situation more critical, the public health program instituted by the British, the elimination of malaria and epidemics, had vastly increased the life span. It was estimated that India's population would increase another 100 million in the next fifteen or twenty years.

Fortunately Japan's new government under Allied military control was encouraging every effort to meet the population problem. Baroness Ishimoto, now Mrs. Shidzue Kato, was rebuilding the Birth Control Association of Japan. Elected a senator in the House of Councillors, she became the spokesman for the movement in the highest places of state. Dr. Kan Majima had reopened his clinics. In the Ministry of Public Health, Dr. Yoshio Koya was preparing a blueprint for public birth control. Significantly enough, the problem was also being brought to the whole country through an enlightened publisher. Mr. Chikao Honda, president of the *Mainichi* papers, had organized the Population Problems Institute—a central clearing house for studying and analyzing population and birth control.

In India, the leaders of the All-India Women's Conference of 1936 were now in the vanguard of the national liberation movement. The India Family Planning Association was being rebuilt under Lady Rama Rau. New clinics were being opened in municipal and state hospitals. There would be a new government soon, a free Indian Government, and many women were already advocating birth control as a basic national policy.

All the elements of a world birth control movement were here— its pivot, as Mrs. Sanger had always predicted, in the Far East. It needed only that indefinable spirit which could weld the separate and disorganized pieces together. This was Margaret Sanger's genius —that she could infuse hope and relentless determination into the bare outlines of an idea, that she could sweep it forward with her strength and courage, that from a few sparks she could stir a flame that would soon begin to move across the earth.

Induce . . . Strive . . . Awaken! "We must induce men and women to strive for a better civilization for themselves and their children's children," she was to say at a Lasker Award dinner. "We cannot give them freedom on a silver platter, but we can awaken in them the demand for a free, self-disciplined life and consciously controlled birth rate and population."

There was not even a formal organization to build on. The Birth Control International Information Centre in London had been disbanded during the war. There was no American committee, not even a budget until Mrs. Stanley McCormick, a devoted supporter of birth control from the pioneering days, gave Mrs. Sanger a check —"for your dreams," she said.

The dream was launched quietly in Stockholm in 1946. Mrs. Elise Ottesen-Jensen, the Swedish birth control leader, had organized a conference on International Birth Control and Sex Education. It was a modest affair. The birth control movement had been destroyed in Germany, Austria, and Italy. Neither India, struggling for its independence, nor Japan, still a prostrated, conquered nation, could send delegates. Even in England and Holland, the movements had been badly disorganized. The Stockholm conference, therefore, attempted only to bring some order out of the chaos of war and to formulate a blueprint for the first large-scale meeting in England in 1948.

An English doctor at Stockholm had taken the responsibility of finding a site for the 1948 meeting and forming an English committee. But after six months he had made little progress; Mrs. Sanger hurried over to England. There was nothing dramatic about this stage of the building of the movement. It was laborious, detailed work. She faced seemingly endless obstacles. She threw her strength against them and, in one fashion or another, gradually battered them down. "It would be impossible to define Mrs. Sanger's work in this period," an associate said. "Almost singlehanded, she created this conference, and those that followed, out of nothing but will power. She was unyielding, relentless, and egotistical in a way that was wonderful to behold. It was the kind of egotism that never asked anything for herself, only for the objectives with which she was completely identified."

At one luncheon that Clinton Chance gave at his club, she rallied some of the key men in England—Lord Horder, Dr. C. P. Blacker, executive director of the Eugenics Society, and others—behind the conference. She searched the area and came up with an exceptional conference site, the lovely town of Cheltenham. She needled Lady Denham into calling a meeting of the British Family Planning Association, and when they complained their participation in the conference would be limited by money, she turned over the balance of Mrs. McCormick's fund.

The Cheltenham conference on Population and World Resources in Relation to the Family raised the curtain on the new era of international birth control. Its roster of speakers was headed by Sir John Boyd-Orr, director general of the U.N.'s Food and Agricultural Organization. Its delegates came from over fifteen countries—not only the older birth control nations like Sweden and Holland, but Egypt, Italy, Czechoslovakia, Germany, British West Africa, Pakistan, India, and North Ireland. Most significant of all, the delegates drew up a concrete plan for a permanent International Planned Parenthood Federation which would be formed at the next conference in 1952.

The Japanese movement was now at a turning point. In 1948, with an improved amendment in 1949, a Eugenic Protection Law had been passed which legalized abortions, not just for medical reasons but at the free discretion of the mother who wished to limit her family. Japan had thus become the first major government to adopt a eugenic policy. Although contraception too was legalized under the amendment, Japan's birth control leaders feared this emphasis on abortions. A concentrated crusade was needed to encourage the spread of birth control clinics—a crusade that Mrs. Kato and Dr. Majima wanted Margaret Sanger to lead. Mrs. Kato, therefore, as president of the Birth Control Association of Japan, sent Mrs. Sanger a formal invitation. It was backed up by the invitation of Mr. Tsunego Baba, president of the *Yomiuri Shimbun,* the country's largest daily newspaper. "We Want Mrs. Sanger" meetings were staged at Dr. Majima's clinics. Thousands of Japanese women put their names to petitions of invitation.

But when Mrs. Sanger applied for a visa an unexpected obstacle arose. General Douglas MacArthur, Supreme Commander for the Allied Powers, rejected her request. In 1922, it had been the Japanese militarists who had tried to block her entry. Now it was an American!

What was the reason behind MacArthur's action? A book by Professor Edward A. Ackerman of the University of Chicago on Japan's population problem and resources had just been withdrawn from circulation by occupation authorities after protests by the Catholic Women's Club of Tokyo. In addition, favorable references to birth control had been eliminated. In its story of February 12, 1950, the *Yomiuri Shimbun* explained that, "In view of the pressure from Catholic Church groups, it was believed impossible for General MacArthur to allow her to lecture to Japanese audiences without appearing to subscribe to her views."

Amazingly enough, these Catholic groups comprised only 130,000 people out of a total population of 80 million!

This was the kind of fight Margaret Sanger relished. The intervention of the highest military authority would only dramatize the necessity for birth control among the Japanese people. "That an American can be barred from a perfectly proper mission by the bigotry or whim of other Americans is intolerable," she cried. ". . . In 1922, the angry protests of the people forced the lifting of the ban. I am confident that something of the same sort will occur in 1950."

The case soon became something of a *cause célèbre.* "Mrs. Sanger was the obvious person to consult," Mrs. Eleanor Roosevelt wrote in her newspaper column, "and why our occupying forces should interfere with the wishes of the Japanese people in this respect is a little

difficult to understand." Dr. John Haynes Holmes, leading a protesting group of clergymen, stated, "It is tragic that such an exhibition of
bigotry should be displayed to the Japanese people at this critical
hour."

The fight was carried by Mrs. Sanger and the Planned Parenthood
Federation directly to Secretary of Defense Louis Johnson. For
months, eloquent and often acid letters went back and forth between
New York, Washington, and Tokyo. Then suddenly the whole im-
passe was resolved by the most dramatic event of all—General Mac-
Arthur's removal from command.

Instead of leaving immediately for Japan, however, she decided to
combine the trip with the first conference of the International
Planned Parenthood Federation in 1952. She called a meeting of the
planning committee in London. The new Indian Government under
Premier Nehru had just come out in support of birth control. The
Indian Planning Commission was considering the establishment of
clinics throughout the country as part of its Five-Year Plan. With
international attention focused on this great experiment, why not
hold the conference in India? Mrs. Sanger's committee agreed. She
immediately telegraphed Lady Rama Rau and asked if India would
act as host to the conference. The Indian Family Planning Associa-
tion·was being reorganized; it was short of money. "We'll get the
money," Mrs. Sanger wired back. It was all settled. The conference
would be held in Bombay in November 1952. A month before that
Mrs. Sanger would arrive in Japan for her nation-wide tour.

That summer she spent at Santa Barbara, California, working day
and night with four secretaries, dictating letters, memorandums,
directives. It was essential that this conference have the finest pos-
sible support. She secured a list of sponsors that included Mrs.
Eleanor Roosevelt, Mrs. Eugene Meyer, Albert Einstein, Professor
Robert A. Millikan, Dr. Frederick Osborn, and Dr. Paul Popenoe.
She lined up delegates from every corner of the world—Hong Kong,
Israel, Australia, South Africa, Canada, Pakistan, Japan, and West
Germany. With painstaking labor, she collected that most important
ingredient, money.

"She never asked for a penny outright," a friend said. "But where-
ever she went—and she was invited so many places she was like the
'debutante of Santa Barbara'—she kept her work at the forefront.
Her spirit, her very presence seemed to command people to help."

Her technique was to stir interest by producing results. At one

Santa Barbara meeting, she told a group of women that after in- numerable obstacles she had secured a delegate from Israel. One woman immediately said, "Wouldn't it be fine if we could raise the money to send that doctor to India?" It was raised on the spot. At a Tucson party, she described how urgent was the need for a research clinic in Bombay. A week later a group of these women turned over a $1,500 check to her for the Indian delegation.

The strain of organizing the conference and preparing for the Japanese tour had taken their toll. The year before Mrs. Sanger had been hospitalized by a coronary thrombosis. Since then, she had suffered a heart condition. Four Tucson doctors and her own son, Dr. Stuart Sanger, flatly opposed her making the trip. One doctor in Santa Barbara warned her that if she insisted on going he did not expect to see her back again.

Mrs. Sanger laughed off their warnings. She drove herself relent- lessly, ignoring the ills of her own body. "Do not pity her. Pity the doctors," Mrs. Brush once said. ". . . The one way to make her mad is to be sorry for her and to try to take care of her." Despite her heart attack the year before, Mrs. Sanger insisted on moving into her new house as soon as she was out of the hospital. Mrs. Brush rushed out to Tucson, theoretically to relieve her of this ordeal. "The only result," she stated, "was that we moved in twice as fast, for she worked right along beside me every moment, stretching, lifting, opening boxes, and indignant at even the most timid suggestion that I do it instead."

What was the source of this strength? It seemed to spring from a deep mystical reservoir, an exaltation of the spirit in its devotion to the final quest. In 1949, Mrs. Sanger was honored by Smith College with the degree of Doctor of Laws. Mrs. Brush drove her to the ceremonies. "Then just as we were leaving," she described the inci- dent later, "something terrible happened. I accidentally slammed the car door on her fingers! She slumped down in the front seat and I begged her to let me take her right to a doctor. She absolutely refused and said, 'Just don't talk, don't say a word. My hand isn't broken, and if you'll just keep still I can work this out myself.' Well I couldn't keep still but she did work it out herself. Presently she said the pain was gone. I opened her hand gently and there were five big blood blisters. Again she would not hear of a doctor, and she said those too would be gone soon. I said, 'You are a miracle worker, I know, but you can't do that.' Nevertheless, she really did.

"Later I asked her how she could do that. I could understand getting rid of the pain, perhaps, but not the blisters. She said she thought it was because she had been so happy over the degree; that there had been inside her a great white light of burning joy."

3

It was this same strength, this exaltation of the spirit that carried Mrs. Sanger through the trip to Japan and India—probably the most taxing ordeal and greatest triumph of her life. Stopping off at Hawaii on the way to Tokyo, she was stricken again after an intensive day of receptions. There had been a large tea at Mrs. Walter Dillingham's villa, a reception for her at the country club given by the American Association of University Women, and Mrs. Ellen Wattamull's *luau*, an authentic Hawaiian feast and dance. But the strain of shaking hands with hundreds of guests that night was too much.

Convinced that no one on earth could make her turn back to Tucson, her friends decided that the next best thing was to have a doctor accompany her on the boat to Japan. Mrs. Brush, a member of the delegation, therefore, gave up her stateroom to another member of the party, who was a doctor, and went on to Tokyo by plane. But as soon as Mrs. Sanger discovered the plot she showed her disdain for such coddling by getting out of bed to throw a huge dinner party for all her Hawaiian friends the night before the sailing.

Margaret Sanger's arrival in Japan was described by an awed army officer at the dock as "the closest thing to a Hollywood opening night I'd ever seen out here." At seven in the morning, when the S.S. *Cleveland* entered Yokohama harbor, her stateroom was already packed with forty reporters who had come aboard on the pilot boat. Another hundred reporters and photographers waited for her as she came down the gangplank. Fifty Japanese women, representing the unions and working women of Yokohama, dressed in their most resplendent ceremonial kimonos, stood in a welcoming line, bowing to her with that meaningful Japanese bow that bespeaks respect, reverence, and love. A Japanese girl, representing Mrs. Kato and the Birth Control Association, placed a corsage of flowers in Mrs. Sanger's arms. Then an officer of the *Mainichi* press, Japan's largest group of newspapers, which was sponsoring her trip, stepped forward with a chrysanthemum wreath. Photographers crowded around, demanding picture after picture until she was finally taken to a waiting limousine and driven to the Imperial Hotel in Tokyo.

That first afternoon was typical of her whole frantic schedule in Japan. A welcome by President Honda of *Mainichi* at one o'clock. A broadcast over Radio Tokyo at two. A reception by the *Mainichi* press at four climaxed that evening by a large dinner-party in her honor.

The *Mainichi* press had established her in a large suite at the Imperial and assigned a husky interpreter and bodyguard, Mr. Mahara, to look after her comfort and maintain some privacy. Mr. Mahara arrived each morning promptly at eight. But an hour earlier, before she could even finish her morning coffee, the sitting room was often crowded with reporters. Writing home at the end of the week, she admitted to her friends that "I was tired enough to die." But she steadfastly refused to curtail her schedule. At Osaka, she made a major speech. After each sentence, the interpreter had to translate her words into Japanese. Yet she insisted on standing the whole two hours in the cold, drafty meeting hall, refusing to sit even during the periods of interpretation.

In the rain at Osaka, hundreds of women, many with their husbands, waited for her at the station platform. At the hotel, the maids stopped work for an hour to visit her in her room. One peasant woman traveled hundreds of miles to Tokyo to bring a few small gifts. Wherever she went, by train or car, women recognized her. The front pages of the newspapers carried her picture day after day. "Women reached out to touch her and kiss her hand," one member of the American delegation said, "as if they knew instinctively that she was bringing a new hope and promise into their lives."

When she visited Kamae village outside of Tokyo, where Dr. Majima maintained a birth control clinic, the whole town turned out as if it were a national holiday. Hundreds of children in ceremonial costume stood in the courtyard of the school, waving Japanese and American flags. The mothers had prepared a special party of tea and cakes. They flocked around Mrs. Sanger and sang a tender, haunting song of triumphant motherhood:

> *We hope to build a strong new world,*
> *Like the graceful plum blossoms in our heart,*
> *We hope to keep the high ideal of mothers*
> *Forever and ever.*

At the end of one of her Tokyo speeches, Dr. Koya of the Ministry of Health came up to Margaret Sanger and grasped her hand. There were tears in his eyes. "You have come like an emissary of peace," he said.

Her reception by crowds on the street, by distinguished audiences at overflow meetings, all had that outpouring of adulation given in the United States only to heroes of conquest, adventure, or sport. In Japan, Margaret Sanger was hailed as a prophet. On her 1922 trip, when the population stood at 60 million she had predicted that war was inevitable if the population should reach 75 million. It reached that in 1940. Now the population was still rising. It would reach 100 million in 1970, she said. She warned against another catastrophe.

Against this pessimistic future, Margaret Sanger and birth control stood like a pinnacle of hope. Japanese women were just winning political and economic freedom. Mrs. Sanger touched them with the meaning of a deeper freedom—the freedom to plan their lives as mothers, to bring new beauty into their family life.

It was this treasuring, this reverence of life that was basic to her philosophy. Abortions! Here was the most cruel and colossal waste, the sapping of the strength of motherhood. The recent Eugenic Protection Law resulted in over a million abortions in Japan in 1951, over a million and a half in 1952. Wherever she went, she spoke out against the barbarity of this practice.

One morning Mrs. Kato organized a procession of trucks with loud-speakers and platforms to take Mrs. Sanger through the working-class districts of Tokyo. As the trucks moved through the streets, the loud-speakers cried, "Sanger is here! Sanger says no abortions!" Women gathered at every corner to watch her pass. When the trucks stopped and Mrs. Sanger climbed to the platform to speak, hundreds of them crowded around her. She knew that they understood. She had touched one of the fundamental truths of motherhood.

Crowded into her schedule were long hours of consultation with the leaders of the birth control movement. She studied the progress of the tests being made in three rural villages by Dr. Koya. She analyzed the work in Dr. Majima's clinics, met with Mr. Honda, Mrs. Kato, and government officials about an extension of the birth control program of the Health Ministry. She drew up a five-year plan for their approval—a teaching center clinic, an educational program, hospitals and health centers, and research into the statistics of maternal health. All these technical discussions were essential to the scientific development of the movement. Yet in the final analysis, it was Mrs. Sanger's triumphant tour that swept Japan with the flame of birth control. In these ten short days, she had aroused a nation more effectively than she had ever done in America with years of relentless labor.

4

She arrived in Bombay for the conference on November 24. It was to be a new kind of triumph. In Japan, it had been the people behind her. Here, for the first time in any country, it was the government. On the opening day of the conference, she was seated on the dais in the place of honor next to the Vice-President of India, Dr. S. Radhakrishnan. When a garland of rare flowers, India's most meaningful tribute, was draped around her neck, the audience in the huge hall rose in a standing ovation.

That night at a dinner at the Cricket Club, given by Lady Rama Rau and Madame Kamiladevi Chattopadhyay, leader of the Indian Co-operative Movement, she was seated again next to the Vice-President. The next day she was the guest of honor at a special dinner given by the Mayor of Bombay. A thousand people packed the lawns of the beautiful hanging gardens of Malabar Hill overlooking the city's main park. The Mayor welcomed her in his opening address. It was the first time that the top official of a major city had given full, official honors to the birth control movement.

For India had now made birth control an instrument of national policy. It had established two hundred clinics in twenty-eight cities, seventeen in Bombay alone. At military posts, the Army had set up an additional 106 clinics. Premier Nehru had issued his long-awaited Five-Year Plan, and birth control, with 1.3 million dollars specifically allotted for government clinics, was one of its major planks.

Doctors, nurses, and delegates—many of them old friends from her 1936 trip—flocked to Margaret Sanger's room at conference headquarters. They urged her to visit their cities and towns to speed the development of the movement; they begged for new contraceptive supplies, new teaching techniques. One doctor, who had come hundreds of miles to see her, had so little money left that the basket of fruit on Mrs. Sanger's table made his principal meal that day. Over half the Indian delegates were under thirty-five, many so poor they had walked miles to Bombay and could not afford even the cheapest hotel rooms. The American delegation had taken a special bedroom at the hotel where the conference sessions were being held.

Its principal purpose was to give Mrs. Sanger a hideaway for occasional rest. "But she was the only one who never used it," said Dr. William Vogt, national director of the Planned Parenthood Federation. "She was always in conference with delegates or dashing off to inspect one of the local clinics."

Every minute in Bombay was precious. Here was the dream taking shape on an unprecedented scale, a great new nation struggling to check its soaring population and extend the teachings of birth control to the most remote villages! "There is no time left for half-way measures," she warned. "Magnificent as the economic and agricultural results of India's Five-Year Plan may be, they cannot increase the standard of living or provide enough food and housing for 20 million additional people."

Always she cried out for action. The search for the new, simple contraceptive—this was the principal hope of bringing birth control to those vast sections of the population which had not been reached. "It seems unbelievable," she stated, "that in an age when we have harnessed the tremendous potentialities of the atom we still cannot perfect a simple method of biological contraception."

The final session of the conference was held in Sir Cowasji Jehangir Hall, filled now to overflowing. The delegates of six national birth control organizations were represented here. Dr. C. P. Blacker of Great Britain stood up and proposed that they should be joined together permanently into a new world organization, the International Planned Parenthood Federation. The motion was seconded and adopted. Then Mrs. Ottesen-Jensen of Sweden moved that Margaret Sanger and Lady Rama Rau should be elected honorary presidents of the new federation. The motion was passed; the traditional garlands of flowers hung around the necks of the two women.

Margaret Sanger stood on the dais, frail, almost diminutive in a simple black dress. From every corner of the hall, waves of applause rolled toward her. She had gone to jail nine times. She had worked a lifetime for this moment. It was almost thirty-eight years to the month since she had sailed from Montreal, an exile from her own country. Since then, she had won the fight for birth control in the United States; now she was winning the world.

CHAPTER 28

She had sold the house at Willow Lake after the war and made Tucson her permanent home. She had loved this place, its manorial solidity, its flaming gardens, the endless serenity of its woods and lake—almost every brick and path the product of her own design. Her granddaughter, Margaret, who had spent many months of childhood there, said tearfully, "When I grow up, I'm going to marry a rich man so I can buy Willow Lake back."

No, Mrs. Sanger said, it was the moving forward that counted, the eternal quest of what was ahead. The new house in Tucson symbolized her outlook. It was vibrantly modern. She had worked on the plan with the architect and decorated the interior herself after spending months studying modern design. It was built on one level, with the rooms radiating out from the entrance way and central, circular dining room. From the air, it looked like a fan. The roof was aluminum, polished aluminum that shimmered in the bright desert sun.

The living room was the main spoke of the fan—spreading dramatically from a width of about thirteen feet at the entrance to over forty feet at the far end, with floor-to-ceiling windows that looked up into the mountains. A large steel fireplace stood in the center of one side wall. In front of it was a gracefully curving pool of water on whose surface in wintertime the reflection of the flames made a riotous dance. At other times, flowers floated on the pool, and at Halloween, it was filled with apples and the neighborhood children came in to bob for them.

The stark white walls, the couches and chairs covered in white fabric set off the classic splendor of her Aubusson rug and the two dark wood chests, trimmed with burnished brass, that she had brought back from Korea. The Oriental theme was accentuated in the two huge Chinese portraits on the wall, priceless gifts that had been given her on her first tour of the Far East. "The ancestors," she liked to call them, a phrase that obviously confused the workmen who were painting the house. "Funny, isn't it?" one of them protested to the maid. "Mrs. Sanger doesn't look at all Chinese."

There was an enclosed porch, large enough for her largest dinner parties, opening out on the terrace and gardens. Here she liked to sit with her friends at the end of the day, sipping cocktails, watching the sun brush the whole valley with fire and turn the stainless steel birds on the garden fountain into pinwheels of color.

Fittingly enough, the kitchen and pantry had the spaciousness to accommodate her love of entertaining and her constant experimentation with new dishes. Before she left on one trip to Japan, she invited eight of her closest friends to a suki-yaki feast for which she had hunted the proper ingredients all over town. The guests had to take off their shoes at the door, don slippers and kimonos, and make the appropriate Japanese bows. The menus were typed on beautiful Japanese cards. The guest who came closest to guessing the name and ingredients of each dish was given a special prize.

Dr. Stuart Sanger lived in the house next door. On Thursdays, when her cook and houseman were off, she prepared a series of foreign dinners for her son's family. One week it was Indian, one French, one Chinese, and so on around the world. The dinners were completely authentic—even to the clothes. She had brought her boxes of costumes from Willow Lake, and after school, Margaret and Nancy would rush over and raid the boxes. The house was always filled with shouts and laughter—the way Mrs. Sanger liked her house. The grandchildren called her "Mimi." An associate of hers, who had never called her anything more familiar than "Mrs. Sanger" or "M.S." in the decade since she had known her, was startled to hear the neighborhood children shout to her as she passed, "Hi, Mimi." . . . "Where are you going, Mimi?"

One winter she gave Margaret, Nancy, and three of their friends ballet lessons, and together they composed a play with dancing, *The Sad Princess.* She made a stage at the entrance of the living room, using the brightly colored Haitian screen that swung from a track over the door as the curtain of the stage. The play proved so popular they had to give it three times. All the children came from blocks around; then their parents insisted on coming too. Mrs. Sanger in a fanciful peasant hat stood at one corner of the stage and introduced the scenes, occasionally plunging exuberantly into one of the roles when an actress forgot her lines.

At Christmas, she always went to Mt. Kisco, New York, where Dr. Grant Sanger and his wife lived. They had a handsome house in the hills, almost as large as Willow Lake—they needed it now with five boys and a girl racing up and down the stairs. The children had their own dining room, and Mrs. Sanger, an accomplished painter, did the murals herself—six gay and elfin scenes, each dedicated to one of the grandchildren. Here she was called "Domah," which is similar to the Chinese expression for "second mother." But when they were shouting to her to join them in a game on the lawn she was "Dommie" or "Dom." "No reverence in this younger generation," she once complained smilingly. But then she was almost part of this generation, part of the bedlam of Christmas mornings, pushing the younger boys on fire trucks through the hall, guiding her granddaughter's baby carriage through the litter of opened packages. Effortlessly she could touch at the same time the hearts of children and the minds of some of the greatest men of her day. It was a rare fusion, "a delicious blend," as De Selincourt had said, "of great queen and shy little girl."

2

Like the rest of the birth control movement, Mrs. Sanger's own center in New York has undergone drastic transformation in the last decade. In 1942, its name was changed to the Margaret Sanger Research Bureau. Mr. Slee had bought the building on Sixteenth Street and given it to her, but since a large proportion of the patients were treated without charge or at minimum fee, he had, in addition, made up the clinic's deficit every year. Since his death, it had become harder and harder for her to meet these financial burdens. Further, once she had made her permanent home in Tucson it was impractical at that distance to remain in active direction. In 1950, therefore, the building was transferred to a group of supporters. Dr. Abraham Stone was elected director of the bureau for a five-year term. Mrs. Sanger became co-director and a member of the board of trustees.

By August 1954, with a staff of forty-five physicians, each giving a few hours a week, the Margaret Sanger Bureau had dispensed contraceptive information to over 141,000 women. But significantly enough, a new service, an infertility service for both men and women, is fast becoming almost as much in demand as the contraceptive service. It had originally been thought that infertility was specifically a woman's problem. New research has shown the importance of treating the man at the same time. The bureau's policy today is to accept only couples for joint treatment. Not just the physical aspects, but psychical and emotional maladjustments are studied in the total picture. Endocrinological and psychotherapeutic experts are available for the diagnosis of glandular dysfunctions and emotional problems. More than three thousand couples have now been treated at the bureau's infertility service—a service that is also available at some seventy other clinics in the United States.

Once the bureau was a refuge for impoverished, desperate mothers of five or seven children seeking to escape the slavery of constant pregnancies. As late as 1937, a woman could write Mrs. Sanger: "I have recollections of my aunts and mother always in tears—every other month an abortion—and half the time they lay on the deathbed sticking needles into themselves, trying to 'do away with it.' And we had to wait for a Margaret Sanger to appear on the scene to end this utter stupidity and cruelty."

Today the great majority of patients at the bureau are young women who come, not after the agony of repeated abortions, but immediately after marriage to learn how to plan their families. As part of this emphasis on planning, one of the major bureau services is marriage counseling. This service, which had been conducted for many years by Dr. Stone and his wife at the Community Church, was merged with the bureau in 1953. It is now conducted by Dr. Stone and Dr. Lena Levine and incorporates group therapy as well as individual consultations.

3

As much a rebel today as she was in 1913, Mrs. Sanger has continually urged a reformulation of birth control policy in the United States. She had built the movement around a chain of clinics across the country. But the role of the clinic in many areas has changed. The mothers of the middle and lower-middle classes, who were once the clinics' most numerous patients, are now apt to get their contraceptive information directly from their physicians.

On the other hand, the poorest mothers, particularly those in rural areas, have little access to clinics. They are usually burdened with housework, cannot leave the children alone, and are kept from making the lengthy clinic trip by obstacles of time and transportation costs.

Impressed on her last trip to Japan by the effectiveness of midwives and doctors of the Ministry of Health who go directly to the homes of poor fishermen, farmers, and miners, Mrs. Sanger now believes that the American movement must adopt this technique. The poorest strata of our population must be reached in their homes. They must be reached by the program that she pioneered back in 1937—birth control through doctors and nurses of the Public Health Service going to remote rural areas by traveling clinic if necessary.

It is significant that the Planned Parenthood Federation under the presidency of Mrs. Robert L. Ferguson and with Dr. Vogt as national director has already begun to bolster its public health program in the South. This program had slowed down in the last decade because the federation had considered its job done once contraceptive information had been made part of the public health clinics. Now it is recognized that few mothers in the area know of this contraceptive service unless the federation maintains a local chapter to keep up a constant campaign of information and education. Recently the federation organized a committee of Negro and white leaders in Atlanta to stimulate the Georgia program. The federation's chapter in Virginia has its own field director, and the federation has now assigned a national field director to work throughout the South.

In Puerto Rico, the Planned Parenthood Federation is conducting its most determined offensive. This small, forsaken U. S. territory, this island of rampant breeding, contains in microcosm the whole drama of exploding populations. When the United States took it over in 1898, the Spanish had left its feudal society in shambles. American officials introduced the latest miracles of science—hospitals, sanitation, public health medicine—and thus drastically cut the death rate. At the same time, they watched unconcernedly while the population doubled despite the millions of dollars pumped into the island's agriculture and economy. Little was done to bolster the island's agriculture and economy to keep pace with its population. As a result, the per capita income today is only four hundred dollars a year and each Puerto Rican must live off half an acre of arable land instead of the minimum standard of two and one half acres. The island has become a vast slum of our own making. "Our cherished slum," Dr. Vogt has called it.

But significantly enough, although the island is predominantly Catholic, population pressure had become so intense by 1937 that a law was passed and signed by Acting Governor Rafael Menendez Ramos making birth control legal. The result was quixotic. Birth control clinics were opened throughout the island, but due to Catholic pressure no publicity was given them. Many only opened a half day each week, then closed down completely.

Nor was an educational program on the principles of planned parenthood carried to the people. This is essential because of the predominant role played by the husband in the Puerto Rican family. Few men understood the use of contraceptives outside the area of prostitution; fewer still gave their wives the power to use it. It is significant that when they reach New York and come into the range of new social standards and birth control education many Puerto Rican families have taken immediate advantage of the centers here.

In March 1954, Dr. Stone, together with Mrs. Eleanor Pillsbury, one of its past presidents, and Mrs. Dorothy Brush, was sent by the Planned Parenthood Federation to Puerto Rico to launch a vigorous new drive for birth control. The Family Planning Association of Puerto Rico was organized with a membership of distinguished university professors, demographers, and government officials, including former Acting Governor Menendez. The new group is linked directly to the federation, which is supplying not only financial assistance and contraceptive materials but expert medical guidance. It is concentrating specifically on an educational campaign to bring the principles of planned parenthood to the people through the radio, press, and every available medium. Puerto Rico is fast becoming one of the world's significant test tubes of birth control progress. For if the program can succeed in this Catholic island it may be the opening wedge to South America.

4

At least two thirds of the world today is fast approaching a biological bursting point. Population has increased from 470 million in 1650 to 2.5 billion in 1953. A further increase of 1.5 billion by 1980 is predicted by a U. N. Department of Social Affairs Study if the trend continues at the highest expectancy. Forty nations or colonies, including Costa Rica, Cuba, Dominican Republic, Egypt, El Salvador, Mexico, Puerto Rico, and Hawaii, will double their population

within the next thirty years, says Dr. William Vogt. In the meantime, "better than fifty per cent of the world's population is slowly
starving or being exposed to death," according to a leading food
economist, Dr. Robert White-Stevens of Lederle Laboratories. Each
day there are at least seventy thousand more mouths in the world
to feed. "These extra mouths may be a danger for the future com-
parable to the danger of the hydrogen bomb," concludes Britain's
Lord Simon of Wythenshawe.

In the United States, a relatively stable population has nevertheless increased from 151.7 million in 1950 to 160 million in 1953. Birth
control, comparatively speaking, has ceased to be an issue for at
least a decade. But it is still being vigorously fought by the Roman
Catholic hierarchy; it is still legally prohibited in two states, Connecticut and Massachusetts.

The Catholic position, in fact, remains puzzlingly ambiguous.
Certainly the majority of lay Catholics have long accepted birth
control. In 1938, when the *Ladies' Home Journal* asked its readers
if they believed in the right to disseminate contraceptive information to married couples, 51 per cent of the Catholic women answering the poll said yes. In *Fortune's* 1943 poll, 69 per cent of the
Catholic women supported this same position. In its 1948 poll, the
Woman's Home Companion reported that almost 80 per cent of its
Catholic readers accepted the belief that "birth control information
should be made available to some extent; only one-fifth think that
it should be legally forbidden to everybody."

Vatican policy, of course, is the fount of all Catholic dogma. Yet
Vatican policy itself has been somewhat indecisive. The rhythm
method—certainly an attempt to combat the growing acceptance
of birth control by church members—has been sanctioned since the
early 1930s. But Pope Pius XII unexplainably seemed to weaken
this sanction in a speech of October 29, 1951, to Italian midwives
when he said:

*If the carrying out of this theory means nothing more than that
the couple can make use of their matrimonial rights on the days of
natural sterility too, there is nothing against it . . . If, however, it
is a further question—that is, of permitting the conjugal act on those
days exclusively—then the conduct of the married couple must be
examined more closely.*

But in his speech a few weeks later to the Congress of the Italian
National Family Front, the Pope contradicted his previous narrow

interpretation of the rhythm method. The New York *Times* on November 28, 1951, quoted the Pope as saying:

> . . . that the Church considers *"with sympathy and understanding"* the difficulties of the married state in our day and therefore recognizes the legitimacy of *"a regulation of offspring"* by having recourse to periods of natural sterility of woman within limits—which he described as *"in truth very wide"*—set by the Church.

"One may even hope," stated the Pope with what seems like almost enthusiastic sanction of the rhythm method, "that science will succeed in providing this licit method with a sufficiently secure basis. The most recent information seems to confirm such a hope."

In line with this inconsistency, the American hierarchy has combined periods of relative peace with sudden and virulent attacks against planned parenthood organizations. One recent attack occurred in New York in 1952 when the Health Council and the Welfare Council, totaling almost four hundred medical and social agencies, united into the Welfare and Health Council of New York City. For many years previously, planned parenthood groups had belonged to the separate councils without protest from any of the Catholic member agencies. But at the merger, the Catholic Charities of New York and Brooklyn suddenly announced that they would withdraw if planned parenthood was admitted—a quixotic situation indeed, especially since the council's board, including Catholic members, had just approved the planned parenthood program.

Despite the loss of revenue to the council if Catholic agencies resigned, twenty-five of the member agencies recognized the seriousness of the issue of religious domination of a welfare organization. They stood firmly behind planned parenthood. At the election of the council's new board in May 1953, the pro-birth control slate was elected. Planned parenthood was admitted to membership in the council. As they had threatened, the Catholic Charities resigned.

Another line of Catholic attack has been aimed at hospitals. In March 1953, for instance, Catholic pressure in Parkersburg, West Virginia, tried to block the opening of a planned parenthood clinic at the city-owned Camden-Clark Memorial Hospital—without success. More ruthless was the ultimatum delivered in 1952 to seven physicians on the staff of Catholic-run St. Francis Hospital in Poughkeepsie, New York. The hospital said: Either resign from the staff or resign from the Dutchess County League of Planned Parenthood. Three of the seven doctors, explaining that the interests of their patients, then in the hospital, necessitated this unfortunate step, gave way to the intimidation.

The hospital authorities, however, quickly met a barrage of criticism from the press and public. In addition, a movement was quietly started to form a solid front of all non-Catholic doctors in the area who agreed to resign from any Catholic hospital if a single doctor was attacked because of planned parenthood affiliation. As a result of all these factors, St. Francis Hospital backed down. The staff privileges of the seven original doctors were all renewed when their appointments came up some months later.

Roman Catholic opposition to birth control, of course, involves far larger issues than these skirmishes in the United States. It has effectively blocked any planned parenthood program in South America, and parts of Europe where the Catholic religion dominates—areas whose exploding populations desperately need birth control. Worst of all, the Vatican has used its influence over Catholic countries in the United Nations—logically the U.N. should be the leading force behind a world population policy—to destroy almost every attempt at facing this critical problem.

In May 1952, when Norway, in the Assembly of the World Health Organization, introduced a resolution calling for a study of the relationship between rapid population growth and health, it was opposed by a block of seven Catholic countries and Lebanon. The Belgian representative even introduced a counterresolution which would have forbidden the U.N. to aid any member nation with family planning—even though that nation had requested it! The resolution was finally shelved.

The W.H.O., to all intents and purposes, thus seems to have come under Vatican domination. "What the Roman Catholic bloc has done," stated Dr. Vogt, "is to deny such aid, through W.H.O., to the vast majority of the world's people, who are not Catholics."

It is doubtful that the speech of Reverend Stanislas de Lestapis at the World Population Conference under U.N. auspices in 1954 in Rome represents any decisive change in the Vatican's stand. The speech, reported the New York *Times*, "was understood to have been cleared with the Vatican." Although reiterating strongly that only the rhythm method could be tolerated, and denying Vatican clearance, Father de Lestapis, according to the *Times*, "said that in underdeveloped countries with a high birth rate, it was the duty of the government to inform citizens of the consequences that an excessive rise in the population might have."

Mrs. Sanger still insists that only one possible solution exists—that the Vatican must revise its encyclical against birth control; that it must make a scientific statement that life begins not at conjugal union but at the moment of conception.

5

Only one objective, one theme like an enormous orchestral crescendo, dominates Margaret Sanger's work today—the search for the birth control "pill." She is so convinced of its absolute necessity as the next step in world birth control that in her opinion the American movement is wasting its time with halfway measures and should concentrate all its resources and money on research. The discovery of the "pill"—the climactic dream of her life—will undoubtedly prove one of the revolutionary events of this century.

The money behind birth control research has been shockingly small. In 1953, the Federal Government spent 30 million dollars in an attempt to control hoof-and-mouth disease. The Atomic Energy Commission had at its disposal 2 billion dollars to develop nuclear fission and atomic weapons. But the study of fertility control, including work by the commercial pharmaceutical houses, probably received no more than five hundred thousand, according to Dr. John Rock of Boston, a leader in the field.

Although Mrs. Sanger has played no technical role in the development of the "pill," she has been its prophet, its driving force. She has goaded scientists, hammered at organizations, preached and shouted the urgency of this cause throughout the land. Her vision has been deep and unprejudiced. Every clue, every grain of hope uncovered by a reputable scientist she has given her unstinted support. Not the least important, she has raised, in co-operation with the Planned Parenthood Federation, a continuous stream of money for the work, including the fund from Mrs. Stanley McCormick for research into synthetic, hormone-like substances carried on by Dr. Rock, and Dr. Gregory Pincus of the Worcester Foundation for Experimental Biology.

What is the status of the "pill" today? Actually there is no single "miracle pill." The very diversity of problems and needs in each country make it essential that a variety of new methods must eventually be perfected.

Even the word "pill" is a misnomer. Some new agents are taken orally, others by injection. Some can be used either way. Mrs. Sanger herself favors the use of an injection. First, in underdeveloped areas of the world, it can conveniently be included in the public health program under careful medical supervision. This would permit the keeping of accurate records. Second, the injection method would have the additional advantage of giving protection to a mother for a longer period of time—one injection lasting for three months to a year or more. A pill, on the other hand, would have to be taken at more frequent intervals—one a day, three times a week, or once each menstrual cycle.

There is a further disadvantage to the pill. The user may wander from the strict dosage schedule by forgetfulness. An injection, administered by public health authorities, becomes a scientific act. It is never subject to the temporary mood or passion of the user. Once the social climate of a country has been conditioned, the injection becomes part of the mores of the people. Far sooner than imagined, one Indian woman may casually say to another, as casually as if she were discussing a typhoid shot, "I just came back from the clinic. They're giving birth control inoculations this week."

At least five major approaches to biochemical birth control are being studied and developed in the laboratories today. But the one on which most attention is focused is the work in hormonal agents and hormone-like synthetic substances under Dr. Pincus at the Worcester Foundation. The final development and testing of this approach is the setting for the most dramatic period in Margaret Sanger's life, a moment toward which she has built for almost twenty-five years.

Just when will this moment come? With such intense energy and enthusiasm concentrated on this quest, Mrs. Sanger is naturally optimistic. She predicts that it is not more than a year or two off. Scientists, however, are apt to be more cautious. They point out that the side effects of hormone-like synthetics may be complex and difficult to control. They estimate a testing period of from three to five years.

Tests are now under way at the Margaret Sanger Research Bureau under the supervision of Dr. Stone. They must continue for at least a year to eliminate all possible doubt that the female reproductive cycle will not be altered or inhibited. More than anything else, however, the new contraceptive needs one great dramatic test to put it in the world spotlight. With her keen grasp of the currents of history, no one understands this better than Mrs. Sanger. It is Japan that may offer the decisive setting. The Japanese Family Planning Association is hoping to send a Japanese doctor to the United States to study with Dr. Pincus at the Worcester Foundation. Japan has already made Margaret Sanger a national heroine. Now it may provide the stage for her long-sought greatest dream.

6

Against this catclysm of overpopulation, Margaret Sanger's great gift has been to give the world a hope and a plan. Its base is the International Planned Parenthood Federation, now grown to fifteen member nations. Of these, India and Japan stand forth as particular symbols of the new era that is coming. Mrs. Sanger, who made the Brownsville center in 1917 the beacon for over five hundred later clinics, is a master of the value of symbolism. Here in India and Japan are the two great repositories of that "feminine spirit" which she long ago described as "the most important force in the remaking of the world."

In a few short decades, India's women, fighting both for their political freedom and their freedom as mothers, have made birth control not only national policy but a proud, affirmative way of life. With birth control integrated into its Five-Year Plan, India is now reaching some of its remotest areas with contraceptive information. Almost thirty new clinics have been added to the previous two hundred. A program of traveling clinics under the Family Planning Association is going to far-flung villages. A test project under the auspices of the Harvard School of Public Health has been established at Khanna. It is studying the most effective psychological and sociological methods of instructing rural mothers—its findings to be extended to other villages.

A plan and a hope—they live as vibrantly in Japan. To make it possible for birth control information to reach the great mass of Japanese mothers, a significant law was passed in 1953. Since it is the nurses and midwives—thirty thousand of them—rather than the doctors who provide maternal care for most rural mothers, the new law for the first time allows them to dispense contraceptive information and materials. In one test project in a rural area where midwives brought birth control right to the women's homes, a survey showed that their advice was welcomed in almost 90 per cent of the cases. Now Mrs. Sanger envisions a major program—thirty thousand midwives trained in birth control techniques, a great army of professional missionaries bringing planned parenthood to the most remote homes of Japan.

To find the best contraceptive methods for the rural areas, four test projects have been conducted in the past few years by Dr. Yoshio Koya, director of the National Institute of Public Health—three in rural villages, one in a coal mining area. In these three villages, the combined crude birth rate was 22.2 per thousand in 1950. Three years later it had been cut to 14.6. In the coal mining area, the pregnancy rate was cut in the twelve months after March 1953 from 37.6 to 28.1.

On April 9, 1954, Margaret Sanger arrived once more in Tokyo to welcome the Japanese Family Planning Association into the International Federation and accept their invitation to hold the next conference there. They received her like a national heroine—fifty cameramen and reporters at the plane, a red carpet laid before her. Among the ancient shrines and pagodas of the Villa Camellia, she was honored at a luncheon by Parliamentary Vice-Minister Nakayama and the lady members of the Standing Committee for Welfare of the House of Councillors. At the Prince Hotel, she was honored with a tea tendered by the Speaker of the House of Representatives and Mrs. Yasujiro Tsutsumi. The guest list was crowded with university presidents, government leaders, justices, bankers, and the major industrialists of the city. Each of them, bowing low, was presented to Mrs. Sanger. She was given a rare scroll, painted for an emperor of the Ming Dynasty—a symbol of national reverence.

Then came the most significant moment of all. Two o'clock, April 15, 1954. The council chamber of the House of Councillors in the Diet Building, once known as the House of Peers. She was escorted by the chairman of the Standing Committee for Welfare to the Speaker's rostrum. It was, in all its deepest ramifications, nothing less than a moment in history. She had come from thousands of miles to address them on the crucial issue of birth control. The first non-Japanese woman ever to address the House of Councillors. It was as if she had come from halfway around the world to speak to the Senate of the United States.

The silvery, soaring voice reached out to these statesmen, who comprised the highest legislative body of Japan. A smiling, almost shy woman, radiating that light and confidence that had set a flame in so many countries.

The most important force in the remaking of the world is a free motherhood . . . She will not stop at patching up the world, she will remake it.

Margaret Sanger had written those words long ago. For forty years, she had lived them herself. Now at this crowning era of her life, she had built a movement of fifteen nations and territories—Australia, Ceylon, Great Britain, Holland, Hong Kong, India, Italy, Japan, Pakistan, Puerto Rico, Singapore, Sweden, Union of South Africa, the United States, West Germany.

Yet she had only started. Always the unknown challenge ahead—the dream of free men and women shaping their own destinies. She had swept away ignorance and prejudice, crushed the defeatists and fatalists. The message that she had stamped ineradicably on her time was that human beings could consciously control the plan and purpose of their lives; that out of the evolutionary process they could raise society to a new level of dignity and beauty.

Always there was a joyous contagion in her spirit. Within forty years, it has spread from the early *Woman Rebel*, with its few thousand readers, to almost every corner of the world. As a personal phenomenon, this spirit was the culminating link in that chain of indomitable women, going back to Mary Wollstonecraft, who won for their sex new vistas of freedom. As a woman, Margaret Sanger brought a new meaning and glorification to love as the most powerful force in our destinies. Her fight was unique in that it went much deeper than education or suffrage and reached the most fundamental fact of women's lives—the yearning for biological freedom.

But as a crusader, as the leader of a world movement, she has gone even farther. She has made birth control an instrument of social action that now holds in its grasp the future of many nations.

The social revolution she brought in her own country has been so sweeping and decisive in the space of a few decades that, paradoxically enough, most young mothers today take birth control as much for granted as if it were incorporated in the Bill of Rights. Yet in vast areas of the world the force of her revolution is only taking hold. The spirit she unleashed is just beginning its march. The impact of birth control on family life, on the relations of husbands and wives, on the happiness of children is so profound that it may never be fully grasped in our time.

In the economically underdeveloped countries that cover so much of the world from Puerto Rico and South America to the Middle and Far East, she has brought far more than a social revolution in the family. Through birth control, she has provided the most constructive means of national survival. She has fused in one great historical force the power of love and biological control of the human race.

H. G. Wells early recognized the scope of this concept. "Alexander the Great changed a few boundaries and killed a few men," he wrote. "Both he and Napoleon were forced into fame by circumstances outside of themselves and by currents of the time, but Margaret Sanger made currents and circumstances. When the history of our civilization is written, it will be a biological history and Margaret Sanger will be its heroine."

APPENDIX 1: ACKNOWLEDGMENTS AND SOURCES

It was the author's good fortune not only to have the opportunity of hundreds of hours of interviews with Margaret Sanger over a period of two years but also to talk with scores of her friends and associates. Many of these knew her from the earliest days of the birth control movement and thus offered a rare source of personal anecdote and reminiscence.

Mrs. Sanger also made available to the author the two most important collections of material on her life and the movement—one at the Library of Congress, the other at the Smith College Library. This book, therefore, is based to a large extent on these original and, in many cases, unpublished documents. Both collections are a vast storehouse for the social historian and biographer. They contain not only a complete file of all printed material from the birth of the movement, but also invaluable memoranda and correspondence with such key personalities as William Sanger, Ethel Byrne, Hugh De Selincourt, and other members of Mrs. Sanger's intimate circle whose use in this volume was by necessity limited.

In working with the Library of Congress collection, the author is indebted to Mr. David Mearns and his staff in the Manuscript Division for their co-operation; to Miss Florence Rose for her previous labors in compiling the index of the Sanger collection; and to Mrs. Catherine Hiss for her research assistance.

The author is indebted in his use of the Smith College collection to Mrs. Margaret Grierson and Mr. Frederick Waterman of the library staff.

Smaller but valuable collections of material on the movement are at the Margaret Sanger Bureau in New York, whose executive secretary, Mrs. Estelle Flowers, was a loyal helper; and at the national office of the Planned Parenthood Federation in New York. Here the past and present officers, including Mrs. Robert M. Ferguson, Mrs. Philip Pillsbury, Mrs. Harry M. Montgomery and Dr. Abraham Stone; and members of the permanent staff, including Dr. William Vogt, Winfield Best, Mrs. Mildred Gilman, Miss Hope Spingarn, and Frederick S. Jaffe gave the author continued assistance. In particular, Mrs. Lily Lore, the librarian of the Federation, was untiring in tracking down the most difficult research problem.

A host of Margaret Sanger's friends and associates in the movement gave generously of their time and turned over valuable letters and records. It is impossible to mention all the people to whom the author's debt is large. But Mrs. Dorothy Brush, Dr. Clarence Gamble, Dr. Paul Henshaw, Mrs. Raymond Ingersoll, Dr. Lena Levine, Mrs. Henriette Posner, and Leighton Rollins deserve special thanks, as do the author's friends, Professor and Mrs. Lewis Feuer, for their devoted counsel.

The primary published sources on Margaret Sanger's life are her own writings, four of which have been frequently quoted in this biography:

> *Woman and the New Race.* New York: Brentano, 1920.
> *The Pivot of Civilization.* New York: Brentano, 1922.
> *My Fight for Birth Control.* New York: Farrar, 1931.
> *Margaret Sanger, an Autobiography.* New York: Norton, 1938.

Among other significant books by Margaret Sanger are:

> *What Every Mother Should Know.* New York: Eugenics, 1916.
> *The Case for Birth Control.* New York, 1917.
> *What Every Girl Should Know.* New York: Eugenics, 1922.
> *Happiness in Marriage.* New York: Brentano, 1926.
> *Motherhood in Bondage.* New York: Brentano, 1928.

The files of the following publications are also invaluable to any study of Margaret Sanger and the birth control movement:

> *The Call*
> *The Woman Rebel*
> *The Birth Control Review*
> *Around the World News of Population and Birth Control*

The following books have also provided important sources of material on Margaret Sanger or the social and economic background against which the movement grew:

> Beard, Mary. *Woman as a Force in History.* New York: Macmillan, 1946.
> Broun, Heywood, and Leech, Margaret. *Anthony Comstock.* New York: Boni, 1927.
> Brown, Harrison. *The Challenge of Man's Future.* New York: Viking, 1954.
> Coucke, V. J., and Walsh, J. J. *The Sterile Period in Family Life.* New York: Wagner, 1933.
> De Forest, Robert W., and Veiller, Lawrence. *The Tenement House Problem.* New York: Macmillan, 1903.
> Delisle, Françoise. *Friendship's Odyssey.* London: Heinemann, 1947.
> Ditzion, Sidney. *Marriage, Morals and Sex in America.* New York: Bookman, 1953.

Eastman, Max. *Venture*. New York: Boni, 1927.

Ellis, Havelock. *Impressions and Comments*. London: Constable, 1921. *My Life*. London: Heinemann, 1940.

Goldman, Emma. *Living My Life*. New York: Knopf, 1931.

Himes, Norman E. *The Truth about Birth Control*. New York: Day, 1931. *Medical History of Contraception*. Baltimore: Wood, 1936.

Ishimoto, Shidzue. *Facing Two Ways*. New York: Farrar, 1935.

Luhan, Mabel Dodge. *Intimate Memories*. Vol. 3. New York: Harcourt, 1933.

Vogt, William. *Road to Survival*. New York: Sloane, 1948.